W9-DFH-725

The Bitterest Pills

Also by Joanna Moncrieff

THE MYTH OF THE CHEMICAL CURE

DE-MEDICALISING MISERY (*co-editor*)

A STRAIGHT TALKING INTRODUCTION TO PSYCHIATRIC DRUGS

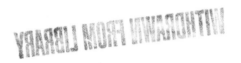

Praise for *The Myth of the Chemical Cure*:

'A revolutionary book written with the calm assurance of someone who knows her subject matter – and the people involved – extremely well. Essential reading for anyone interested in mental health'. Dorothy Rowe, www.dorothyrowe.com.au

'This is a book that should change psychiatry forever'. *Mental Health*

'This book is critically important and should be essential reading for all psychiatrists, politicians, service providers, and user groups. Why? Because Joanna Moncrieff's central tenet is right, and the implications for service delivery are profound. The book is closely argued and well referenced. Even if you disagree with some of it's overall premises, it is not legitimate to dismiss it. I urge you to read it if only as a prompt to a critical evaluation of the status quo, never a bad thing, and almost always an illuminating exercise'. Sarah Yates, Cambridge, UK

'This is a sober and thoughtful book. I found it very engaging and worth the effort to be better informed about a subject that affects many of our clients and impinges on our professional lives as therapists'. *Existential Analysis* (Society for Existential Analysis)

'...Joanna Moncrieff, a practising psychiatrist and academic, has produced a devastating critique of the use of psychiatric drugs... This courageous book has the potential to revolutionise psychiatric practice and the care of people with many forms of mental distress. Many in the therapy professions will, I am sure, celebrate its message'. Rachel Freeth, *Therapy Today*

The Bitterest Pills

The Troubling Story of Antipsychotic Drugs

Joanna Moncrieff
University College London, UK

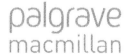

First published 2013 by
PALGRAVE MACMILLAN

Palgrave Macmillan in the UK is an imprint of Macmillan Publishers Limited, registered in England, company number 785998, of Houndmills, Basingstoke, Hampshire RG21 6XS.

Palgrave Macmillan in the US is a division of St Martin's Press LLC, 175 Fifth Avenue, New York, NY 10010.

Palgrave Macmillan is the global academic imprint of the above companies and has companies and representatives throughout the world.

Palgrave® and Macmillan® are registered trademarks in the United States, the United Kingdom, Europe and other countries.

ISBN 978–1–137–27742–8   hardback
ISBN 978–1–137–27743–5   paperback

This book is printed on paper suitable for recycling and made from fully managed and sustained forest sources. Logging, pulping and manufacturing processes are expected to conform to the environmental regulations of the country of origin.

A catalogue record for this book is available from the British Library.

A catalogue record for this book is available from the Library of Congress.

Typeset by MPS Limited, Chennai, India.

To my life-long companions Sarah, Richard and Madeline

Contents

List of Tables and Figures

Tables

Figures

List of Abbreviations

ADHD	attention deficit hyperactivity disorder
APA	American Psychiatric Association
BPRS	Brief Psychiatric Rating Scale
CATIE	Clinical Antipsychotic Trial of Intervention Effectiveness study
CT	computerised tomography
D_1, D_2	dopamine 1 and 2 receptors
DSM	*Diagnostic and Statistical Manual of Mental Disorders*
ECG	electrocardiogram
ECT	electro-convulsive therapy
FDA	Food and Drug Administration
LSD	lysergic acid diethylamide
MRI	magnetic resonance imaging
NAMI	National Alliance for the Mentally Ill
NICE	National Institute of Health and Clinical Excellence
NIMH	National Institute of Mental Health
PACE	Personal Assessment and Crisis Evaluation clinic
PANSS	Positive and Negative Syndrome Scale
PET	positron emission tomography
PIER	Portland Identification and Early Referral programme
PTSD	post-traumatic stress disorder
SSRI	selective serotonin reuptake inhibitor
TIPS	Early Identification and Treatment of Psychosis programme
VA	Veterans Affairs
5-HT_{2a}	5-hydroxytryptamine receptor 2a

Preface and Acknowledgements

I have been interested in the drugs used to treat psychiatric problems ever since, as a junior psychiatrist in the 1990s, I realised how completely drug treatment dominated psychiatric practice, and how inadequate were the current theories for explaining the effects these drugs had on people in real life. Since their introduction in the 1950s, what we now call 'antipsychotics' have become psychiatry's most iconic treatment, symbolising everything that modern psychiatry wishes to portray of itself. They are a simple, easy to administer, seemingly specific medical treatment that, it is claimed, target the underlying biological basis of the most serious and debilitating family of psychiatric conditions, the 'psychoses,' including the most frightening and disabling of all forms of madness, schizophrenia. Discovered by chance, so the story goes, and introduced against resistance from an unwilling and psychoanalytically inclined profession, antipsychotics helped to place psychiatry on a sound medical footing, revealing the true nature of psychiatric disorders as diseases of the brain, and enabling patients to be discharged in droves from the old asylums back into normal life.

This book will challenge this common perception of the revolutionary nature of antipsychotics by setting them in the context of the physical interventions that preceded them, procedures like insulin coma therapy, now mostly discredited, and also by reinstating an understanding of these substances as drugs, in other words as potentially toxic chemicals that change the way the body functions. It will explore the characteristic alterations that antipsychotics induce, particularly their 'psychoactive' effects, that is the way they modify normal processes of thinking and feeling. Exploring the history of antipsychotics reveals that the clinicians and researchers who first prescribed these drugs were interested in these effects and how they impacted on people with mental disturbances of various sorts. As the drugs became transformed in official circles into disease-specific, targeted treatments, however, this knowledge was lost from view. The ideas represented here form an attempt to reclaim this way of understanding the effects of antipsychotic drugs and their potential role within mental health services.

The book also charts the effects of this metamorphosis of antipsychotics into restorative treatments. The belittling of the drugs' serious neurological side effects, the denial of their use to control unwanted behaviour and the lack of interest in properly researching their long-term effects all derive from a bias that sees the drugs as essentially benign because they work by rectifying an underlying disease.

When the limitations of the older drugs started to be acknowledged in the 1980s, a new range of antipsychotics was launched, which was promoted first to people with psychotic disorders and then to a much wider portion of the population with the mantra that the drugs help reverse a 'chemical imbalance' or stop an underlying process of neurodegeneration. This book will show how these claims do not stand up to scrutiny, yet they were successfully utilised by the pharmaceutical industry, aided and abetted by the psychiatric profession, with the result that the new antipsychotics have become multi-million dollar blockbusters, as lucrative as antidepressants and statins.

It is important to state straight away that I am a practising psychiatrist, and that I believe that antipsychotics have a role in helping to suppress the manifestations of severe mental disturbance. I have seen people who are locked into an overwhelming psychotic state, which can sometimes be sufficiently suppressed by antipsychotics of one sort or another that they are able to regain some contact with the outside world again. This suppression comes at a price, however, as other thoughts and emotions are also slowed and numbed, but for some people this price is worth paying, at least initially. The cost–benefit analysis of long-term treatment, especially in people who have recovered from their acute episode, is more difficult to fathom.

One of the problems with writing a critical book on mental health issues is the question of terminology. Commonly used terms like 'mental illness', 'patient,' 'treatment' and, of course, 'antipsychotic' carry connotations that a critically-minded observer might wish to challenge. Yet, as the medical view of mental health problems is so deeply entrenched in the general psyche and forms the basis of the modern mental health system, it is sometimes difficult to make sense if these terms are not used. Alternatives that have general currency and acceptance simply do not exist, and one risks becoming incomprehensible, or at least extremely cumbersome, if one tries to avoid them altogether. I made a decision, for example, to use the term 'antipsychotic' in preference to the more descriptive term 'neuroleptic' throughout this book when a student asked me what a 'neuroleptic' was. Similarly, although I acknowledge that the concept of schizophrenia is highly contested, so much of the research I have looked at accepts this label at face value that it is virtually impossible to avoid the use of the term when looking at this research in any detail without adding endless caveats.

I apologise, therefore, if the language I use is insufficiently critical of concepts and views that I, as well as others, believe are inadequate, misleading, and need dissecting and challenging. Whatever my reservations about current approaches, however, I do accept that some people suffer from severe, disabling and occasionally persistent forms of mental distraction, which can manifest in bizarre, dysfunctional and sometimes dangerous behaviour, whose origins currently remain mysterious and possibly always will. It is for these people above all others that I offer this reappraisal of antipsychotic drugs and their history.

Many other authors have covered parts of the story I have presented in the following pages. I have drawn, in particular, on the work of Peter Breggin, David Cohen, Sheldon Gelman, David Healy, Judith Swazey and Robert Whitaker. I would like to thank Richard Bentall and other anonymous reviewers for their encouraging comments on the initial proposal for this book; Michael King, my head of department at University College London; and Martin Orrell, head of Research and Development at the North East London Foundation Trust for their support; and Sonu Shamdasani and the staff and students of the University College London Centre for the History of Psychological Disciplines for discussing and developing ideas with me. Special thanks are due to all the librarians at the North East London Foundation Trust library for tracing obscure articles; to Doreen, Liz and Irene for help tracking down copyright holders; and to Olivia Middleton and Nicola Jones at Palgrave for their enthusiasm for the project. I am also grateful to all those service users, carers, doctors, nurses, psychologists, social workers and other professionals who have debated with me at meetings and conferences over the last few years, and to all members of the Critical Psychiatry Network for their understanding and assistance. Finally, I would like to thank my mother and father for their hard work proof reading, and for their lifelong support and encouragement.

1
Cure or Curse: What Are Antipsychotics?

Antipsychotic drugs, otherwise known as neuroleptics and sometimes major tranquillisers, were introduced into psychiatry in the 1950s. Many people believe these drugs were the first really effective treatment for the severely mentally ill, and they have been referred to as 'miracle' or 'wonder' drugs that were said to represent a medical advance as significant as antibiotics (Time Magazine, 1954, 1955; Shorter, 1997). Their introduction is frequently credited with transforming the care of the mad or 'insane', enabling the closure of the old Victorian asylums and ushering in the possibility of more humane care based in the community. According to this view, people who would have languished in the back wards of institutions for the whole of their lives could be restored, through drug treatment, to lead normal lives in the outside world. The drugs were said to have brought about the 'social emancipation of the mental patient', and to have changed the nature, purpose and location of psychiatric practice (Freyhan, 1955, p. 84). The introduction of antipsychotics and other modern drugs into psychiatry was heralded as a 'chemical revolution' that constituted one of the 'most important and dramatic epics in the history of medicine itself' (F. Ayd cited in Swazey, 1974, p. 8).

Antipsychotics are not simply believed to be more effective than previous treatments, however. They are believed to be something quite distinct and unique. In contrast to the drugs that came before them, which were regarded merely as a crude means of controlling agitated or challenging behaviour, antipsychotics are thought to work by cleverly targeting an underlying disease or abnormality. They are thought to exert their beneficial or therapeutic effects by counteracting the brain processes that give rise to the symptoms of the most devastating and burdensome of mental conditions—that known as 'schizophrenia'.

1

With the introduction of antipsychotics, psychiatrists believed they could, at last, alter the course and outcome of a major mental illness, and that 'for the first time, public mental institutions could be regarded as true treatment centres, rather than as primarily custodial facilities' (Davis and Cole, 1975, p. 442). The idea that there were proper medical treatments for mental disorders that acted on underlying diseases in the same way as antibiotics or cancer drugs helped to lift psychiatry out of the doldrums, transforming it from a neglected form of social work into what was perceived as a properly scientific activity, and restoring it to its rightful place within the medical arena (Shorter, 1997; Comite Lyonnais de Recherches Therapeutiques en Psychiatrie, 2000). By this account, the introduction of antipsychotics is a story of untainted medical progress.

Yet, for others, antipsychotic drugs are the embodiment of psychiatric oppression, equivalent to the shackles and manacles of previous eras. They have replaced electro-convulsive therapy (ECT) and lobotomy as the main target of criticism of the psychiatric system, and are viewed by detractors as a chemical straight jacket, used to facilitate the control of unwanted behaviour. Many people who have taken the drugs describe the experience as highly unpleasant, like a 'living hell,' 'sheer torture' or being in a 'drug prison' (Breggin, 1993a, p. 57; Anonymous, 2009b). People describe feeling like 'zombies' under the influence of the drugs, with their mental capacities dulled and their emotions blunted (Wallace, 1994). For those who are forced to take antipsychotics against their will, the experience is particularly traumatic. Former patient turned campaigner David Oaks, reflecting on his experience of the mental health system in early adulthood, described how the effect of coerced antipsychotic drug treatment 'felt like a wrecking ball to the cathedral of my mind' (Oaks, 2011, p. 190). Mental health advocacy groups have argued that such activity constitutes a breach of human rights. Demonstrations against forced drug treatment have become a regular occurrence outside major psychiatric conferences in the USA (Mindfreedom, 2012), and campaigns have also been conducted in England (Figure 1.1), Ireland and Norway. Even those who feel the drugs have been helpful often describe the high price they have had to pay for these benefits. 'It makes you sane, but you're not much better off', commented one antipsychotic user on a medication website (Anonymous, 2009a).

Critics from within the mental health professions have also challenged the view that antipsychotic drugs are a restorative and benign medical treatment. Psychiatrist Peter Breggin claims that antipsychotics induce a form of 'chemical lobotomy' and cause permanent brain

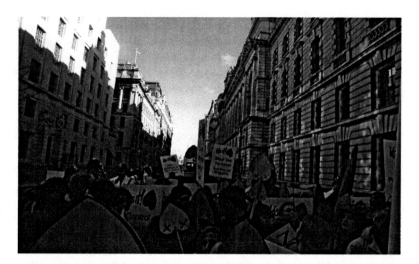

Figure 1.1 'Kissit' demonstration, UK, 2005 (Reproduced courtesy of Anthony Fisher Photography)

damage, leading to a form of drug-induced dementia (Breggin, 2008). Furthermore, Breggin and others suggest that the 'brain disabling' effect of these drugs is not an unintended side effect, but the *intended* consequence of drug treatment. This view of antipsychotics as a chemical cosh that stifles mental and physical activity goes back to the time of their introduction in the 1950s, when many clinicians welcomed the new drugs' ability to suppress normal brain function. Others, however, commented on how the new tranquillisers, later to become known as antipsychotics, had replaced the noise and disturbance of the asylum with the 'silence of the cemetery' (Comite Lyonnais de Recherches Therapeutiques en Psychiatrie, 2000, p. 29; attributed to Racamier or Lacan).

While criticising antipsychotics was once regarded as the territory of a few extremists, the reputation of these drugs has recently become more widely tarnished through revelations about the activities of the companies that market them. In 2009, Eli Lilly reached the record books for incurring what was at the time the largest fine in US corporate history for the illegal marketing of its blockbuster antipsychotic drug, Zyprexa (olanzapine), in situations in which it had not been licenced. AstraZeneca, Pfizer and Johnson & Johnson have also been found guilty of illegally promoting their atypical antipsychotics, and revelations that companies had suppressed or minimised evidence of the serious side effects of these drugs, particularly their propensity to cause weight gain and diabetes, has also come to light (Berenson, 2006). Large settlements have been paid out to people who have alleged drug-induced effects of this sort in North America (Berenson, 2007). Moreover, data have been gradually accumulating from brain imaging studies that confirm earlier suspicions that antipsychotics cause brain shrinkage. Nancy Andreason, a leading biological psychiatrist and former editor of the *American Journal of Psychiatry*, acknowledged these findings in an interview with the *New York Times* in 2008 (Dreifus, 2008). In 2012, British psychiatrist, Peter Tyrer, editor of the *British Journal of Psychiatry*, went even further, admitting that there is an 'increasing body of evidence that the adverse effects of treatment [with antipsychotics] are, to put it simply, not worth the candle'. 'For many', he suggested, 'the risks outweigh the benefits'(Tyrer, 2012, p. 168).

Understanding how a group of drugs, initially understood as powerful nervous system suppressants, came to be regarded as a miraculous medical intervention that could successfully counteract the biological origins of mental disease, helps to illuminate how a motley collection of unpleasant and toxic substances could rise to become modern day blockbusters. Antipsychotics started life in the asylums of the mid-twentieth century, but 50 years later they are being prescribed to millions of people worldwide, including children, many of whom have never even seen a psychiatrist (Sankaranarayanan and Puumala, 2007). Aggressive marketing has driven these powerful chemicals, once reserved for the most severely mentally disturbed, out into the wider community. We all need to be aware now of what these drugs are, and what they can do. Antipsychotics have become everybody's problem.

Use of Antipsychotics

The first drug that came to be classified as an antipsychotic is chlorpromazine, but it is often better known by its brand names—Largactil in the UK and Thorazine in the USA. It was first used in psychiatry in the early 1950s, and it was regarded as so successful that in the following years numerous other drugs aimed at treating psychosis and schizophrenia were introduced. Haloperidol was first marketed in 1958 and, for a long time, it was the biggest selling antipsychotic on the market. Stelazine (trifluoperazine) and perphenazine were also introduced in the 1960s, and Modecate (fluphenazine), the first injectable, long-acting, 'depot' preparation of an antipsychotic, was released in 1969. It was followed by Haldol, a depot preparation of haloperidol, and the still commonly used depot injections Depixol (flupentixol) and Clopixol (zuclopenthixol) (see Appendix 1).

In the 1990s a new generation of antipsychotic drugs was introduced, which are sometimes referred to as the 'atypicals'. These followed on the heels of clozapine, the archetypal atypical antipsychotic, which was reintroduced in 1990, after having been abandoned in the 1970s when its potential to cause life-threatening blood disorders became apparent. The success of clozapine for people who were deemed to have 'treatment resistant schizophrenia', along with problems that became apparent with the older drugs, particularly the drug-induced neuro- logical condition known as tardive dyskinesia, encouraged attempts to develop other clozapine-like drugs for schizophrenia and psychosis. Risperidone, also known by its brand name Risperdal, was duly licensed and launched in 1994, and olanzapine, or Zyprexa in 1996. Quetiapine, marketed under the name Seroquel, was approved by the US Food and Drug Administration in 1994 and in the UK in 1997.

For the first 30 years after their introduction antipsychotic drugs were reserved mainly for the treatment of people with severe psychiatric prob- lems. They were officially recommended for the treatment of people with schizophrenia or psychosis, although they were always administered more widely than this, and were given to many of the inmates of the old asylums, regardless of their diagnosis. Low doses of some of the more sedative antipsychotics were also prescribed to people with sleep problems and anxiety, but such use was not endorsed officially, and they were never regarded as drugs that had a mass market. Since the introduction of the 'atypicals', however, the use of these drugs has widened and aggressive marketing has made some of these drugs into worldwide best-sellers. In 2010 spending on antipsychotic drugs in the USA reached a total of almost $17 billion, only just behind anti-diabetic drugs and statins, and ahead of antidepressants (IMS Institute for Healthcare Informatics, 2011). In England, in 2010, 7.5 million prescriptions were issued for antipsychot- ics in the community alone (excluding the large number of prescriptions issued to patients in psychiatric hospitals)—a 61% increase on the number of prescriptions issued in 1998 (Figure 1.2). The cost of the drugs increased by a dramatic 286% over the same period, with antipsychotics costing the English National Health Service £282 million in 2010. By 2007, they became the most costly class of drug treatment used for mental health problems in England, overtaking antidepressants, which had enjoyed this dubious honour for a decade or more (Ilyas and Moncrieff, 2012).

The success of the new generation of antipsychotics was achieved in two ways. First, marketing campaigns attempted to convince prescribers

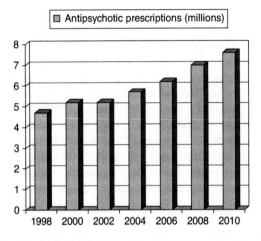

Figure 1.2   Trends in prescriptions of antipsychotics issued in the community in England (data from the National Health Service Information Centre for Health and Social Care, 1998–2010)

that the atypical antipsychotics should replace the use of the older antipsychotics for the treatment of people with schizophrenia or psychosis. By 2002, atypical antipsychotics represented more than 90% of all antipsychotics prescribed in the USA (Sankaranarayanan and Puumala, 2007), and, by 2009, they had captured 73% of the community prescription market in the UK (NHS Prescription Services, 2009). A few blockbusting drugs now occupy the majority of this market, particularly olanzapine, quetiapine and risperidone (Zyprexa, Seroquel and Risperdal). In 2010 these three drugs accounted for 63% of community prescriptions of antipsychotics in England, and olanzapine and quetiapine alone made up 76% of the costs of all antipsychotic drugs.

Second, there has been a concerted effort to expand the indications for the use of antipsychotics in general, so that the atypical antipsychotics could be targeted at the wider population in the way that had proved so successful for modern 'antidepressant' drugs like Prozac and Seroxat (Paxil). Companies promoted antipsychotics for use in elderly people with dementia, targeting the staff of nursing homes and pharmacies, despite the fact they had no licence for the treatment of dementia, or agitation in people with dementia, and regardless of accumulating evidence that the use of antipsychotics in dementia shortens people's lives. Atypical antipsychotics were also promoted for the treatment of common problems including anxiety, depression, irritability, agitation and insomnia (United States Department of Justice, 2009, 2010), and data from the USA and the UK suggest that the majority of prescriptions of atypical antipsychotics are now issued to people who are diagnosed with depression, anxiety or, more recently, bipolar disorder rather than schizophrenia or psychosis (Kaye et al., 2003; Alexander et al., 2011).

The expansion of the concept of bipolar disorder has been one of the key strategies employed to expand antipsychotic use into the wider population. Atypical antipsychotic manufacturers successfully transformed perceptions of the condition from being a rare and highly distinctive form of severe madness, to the common and familiar experience of intense and fluctuating moods. In this manner they were able to capture some of the large population that had previously identified themselves, or had been identified, as depressed (Spielmans, 2009).

Most worryingly, antipsychotics have been prescribed to increasing numbers of children over the last few years, especially in the USA (Olfson et al., 2006). Much of this prescribing has also been justified by giving children the newly fabricated diagnosis of paediatric bipolar disorder, but the drugs are also prescribed, often in combination with other drugs, to children diagnosed with attention deficit hyperactivity disorder (ADHD), autism and 'behavioural problems'. Although parents and academics have been at the forefront of the trend to label children with bipolar disorder and medicate them with antipsychotics, drug company money has helped to lubricate this activity and give it respectability by funding research programmes and cultivating leading academics as allies with generous payments for services rendered (Harris and Carey, 2008).

What Are Antipsychotics and What Do They Do?

This expansion in the use of antipsychotic drugs has been dependent on a theoretical framework that casts psychiatric drugs as specially targeted treatments that work by reversing or ameliorating an underlying brain abnormality or dysfunction. The nature of the abnormality is often referred to as a 'chemical imbalance', and drug company websites repeatedly stress the idea that psychiatric medication works by rectifying a chemical imbalance. The website for the antipsychotic Geodon (zisprasidone—an antipsychotic used in the USA, but not in the UK), stated in its information about schizophrenia in 2006 that 'imbalances of certain chemicals in the brain are thought to lead to the symptoms of the illness. Medicine plays a *key role* in balancing these chemicals' (my emphasis) (Pfizer, 2006). Similarly, Seroquel is 'thought to work', said its manufacturers in 2011, 'by helping to regulate the balance of chemicals in the brain to help treat schizophrenia' (AstraZeneca, 2011). Antidepressants like Prozac and Paxil are also said to 'balance your brain's chemistry' (GlaxoSmithKline, 2009) and information on bipolar disorder, or manic depression, suggests the condition is triggered by 'an imbalance in some key chemicals in the brain' that antipsychotics can help to 'adjust' (Otsuka America Pharmaceutical, 2012).

Information produced by professional organisations makes similar statements. The American Psychiatric Association's 1996 leaflet on schizophrenia suggested that antipsychotic drugs 'help bring biochemical imbalances closer to normal' (American Psychiatric Association, 1996). The UK's Royal College of Psychiatrists claims that there is an 'imbalance in brain chemistry' in people with psychosis or schizophrenia (Royal College of Psychiatrists, 2004) and antidepressants are said by the American Psychiatric Association to 'correct imbalances in the levels of chemicals in the brain' (American Psychiatric Association, 2005).

What sort of drugs antipsychotics are thought to be, and how they are understood to work in people with schizophrenia and other conditions, is fundamental to the debate about their merits and how to use them appropriately. These descriptions of the action of psychiatric drugs as reversing chemical imbalances embody a particular way of understanding the action of drugs, which I have called the 'disease-centred' model of drug action. The disease-centred model can be contrasted with an alternative 'drug-centred' model, and some of the features of the two models are outlined in Table 1.1 (Moncrieff and Cohen, 2005; Moncrieff, 2008a).

The disease-centred model of drug action is based on the idea that drugs work by acting on the aberrant biological processes, be it chemical imbalances or other abnormalities, which are assumed to produce the symptoms of a particular disorder. According to this view, drugs make the body more 'normal' by helping to reverse an underlying

Table 1.1　Models of drug action

Disease-centred model	Drug-centred model
Drugs correct an abnormal brain state	Drugs create an abnormal brain state
Drugs as medical treatments	Drugs as psychoactive substances
The beneficial effects of drugs are derived from their effects on a presumed disease process	The drugs alter the expression of psychiatric problems through the superimposition of drug-induced effects
Example: insulin for diabetes	Example: alcohol for social anxiety

disease or dysfunction. This action on the disease process is the drug's 'therapeutic' action, and all its other actions are designated as 'side effects' and considered to be of secondary importance.

The disease-centred model is borrowed from general medicine, where most modern drugs act on the physiological pathways that produce the symptoms of a disease. Insulin treatment for diabetes helps correct the insulin deficiency that leads to the symptoms of diabetes, for example. Drugs used for asthma, such as salbutamol, expand the airways, reducing the constriction that causes wheezing. Steroids and other anti-inflammatory drugs reduce the over-active inflammatory response that produces the symptoms of various conditions such as eczema and rheumatoid arthritis. None of these drugs reverses the underlying cause of the disease, but they all act on biological processes that produce particular symptoms. In this sense the disease-centred model could be referred to as a 'symptom-centred' model in most cases. Even clearly symptomatic treatments like the painkillers aspirin and paracetamol can be understood in this disease- or symptom-centred manner, as they work by acting on the neurophysiological pathways that produce pain.

The disease-centred model of drug action has become the dominant way of theorising what drugs do when they are taken by someone with a mental health problem. It is so influential that people are not aware that there are other ways of conceptualising how drugs affect people with mental disorders, or whether the disease-centred model is supported by scientific evidence. But the idea that psychiatric drugs work by targeting underlying biological processes that are specific to certain sorts of mental health problems or symptoms is central to the way that psychiatric treatment is administered and presented, and to the way that research on drug treatment is designed, conducted and interpreted. The latest edition of the principle American textbook of psychiatry (which, interestingly, opens with a four-page colour spread of different drugs listed alphabetically under their trade names), stresses that 'mental disorders are true medical conditions that can benefit from drug therapy in the same way that diabetes, asthma and hypothyroidism, and other chronic disorders are responsive to medication' (Sussman, 2009).

As we shall see in the following chapters, however, this conception of how psychiatric drugs work is relatively recent. Prior to the 1950s the drugs that were prescribed to psychiatric patients were understood quite differently, according to what I have called the drug-centred model of drug action. This model is so named because it suggests that psychiatric drugs need to be understood first and foremost as *drugs*, that is as chemical substances that alter the way the body functions. Moreover, psychiatric drugs are a special type of drug known as *psychoactive* drugs, which are substances that affect brain functioning, and which, as a consequence, alter mental experience and behaviour. According to the drug-centred model, rather than reversing some underlying brain abnormality, psychiatric drugs themselves create an abnormal or altered state of physical and mental functioning.

Psychoactive drugs, by definition, are chemicals that act on the body's central nervous system and by doing so produce changes in perception, mood, consciousness and behaviour. The most familiar psychoactive substances are recreational drugs like alcohol, nicotine, heroin, cannabis and LSD. When we think of recreational drugs we refer to the altered mental states they produce as 'intoxication'. Some drugs, such as alcohol, produce profound and easily identifiable states of intoxication, whereas the intoxication produced by drugs like nicotine and caffeine is more subtle. Psychiatric drugs also produce states of intoxication whose features vary according to what sort of drug is taken. Just as the effects of cannabis differ from those of alcohol or heroin, so the effects produced by 'antipsychotics' are different from those produced by drugs like Valium, which differ again from the effects of the so-called antidepressant drug Prozac, for example. The characteristic features of the intoxicated or drug-induced state depend on the chemical structure and nature of each drug. Recreational drugs produce effects that some people find pleasurable or enjoyable. Many other psychoactive drugs, however, including the antipsychotics, produce effects that most people find unpleasant.

One of the many and varied effects of antipsychotic drugs is their ability to oppose the actions of the brain chemical called dopamine by blocking certain types of dopamine receptors.[1] At least five types of dopamine receptor have been identified so far, but it is the ability of antipsychotics to block one particular type of dopamine receptor, the D_2 receptor, that gives rise to their characteristic neurological effects and is thought, by many, to produce their therapeutic effects. However, both the first and second generation of antipsychotic drugs come from a number of different chemical classes, and none of them act solely on dopamine receptors. Many antipsychotics, including chlorpromazine, thioridazine, clozapine and olanzapine, have an extremely broad range of actions on a large number of the brain's chemical systems, and some of them, such as clozapine and olanzapine have relatively weak actions on the D_2 receptor. Even those drugs that target the dopamine system more precisely, like haloperidol, have a variety of actions on other systems. Despite decades of research and speculation, we do not fully understand the chemical basis of the actions of antipsychotics, or whether, as a group, they act on symptoms through the same mechanism or through a variety of different mechanisms.

Although there is variation in individuals' response to all drugs, psychoactive drugs produce their characteristic range of effects in anyone who takes them, regardless of whether or not they have a psychological problem. Most psychoactive drugs also have physical effects, and the physical and mental effects are often inextricably linked. Alcohol and benzodiazepines, for example, produce a state of both physical and mental relaxation, and stimulant drugs, like amphetamines and cocaine, stimulate mental processes like attention and alertness, as well as physical processes like increasing heart rate and blood pressure. The physical and mental effects of antipsychotics are also intimately linked, as we shall see, and it is impossible to understand one without an appreciation of the other.

The drug-centred model suggests that drugs can sometimes be helpful because certain drug-induced psychoactive effects can replace or suppress the manifestations of mental disorders. An example of this is the long-accepted benefits of alcohol in people with social phobia or social anxiety. Alcohol is not thought to be helpful because it corrects a deficiency of alcohol within the brain, or because it corrects another chemical imbalance. It is thought to help because one of the characteristic features of alcohol intoxication is that it reduces social inhibitions, which may be helpful for someone who finds social situations anxiety-provoking.

Following the drug-centred model of drug action, the barbiturates and other sedative drugs that were used in psychiatry prior to the advent of antipsychotics were understood to be acting as chemical restraints, which sedated people and rendered them more manageable, without affecting the underlying problem. As we shall see, the antipsychotics themselves were also viewed in this manner at first. Perceptions changed over the course of the 1950s and 1960s, however, and the group of chemicals that were first known as neuroleptics or tranquillisers, came to be viewed as a specific treatment for the symptoms of psychosis or schizophrenia. First thought of as special sorts of sedatives, they were transformed in the minds of those who prescribed them into psychiatry's first real 'magic bullet'.

Evidence for the Action of Antipsychotics

This transformation was not, however, as we shall see in more detail in Chapter 3, the result of an accumulating body of compelling scientific evidence, or even of persuasive and informed debate. No studies were set up to evaluate whether antipsychotics or antidepressants really targeted a disease process, and whether their mind-altering properties could be deemed irrelevant to their impact on mental health problems. When the disease-centred model of drug action was adopted, the fact that there was another way of thinking about drug action was swiftly forgotten, and so almost no research was conducted to attempt to confirm or refute the idea that psychiatric drugs worked in a disease-specific manner. Elsewhere, I have reviewed in detail the little evidence that exists on all types of psychiatric drugs (Moncrieff, 2008a) and, in the course of this book, we shall see what research has been conducted that might illuminate the mode of action of antipsychotics. I shall argue that none of the evidence justifies the presumption that antipsychotics act in a disease-specific manner in schizophrenia or psychosis, and that the drug-centred model remains a more compelling approach for explaining the full range of actions of antipsychotics— both those that are intended and those that are not.

It is important to realise at the start that no chemical imbalance or other biological process that might explain drug action in a disease-centred way has been substantiated for any psychiatric disorder. The serotonin theory of depression and the dopamine hypothesis of schizophrenia, which appear to suggest that drugs act in this way, remain merely hypotheses. Most authorities now admit that there is no evidence that depression is associated with abnormalities of serotonin or noradrenaline, as used to be believed (Dubovsky et al., 2001). There is also little empirical support for the dopamine hypothesis of schizophrenia, as we shall see in Chapter 4, and many psychiatric researchers acknowledge it is at least inadequate as an explanation for the aetiology of schizophrenia. The fact that the theory will not die, despite decades of contradictory findings, illustrates the importance of portraying the action of antipsychotics in disease-centred terms. By helping to establish the idea that antipsychotics exert a disease-specific action in schizophrenia and psychosis as unquestioned fact, the dopamine hypothesis has helped to create the impression that antipsychotics might have disease-specific actions in the many other circumstances in which they are now employed.

The Zyprexa website boldly suggests that 'antipsychotic medicines are believed to work by balancing the chemicals found *naturally* in the brain' (my emphasis) (Eli Lilly, 2011). The statement demonstrates the utility of adopting the disease-centred model of drug action. By taking Zyprexa it is implied that you will restore some imagined chemical harmony, whose disruption is suggested to be the origin of your problem or symptoms. This appealing, but entirely hypothetical, proposition conveniently disguises the fact that drugs consist of foreign chemical substances that would be expected to alter and disrupt the body's normal chemical functioning, rather than restore or enhance it.

The Nature of Psychosis and Schizophrenia

Although antipsychotics are used more widely, their most well accepted use continues to be what they are named for—the treatment of psychosis, or what generally used to be called schizophrenia. Schizophrenia is a highly contested concept, of course, and even mainstream psychiatrists would acknowledge that the label is applied to people with a variety of different problems. The German psychiatrist, Eugene Bleuler first coined the term schizophrenia, and described what he saw as the characteristic 'splitting,' disintegration or fragmentation of psychic functions (Bleuler, 1911). He also drew attention to the withdrawal from reality that people with the disorder show, which he referred to as 'autism'—a term that has now, of course, been used to designate another proposed, but also disputed, psychiatric condition (Timimi et al., 2011). Bleuler also divided the symptoms into 'positive' symptoms, which consist of bizarre thoughts and experiences, including delusions and hallucinations, and 'negative' symptoms. The latter denote a state of demotivation and apathy, a loss of interest in participating in the normal activities of life, and the blunting of emotional responses (Table 1.2).

The term 'psychotic' is usually applied to the positive symptoms of schizophrenia, and an episode of 'psychosis' refers to an episode characterised by symptoms such as delusions and hallucinations that indicate a loss of contact with reality. In an extreme psychotic state people appear to be locked into an internal mental world. As Bleuler put it: 'one of the most important symptoms of schizophrenia is the preponderance

Table 1.2 Positive and negative symptoms of schizophrenia

Positive symptoms	Negative symptoms
• Hallucinations (usually auditory, 'hearing voices') • Delusions • Feelings of being controlled • Feelings of having thoughts read, broadcast or interfered with • Incoherent or tangential speech	• Reduced speech • Apathy or inactivity • Social withdrawal • Blunted emotions

of inner life, with an active turning away from the external world. The most severe cases withdraw completely and live in a dream world; milder cases withdraw to a lesser degree' (Bleuler, 1951, p. 397).

The pattern thought to be most characteristic of schizophrenia is where a young person, usually a young man, withdraws from the world, develops 'positive,' psychotic symptoms, and then sinks into a state of apathy, decline and withdrawal, sometimes punctuated by recurrent psychotic symptoms. This was the trajectory described by Kraepelin, the German psychiatrist who described the condition he called 'dementia praecox', generally considered to be the forerunner of schizophrenia. This pattern is actually rare, however, at least in modern day mental health services. Many people experience episodes characterised by various 'positive' symptoms only, which eventually abate,and they return to their previous roles. A few display only 'negative' symptoms, although often there is a suspicion that they might be having some unusual internal experiences, which they cannot articulate. Others present an array of challenging behaviour and strange thoughts, but do not conform neatly to the characteristic pattern of symptoms labelled as schizophrenia.

To illustrate the variety of ways that people can manifest what is called psychosis or schizophrenia I have summarised some accounts written by people who have had this experience (or their carers) in Appendix 2. As these stories demonstrate, for some psychotic symptoms are frightening and distressing and clearly unwanted, but for others psychotic reality can be enjoyable and exciting. For others it is both of these things. Some people take years to reach a state of stability, and for many this involves a long and arduous process of coming to terms with the unpleasant and stifling effects of antipsychotic medication. Even then, some people continue to experience psychotic symptoms and struggle to function independently. The final story, however, illustrates that it is possible to make a full recovery from severe and prolonged psychotic episodes without modern drug treatment, and to derive benefit from the experience.

There has, of course, been a vast amount of research and debate into the nature and causes of schizophrenia. On the one hand, mainstream biological psychiatry asserts that it is a brain disease caused by a specific, but not yet fully identified, abnormality of brain function, which may, in turn, be the result of a particular genetic make-up. On the other hand, the critics of biological psychiatry have questioned the validity of the whole concept of schizophrenia. Thomas Szasz, for example, the psychiatrist famous for denouncing psychiatry, views all psychiatric diagnoses, including schizophrenia, as disguised moral and political judgements about deviant behaviour (Szasz, 1970). Others have suggested that psychotic breakdowns are reactions to traumatic situations, and recent research reveals high levels of previous physical and sexual abuse and victimisation in people diagnosed with psychotic disorders (Read et al., 2003; Gracie et al., 2007). This view overlaps with theories advanced in the 1960s and 1970s by 'antipsychiatrist' R.D. Laing and colleagues, who suggested that psychotic experiences could be understood as meaningful responses to the circumstances of an individual's upbringing and environment (Laing, 1965). In his later writings, influenced by the 1960s counterculture, Laing suggested that psychosis might even represent a 'sane response to an insane world' (Laing, 1967).[2] Other psychological analyses, without necessarily contradicting the possibility of understanding the condition at a biological level, have underlined the relation between psychotic symptoms, like hearing voices and paranoid delusions, and normal mental processes (Freeman, 2007; Waters et al., 2010).

Szasz and other writers have emphasised the difference between a 'mental illness', such as schizophrenia, and an ordinary bodily disease. British psychiatrist Alec Jenner described schizophrenia, as 'closer to a life process than to an illness' (Jenner et al., 1993, p. 61). According to this view, the tendency to have psychotic breakdowns or a longer lasting mental condition can be understood as part of the variety of human nature or a set of 'ways of being human' (Jenner et al., 1993). This does not mean that it is a desirable state of affairs, but it does mean that, like other aspects of human character and behaviour, madness or mental disorder results from a complex interaction of biology, environment and agency, and that disentangling the precise contributions of these different factors may well be impossible.

In this book I wish to largely side-step the question of the nature of schizophrenia, as it is already the subject of many other books. Nor is it immediately relevant to the subject of what antipsychotics do and how they do it. The analysis of antipsychotic drugs presented here is applicable whatever position you take on the nature of schizophrenia. A drug-centred model of drug action is compatible with the idea that schizophrenia is a brain disease, as well as with other models of the nature of schizophrenia. The drug-centred model merely suggests that current psychiatric drugs do not work by acting on an underlying disease process. It does not necessarily deny that there is an underlying disease, although it does weaken the current case that such an entity exists because the idea that antipsychotics have a disease-specific action has long been an important part of the evidence for this position.

It is necessary to point out, however, that despite the claims of much official information, current evidence does not allow us to conclude that schizophrenia is a brain disease in the simple sense in which we usually understand the term 'disease'. No biological factor, whether it be a genetic, biochemical or anatomical deviation, has been found that is consistently and specifically related to schizophrenia, despite more than half a century of recognisably modern research efforts. Moreover, what was thought to be one of the most reliable indications that schizophrenia arises from a defective brain, namely the finding that people with the diagnosis have smaller brains and larger brain cavities than people without, turns out, as we shall see in Chapter 10, to be at least partially a consequence of antipsychotic drug treatment.

Whatever its nature, however, and whether it is best understood as a brain disease, as social deviance, a response to trauma, a way of being human or a combination of these ideas, schizophrenia, psychosis or madness remains a serious problem for many of the people who go through it, their families and carers, and for society as a whole.

Antipsychotics and Mental Health Policy

Antipsychotic drugs were introduced during a period of transformation in the nature of mental health services in the Western world, when the care of people deemed mentally disturbed moved out of the Victorian institutions and into the community. Whether or not the introduction of antipsychotic drugs facilitated this process, and whether the drugs worked by restoring people to normality or through chemical suppression, has been the subject of much debate, but they undoubtedly played a symbolic role, if nothing else (Gronfein, 1985).

Psychiatry has changed in other ways over the decades since the introduction of antipsychotics. The once influential ideas of psychoanalysis have almost disappeared from mainstream teaching and practice, and in their place has risen a renewed and increasingly dogged biological psychiatry. In this new psychiatry, people are given medical-type diagnostic labels derived from manuals like the American *Diagnostic and Statistical Manual* (the *DSM*), which are regarded as designating underlying diseases, and treatment is applied according to the label or the diagnosis, with little regard for the personal history and particular circumstances of the individual. The skill of the practitioner, and the importance of the therapeutic relationship, once thought central to being a good psychiatrist, have been relegated to the shrinking specialism of psychotherapy, and replaced with a guideline-driven, shallow imitation of general medical practice. Drugs, especially when understood as acting according to a disease-centred model, fit nicely with this new approach, providing the basis for quick, cheap and apparently evidence-based therapy.

In the following chapters I will describe how antipsychotic drugs have been central to the transformation of the image of psychiatry in the minds of its practitioners and the public over the last few decades. The acceptance that these drugs could target the basis of schizophrenia conferred on psychiatry a level of respect it had never had before. Coupled with the use of technology, such as brain scans, for example, psychiatry acquired all the appearances of being a high-powered, cutting-edge scientific activity in which a variety of brain abnormalities could be detected and rectified with highly specific and targeted interventions. Having a psychiatric diagnosis lost its stigma, and people actively sought to be labelled and treated with the new products of this sophisticated branch of medicine.

The new image of psychiatry is exemplified in the portrayal of the use of drugs for the control of challenging or aggressive behaviour. No longer regarded as the equivalent of the shackles and manacles that were used to restrain the ravings of the mad in times past, the use of antipsychotics to reduce disturbance in psychiatric institutions is portrayed as a benign, therapeutic intervention administered for the health and benefit of the patient. Despite the fact that the same drugs are routinely employed as animal tranquillisers, the view that antipsychotics work in a disease-centred fashion has helped to present psychiatric activities as fundamentally therapeutic rather than coercive.

As early as the 1950s, Thomas Szasz pointed to the dangers of presenting the forcible control of unwanted behaviour as a medical treatment. The use of drugs conceals the power relation that enables one group of people to force their will on another, and removes the natural checks that exist when the reality of the situation is acknowledged. As Szasz observed in 1957, 'restraint by chemical means does not make us guilty; herein lies the danger to the patient' (Szasz, 1957, p. 91). Behavioural control using drugs does engender guilt, however, albeit less directly and immediately than mechanical restraint, and the rise of the disease-centred model of antipsychotic action is a testimony to the persistence of that guilt into the modern pharmacological era. As long as antipsychotic drugs were understood according to a drug-centred model, the qualities that made them useful restraints could not be ignored. It was only with the disease-centred model that forcible drugging could be presented as a treatment for the patient's underlying disease, and the guilt could truly lift.

The introduction of a legal framework for enforced community treatment in many Western countries, including the UK, means that people can now be compelled to take prescribed psychiatric drugs, even when they have fully recovered. Just as Szasz would have predicted, the idea that antipsychotics represent a restorative medical treatment has enabled the power that was located in psychiatric institutions to spread its tentacles out into the community. For increasing numbers of people with mental illness, there is no longer any choice over whether they take antipsychotics or not (NHS Information Centre for Health and Social Care, 2010). Although many psychiatrists would argue that enforcing drug treatment after recovery helps people to remain well or sane, others have a different view. In the words of David Oaks 'the monster that is forced drugging' has migrated from the 'back wards of locked psychiatric institutions to the front porch of our own homes in our own neighbourhoods' (Oaks, 2011, p. 189).

An Alternative View of Antipsychotics

The account I offer in the rest of this book suggests that antipsychotic drugs can be regarded as implements of social control, but that they can also help individuals gain relief from intense and intrusive psychotic experiences or destructive emotional states. The neurological inhibition they induce helps to reduce psychotic thought processes, and calm an agitated mind and body. Sometimes, when people are locked into an internal reality they cannot escape, this chemical suppression can bring them back into contact with the real world, and enable them to resume some normal activities and re-establish relations with other people. These benefits come at a price, however. Some people simply feel a little sedated, or numb or stiff. But others complain that their whole personality has been altered by the drugs. They feel they have lost their motivation and interest in the world, their originality, their emotional intensity; in short, the very things that make us human.

The same pharmacological properties that suppress psychotic experiences are what make antipsychotic drugs effective in tranquillising the challenging, aggressive patient and subduing the frenzied activities of the individual gripped by mania. In the long term the drugs can be used to modify behaviour that others find threatening, disturbing or anti-social. Taking a drug-centred approach to the nature of antipsychotics therefore reveals how they can be both effective chemical restraints and useful, therapeutic interventions.

By suggesting that social control is still at the heart of psychiatry, the drug-centred model of antipsychotic drugs opens up issues that the psychiatric profession had hoped to close, however. This book will chart the way that this mode of understanding was successfully buried, and how its replacement with the disease-centred model of drug action helped to divert attention from the pharmacological properties of psychiatric drugs and their potential application for the modification of unwanted behaviour. I hope the book will enable readers to re-evaluate the story of antipsychotic drugs as it is usually told, and appreciate the many dangers they present, as well as the opportunities they provide some people in the grips of a severe mental disorder. It is intended to throw a sceptical light on the acres of research literature and marketing material that presents these drugs as a practically untarnished boon to humankind, but also to show, through first-hand accounts, how the drugs might be distinctively helpful in some situations. It should also raise questions about the consequences of long-term treatment, and why, six decades after their introduction, we still cannot be sure if antipsychotics help or harm people who take them for long periods of time.

2
Chlorpromazine: The First Wonder Drug

Since the 1950s, drugs have been regarded as the principle form of treatment for people with psychiatric conditions. Alongside the introduction of chlorpromazine and other so-called 'antipsychotics' in the 1950s, lithium was suggested as a treatment for people diagnosed with mania or manic depression, drugs that are referred to as 'antidepressants' started to be used and, in the 1960s, the benzodiazepines—a class of sedative drugs that includes such household names as Valium, Librium and Ativan—were developed for the treatment of anxiety. Nowadays, the central, and often the only, aspect of treatment most people with mental health problems receive is drug treatment. When one drug fails to resolve a person's difficulties, another one is started, and then another, and then drugs are needed for the side effects of the first drugs and so on. Many people end up taking multiple substances in what is often an endless quest based on the belief that the right drug or drug combination can reverse the underlying problem.

A large proportion of psychiatric research and theory has also been inspired by the introduction of new drug treatments. When the disease-centred theory of drug action took hold, newly discovered drug-induced effects were interpreted as a clue to the underlying basis of the mental disorder the drug was thought to treat. So when antipsychotics were found to block dopamine receptors, acres of research were devoted to locating dopamine abnormalities in people with schizophrenia, as we shall see in Chapter 4. In a similar fashion, the effects of stimulants and some early 'antidepressants' on noradrenaline, and later the effects of drugs like Prozac on the serotonin system, inspired a vast research effort to investigate levels of noradrenaline and serotonin in people with depression—research that has yielded even less that is conclusive or enlightening than the research on dopamine in schizophrenia.

Although critics consider this research activity a waste of resources and a dangerous distraction from the real nature of psychiatric drugs (Breggin, 2008; Kirk et al., 2013), many scientists believe that modern drug treatments are helping them to unlock the secrets of mental illness.

Psychiatry in the Early Twentieth Century

The use of drugs has a long history in psychiatry, but the idea that they are an important intervention and that their action relates to the nature of the underlying condition is more recent. In the early twentieth century there was plenty of interest in the possible biological factors underlying mental disorders, with frequent articles discussing their proposed hereditary, biochemistry and histology, but there was little focus on treatment. At this time, psychiatric care took place in large state asylums that catered for 'pauper lunatics'—that is people whose families had no money to pay for their care—and smaller private asylums for private patients. There was no care or follow up once people left the asylum. Many of the pauper lunatics came from, and returned to, the local workhouse—the institution that provided a minimal level of subsistence for those who had no other means.

The usual account of early psychiatry suggests that few people recovered and that, after being admitted to an asylum, people were rarely discharged. This picture has been challenged, however, by a considerable amount of historical research, which shows that 40–60% of people admitted to asylums in England and Wales were discharged within a year. By the last years of the nineteenth century, two thirds of patients admitted stayed less than two years (Wright, 1997; Ellis, 2006).

As far as there was any conception of 'treatment', it consisted of fresh air and the structured routine of the asylum, which included jobs within the asylum system that patients were set to do as soon as they were thought fit (Henderson and Gillespie, 1927; Anonymous, 1990). There was experimentation with various physical procedures, like surgery, to remove potential sites of infection, which was thought, at one point, to be a cause of chronic mental disturbance (Scull, 1994), but there were no widely accepted interventions for particular conditions. Various sedative drugs were prescribed liberally during this period; 'doled out by the bucketful', in the words of one retired psychiatrist (Rollin, 1990), but they aroused little interest among psychiatrists, and official recommendations were to use them 'as sparingly as possible' (Henderson and Gillespie, 1927, p. 154). It seems these early drugs were regarded merely as 'chemical restraints', which fulfilled the same purpose as the mechanical restraints—the straight jackets and manacles—which were also in use at the time (Braslow, 1997). Staff of the mental asylums at the beginning of the twentieth century believed they were, at best, helping to promote a natural recovery and, at least, providing a long-term residence for people who required on-going assistance or containment.

Physical Treatments

In the late 1920s, the idea that inducing malaria might cure or benefit people suffering from the severe neurological degeneration seen in some people with late-stage syphilis infection (known as general paralysis of the insane, or GPI) was suggested, and 'malarial therapy' started to be used in asylums. Patients were deliberately infected with malaria using mosquitoes bred in the grounds of the asylums. As it was never subjected to controlled evaluations, it remains uncertain whether this technique had any beneficial effect, although we know that it was hazardous. It was generally accepted as a major medical innovation, however, and its inventor, Austrian psychiatrist Wagner Jauregg, was awarded the Nobel prize for medicine, despite the objections of one member of the committee about the ethics of giving people malaria (Austin et al., 1992). Regardless of its actual efficacy, malarial therapy encouraged the idea that apparently incurable conditions might be treatable, and it gave the staff of asylums a sense of having a truly medical purpose (Braslow, 1997).

From the early 1930s onwards a range of other physical techniques, including insulin coma therapy, chemical and then electrically-induced shock therapy and lobotomy, were introduced into psychiatry and all became standard and accepted forms of treatment. Like malarial therapy, these interventions were based partly on the prevalent belief that there was a mutual antagonism between certain diseases and that some mental conditions could be reversed or eliminated by inducing another sort of disease.

Insulin coma therapy was the first physical procedure to come into widespread use that was aimed at people who would conventionally be said to suffer from a mental disorder, rather than a neurological disease like neurosyphilis. It was proposed and promoted by Manfred Sakel, an Austrian psychiatrist, who had started experimenting with the use of insulin in people addicted to morphine. Insulin was isolated in 1922, and its discovery, along with the synthesis of thyroid hormone in 1927, inspired interest in the role and use of hormones in many areas of medicine. When Sakel noticed that insulin induced a state of calm in his morphine-addicted patients, he started to try it out in patients diagnosed with acute schizophrenia. In these patients he devised a regime that consisted of using insulin to induce hypoglycaemic comas. The patient was kept in the state of coma for 2–3 hours, and then dramatically awakened by an injection of glucose. The comas were given every week-day morning and continued for weeks at a time. The procedure was both degrading and dangerous. Patients sweated profusely during the comas, and were often doubly incontinent. Afterwards they would be confused and disorientated, with the confusion lasting for several days after prolonged treatments. The death rate was between 5 and 10% (Ebaugh, 1943; Fink and Karliner, 2007).

Although there were never any well-accepted theories about how insulin coma therapy produced improvement, there was a general belief that it did so by acting on the underlying biological basis of schizophrenia. One psychiatric textbook described how 'hypoglycaemic treatment obviously touches the physical basis of schizophrenia more closely than all earlier modes of physical attack' (Mayer-Gross et al., 1954, p. 286). Sakel himself claimed that insulin coma therapy selectively killed diseased brain cells like 'fine microscopic surgery' (Sakel, 1958, p. 334). Others proposed that it worked by correcting faulty brain circuits or correcting hormonal imbalances (Fink et al., 2007). A German psychiatrist, looking back at the introduction of insulin coma therapy from the 1960s felt that it was 'the decisive step from a purely symptomatic to a curative therapy of the "endogenous" psychoses' (Ehrhardt, 1966, p. 838).

In 1953 Harold Bourne, a young doctor from New Zealand, published an article in *The Lancet* entitled 'The Insulin Myth'. He pointed out that the effects of insulin coma therapy were likely to be due to a placebo effect produced by the particularly dramatic nature of the procedure. A subsequent randomised controlled trial that compared insulin-induced comas with an anaesthetic procedure using barbiturates, found no difference between the two (Ackner et al., 1957). However, a comparison between insulin coma therapy and chlorpromazine, the first antipsychotic drug, also showed no difference (Fink et al., 1958). The author Robert Whitaker has suggested that, like lobotomy, insulin coma therapy may have been effective in calming patients by inducing a form of brain damage, which may explain its similarity to antipsychotic treatment (Whitaker, 2002). In the end insulin coma therapy faded out of use and was replaced by the new antipsychotic drugs in the 1950s. Psychiatrists, 'like a large shoal of fish...simply switched direction to follow the lights of the more fashionable pharmacotherapy of schizophrenia', according to British psychiatrist Michael Shepherd

(Shepherd, 1994). Today, insulin coma therapy is almost entirely forgotten. It stopped being recommended in the 1960s and is no longer regarded as effective.

Following the proposal that hypoglycaemic comas might cure or improve schizophrenia, came the idea that inducing epilepsy might relieve people of their madness. 'Convulsive' therapy reflected not only the idea that mental disorders might be cured by the presence of a physical disease, it was also a product of a longstanding notion that people could be shaken out of their mental disturbance by violent shocks (Frank, 1978). At first, epileptic convulsions were induced using chemical agents, but this technique was later replaced by the use of an electrical current applied to the brain in a procedure known as electro-convulsive therapy (ECT). As it was easier and quicker to administer than insulin coma therapy, and considerably less dangerous, it became the mainstay of treatment for people with schizophrenia in the asylums of Europe and north America in the 1940s. Although the majority of people to whom it was administered were diagnosed with schizophrenia, it was later suggested that ECT was most effective in people with 'involutional melancholia' (severe depression of old age) or manic depression. In these conditions it was suggested that it might rectify underlying abnormalities, such as reversing dysfunctional 'brain circuits' (Paterson, 1963) or an underactive pituitary gland (Sadler, 1953), but there was, and remains, no consensus about its mechanism of action.

Treatments like insulin coma therapy, ECT and, subsequently, lobotomy ushered in a transformation in attitudes towards the treatment of mental health problems, and marked the beginning of a sustained period of therapeutic zeal. Suddenly, 'treatment' became a topic worthy of discussion, with textbooks and academic papers describing the application of the new physical procedures (Moncrieff, 1999). Mental hospitals established ECT and insulin suites; X-ray facilities and pathology laboratories were introduced; and neurosurgeons appointed to the staff to conduct lobotomies (Anonymous, 1990). The asylums of the nineteenth century were at last believed to be becoming true hospitals, where people would be restored to sanity by real medical procedures. The days of waiting for nature to take its course, and trying to limit the damage on the way, were thought to be past.

Moreover, psychiatrists believed that their new treatments could, at last, alter the course of mental disturbance. Insulin coma therapy and ECT, in particular, were thought to represent effective and specific treatments for the two major psychiatric disorders that had been defined by Kraepelin at the end of the nineteenth century and that structured mid-twentieth century psychiatric thinking: schizophrenia and manic depression.

The Introduction of Chlorpromazine

Chlorpromazine, otherwise known by its trade names Largactil and Thorazine, was the first of the drugs now referred to as 'antipsychotics' or neuroleptics to become an established psychiatric treatment. It was not developed with psychiatric uses in mind, however, and the circuitous manner in which it arrived in psychiatry has led to it being dubbed a 'drug in search of an illness' (Lickey and Gordon, 1986, p. 78). It was originally synthesised as an antihistamine; it was first used clinically in some dubious anaesthetic procedures; it was promoted as an anti-sickness agent, probably for morning sickness; and it was named Largactil after its 'large action'. But it landed in psychiatry at a propitious moment, and that is where it stuck.

The story of chlorpromazine's introduction into psychiatry has been well told by a number of historians (Swazey, 1974; Healy, 2002), but the story is worth retelling in order to highlight a number of issues that are not well recognised. The adoption of insulin coma therapy, ECT and lobotomy already illustrates that psychiatry was ready to embrace highly intrusive and dangerous procedures in the name of providing mental patients with what seemed like medical 'treatments'. The use of chlorpromazine in psychiatry also emerged out of a bizarre and dangerous experimental technique for the prevention of surgical shock, known as 'artificial hibernation', based on long-outmoded theories about the origins of shock that contradicted conventional treatment practices both then and now. Confidence in physical treatments in general encouraged psychiatrists to embrace the new chemical approach to treatment, which also happened to promise an alternative for the containment of the mentally ill that was cheaper than long-term confinement in the asylum system.

Chlorpromazine's early history also illustrates the drug-centred framework within which drugs were understood at this time. The clinicians who used chlorpromazine in its early years were fascinated by the peculiar way the drug modified human emotions and behaviour, and recorded their observations in detail. Simultaneously, however, the story indicates the circumstances that lead to the transformation of ways of understanding the new drugs. The seeds of the disease-centred view are already apparent in the enthusiasm with which they were greeted and the desire to view them as something quite distinct from the sedatives that were in use before their arrival.

The Antihistamines

After the demonstration in 1910 that histamine could produce an acute allergic shock reaction when injected into mammals (Dale and Laidlaw, 1910), work began to develop a drug that could counteract the effects of histamine. A group of chemicals called the phenothiazines, which had first been synthesised and used as dyes in the chemical industry in the late nineteenth century, were found to have this effect and, by 1941, Rhône-Poulenc, the French pharmaceutical and chemical company patented the first antihistamine for clinical use in humans, phenbenzamine, known as Antergan. It was closely followed by several more, including promethazine (Phenergan) and, by the mid-1940s, antihistamines were in widespread use for the treatment of mild allergic conditions, including hay fever and allergic rashes. By 1950 there were at least 20 antihistamines on the market (Emanuel, 1999).

It was immediately recognised that one of the main effects of antihistamines was drowsiness or sedation, and several groups of researchers began to look at these effects in more detail. Scientists at Rhône-Poulenc identified that promethazine and other antihistamines could prolong the sleep-producing effects of barbiturates in rabbits, and work in the USA showed that antihistamines could also inhibit animals' ability to learn new behaviour. Rhône-Poulenc started to search for antihistamine compounds with a stronger ability to suppress the activity of the central nervous system, which they referred to as a 'depressant' action, although the company was not yet sure what clinical applications such drugs might have (Swazey, 1974).

The 'depressant' or sedative actions of antihistamines lead to some of them being put to use in psychiatric practice during the 1940s. Phenbenzamine and promethazine were tested in patients with manic depression by French doctors who concluded that they were promising treatments. Promethazine was described as producing helpful sedation and drowsiness in agitated psychotic patients, and reducing the duration of manic episodes (Guiraud and David, 1950).

The Contribution of Laborit and His Theory of Shock

Henri Laborit was a surgeon who worked for the French navy and, like many of his colleagues, he had an interest in the physiological state known as 'shock'. Shock is a condition that occurs when blood circulation fails and bodily organs are deprived of oxygen, and as it can occur after surgery and wounding, it has been a concern of doctors and surgeons throughout history. We know now that this sort of shock is a consequence of blood loss, even if the source of the loss is not immediately apparent, but this was not always obvious and, for much of the nineteenth century, the cause or mechanism of shock was believed to lie in the nervous system (Manji et al., 2009). Various contradictory theories circulated, such as ideas that the symptoms of shock resulted from either overstimulation or understimulation of various nervous pathways, but the most influential proponent of the nervous theory of shock, the American George Crile, suggested that shock was due to overstimulation of the sympathetic nervous system, the system that increases heart rate and blood pressure, leading to exhaustion and failure of the nervous mechanisms controlling blood circulation (Moffat et al., 1985).

From the beginning of the twentieth century it became clear that blood or fluid loss was the primary mechanism of all traumatic shock, and it was believed that blood was lost because the fine blood vessels—the capillaries—became overly permeable, but it was still believed by some that the underlying mechanism was dysfunctional nervous impulses. Linked with these theories was the idea that an as yet unidentified toxic substance mediated the abnormal nervous activity that caused the increased capillary permeability (Moffat et al., 1985). After identifying histamine as the cause of severe allergic reactions, the famous physiologist Henry Dale proposed that histamine might be this substance (Dale and Richards, 1918; Dale and Laidlaw, 1919).

Following World War I, when the role of blood loss became clear and most attention was directed to producing effective blood and fluid replacements for people experiencing traumatic shock (Gurd, 1955), several experiments were conducted which contradicted the nervous stimulation hypothesis. It became more generally accepted that the activity of the sympathetic nervous system was not the mechanism underlying shock, but the body's response to it (Manji et al., 2009). Following this revelation, standard approaches to shock attempted to support the nervous system's reaction to shock, not suppress it.

The old nervous system hypothesis was not abandoned by everyone, however, and in 1950, following on from work by other French researchers, Laborit, who was based in Tunis at the time, elaborated on the idea that shock was the result of prolonged 'nervous irritation' of the sympathetic nervous system, leading to massive dilatation of blood vessels (Laborit, 1950). Laborit proposed that histamine was one of the endogenous chemicals that mediated the effects of this overstimulation (Laborit, 1949), although experiments conducted in the

1930s and 1940s had shown that histamine was not involved in the mechanism of shock (Hunter, 1967). Based on his hypothesis, Laborit devised a complex combination of drugs designed to counteract the effects of the chemicals that produced the nervous overstimulation, and he included antihistamine drugs as part of what he called his 'lytic cocktail' ('lytic' from the idea that they lysed, dissolved or reduced the nerve-stimulating activity of these chemicals). He referred to the overall results of the drug cocktail as 'neuroplegia' owing to its capacity to inhibit nervous conduction.

In 1951, Laborit was transferred to Paris and started collaborating with the anaesthetist, Pierre Huguenard. Together they formulated a technique they referred to as 'artificial hibernation', which was designed to prevent surgical shock by a combination of 'neuroplegia and hypothermia'. The induction of hypothermia by surrounding the patient with ice packs had been proposed as a way of slowing down the body's metabolic rate to enable long and complex operations to be conducted, but it had also been proposed as a method of preventing surgical shock. In this case it was to be combined with the use of Laborit's drug cocktail (Laborit and Hugenard, 1951).

Although some other surgeons experimented with the use of artificial hibernation (Lazorthes et al., 1952), and the fashion for hypothermia was widespread, Laborit acknowledged at the time that his ideas were unorthodox, and that counteracting the action of the sympathetic nervous system went against the prevailing view that one should support the body's reaction to shock, not suppress it (Laborit, 1952). Conventional drug treatment for shock, for example, included sympathetic nervous system stimulants like noradrenaline, which had the opposite effect of that intended by Laborit's cocktail (Gurd, 1955). Experiments in the late 1950s suggested that hypothermia probably worsened shock rather than prevented it (Beresford et al., 1956; Ferguson et al., 1958), and many surgeons were sceptical about the artificial hibernation technique and concerned about its safety. When Laborit was flown to the USA by Smith Kline & French to promote the technique to US surgeons, his tour was a disaster. Most of the animals he used died during the demonstration and US surgeons, thankfully, showed little interest (Swazey, 1974)!

Laborit's legacy is not in surgery, however, but in psychiatry, owing to his observations of the novel sedative quality of the antihistamine drugs he was employing, and his intuition that these might be useful in subduing psychiatric patients. His suggestions may have fallen on deaf ears had psychiatrists had the same attitude to artificial hibernation as the US surgeons, but the parallels between Laborit's technique and the physical treatments in use in psychiatry at the time helped to smooth the passage of chlorpromazine from surgery to psychiatry. The psychiatric procedure most closely analogous to artificial hibernation was 'deep sleep' therapy, sometimes known as 'continuous narcosis'. This highly dangerous procedure was popularised by Swiss psychiatrist Jakob Klaesi in 1920 and involved putting the patient into a state of deep sleep induced by high doses of barbiturates, which could be continued for up to 10–12 days. The rationale behind 'deep sleep' therapy represented a curious blend of biological, psychoanalytical and behavioural theories, with some proponents viewing it simply as a physical intervention, similar to insulin coma therapy, but others suggesting that the prolonged sleep could regress the patient to an earlier stage of development, from which they could relearn more adaptive habits and behaviours (Greenson, 2012). Sleep therapy was particularly popular in France, Switzerland and Russia, but was widely used across Europe and less frequently in North America. In the UK there is evidence that it was being conducted up until the 1970s (Gittins, 1998), and a modified version was used to treat American soldiers in the Vietnam war (Bloch, 1970). Deep sleep therapy was also the precursor to the idea of 'abreaction', the technique that aimed to elicit repressed memories from people during periods of barbiturate-induced intoxication, a procedure that is still occasionally employed to this day. In the 1950s, the fact that deep sleep therapy was a widely accepted treatment meant psychiatrists willingly embraced the idea of artificial hibernation as transferable into psychiatry, along with the drugs used to achieve it.

Laborit was in close communication with Rhône-Poulenc, and the company was persuaded by his ideas that an antihistamine drug with strong sedative properties might be useful in anaesthesia, as well as other areas. In December 1950 company scientists synthesised a new molecule by adding a chlorine atom to the phenothiazine drug promazine to produce what was later called chlorpromazine. It quickly became apparent that the new substance had a strong effect on the central nervous system, as identified by animal screening tests, and, only four months after its synthesis in April 1951, it was tested in humans with a variety of complaints, including some psychiatric patients. It was noted to enhance the effects of barbiturates in these patients, and psychiatric uses were included among Rhône-Poulenc's list of prospective indications. But the company was prepared to try it for almost any purpose, long before its full profile of effects was established, such was the laxity of drug regulation at the time. The proposed indications also included epilepsy and muscle spasm, for example, even though subsequent observations indicated that the drug could induce epileptic fits and that it caused, rather than prevented, muscle spasm and rigidity (Swazey, 1974).

Laborit was given some samples of the drug in June 1951, and started to use it as part of his lytic cocktail in the artificial hibernation experiments he was conducting with Huguenard. In their first report, they were enthusiastic about the new drug's ability to facilitate the state of hibernation, and also noted how the patient, once injected with chlorpromazine, entered a 'twilight state' (Laborit and Hugenard, 1951). In a later paper published in 1952, they commented on how patients who had taken it showed a 'disinterestedness' in the things that were going on around them, and they suggested, on this basis, that it might be useful in psychiatry (Laborit et al., 1952, p. 207).

First Uses in Psychiatry

Intrigued by its psychoactive properties, Laborit urged his psychiatric colleagues to try the new drug and one young psychiatrist agreed to take a dose of chlorpromazine in Laborit's presence to allow further observation of its effects. Cornelia Quarti taped and later transcribed her experiences, describing how the drug gave her an 'extreme feeling of detachment' from herself and others, and 'muted' her sensations and perceptions. Later on she felt tired, weak and lethargic, and had difficulty finding words. Although Laborit was not discouraged, the director of the hospital, who had been told about Quarti staggering about under the influence of the drug, suspended further use of chlorpromazine at the hospital (Chertok, 1982).

Dr Hamon, a colleague of Laborit's and director of the neuropsychiatry unit at the Paris military Hospital Val de Grace, agreed to try chlorpromazine in some of his patients. The drug was duly given to a 24-year-old highly aroused and agitated manic patient, Jacques Lh. Although his case was reported as a demonstration of successful treatment with chlorpromazine (Hamon et al., 1952a), at the same time as he received chlorpromazine at relatively modest doses, he was also being given barbiturates, pethidine and ECT (Deniker, 1989). Hamon and colleagues acknowledged the influence of Laborit's ideas, referring to chlorpromazine as an autonomic 'stabiliser' and its use as constituting 'artificial hibernation', which they proposed could become a useful technique in psychiatry (Hamon et al., 1952b).

The people who are usually credited with introducing chlorpromazine into psychiatry, however, are the psychiatrists Jean Delay and

Pierre Deniker, who were based at the neurology and psychiatry hospital of Sainte Ann in Paris. Jean Delay was a professor and the head of the psychiatric department of the University of Paris, the most prestigious and respected job in French psychiatry. He had trained as a neurologist before entering psychiatry, and he was firmly committed to the idea that psychiatric disorders could be treated by medical or biological means. Much of his early work consisted of attempts to elucidate the mechanisms of ECT, for example, and he and Deniker had been experimenting with the use of a variety of new drugs before they started using chlorpromazine (Swazey, 1974).

Delay was interested in Laborit's ideas about surgical shock because of his own work on shock therapy in psychiatry, and, in 1953, he and Deniker proclaimed 'how enthusiastically we have followed the remarkable work of our friend Laborit and his team' (Delay and Deniker, 1953, p. 347). Deniker had heard about Laborit's observations on chlorpromazine from his brother-in-law, who was a surgeon, and ordered some samples of the drug from Rhône-Poulenc in February 1952 (Swazey, 1974). At first, chlorpromazine was used in conjunction with ice packs to induce the state of 'artificial hibernation' devised by Laborit. A junior psychiatrist who was involved, Jean Thuillier, subsequently described how nursing staff started to use the drug on its own because the pharmacy could not supply the ice packs quickly enough. When this was reported to Deniker, he decided to continue using the drug in this way (Thuillier, 2000). Deniker explained subsequently that he and Delay decided that the artificial hibernation technique was too dangerous (Swazey, 1974).

Between May 1952 and July 1952, Delay and Deniker published six papers outlining their experience with the new drug in patients with various types of 'psychic excitation', and Deniker made several presentations to the 50th meeting of the French Congress of Psychiatry and Neurology in 1952. The paper that is usually cited as being the first to confirm the utility of chlorpromazine described the use of chlorpromazine in 38 patients with excited states of various sorts. The best results were said to have been obtained in people who had 'confusional states'—although this may have included some patients who were psychotic. Only six patients were classified as having schizophrenia in whom results were said to be mixed, although the authors did comment that a few remissions had occurred among some of the most 'refractory cases' (Delay and Deniker, 1952).

Delay and Deniker's early papers also record their observations of the altered state produced by chlorpromazine. In 1952, for example, they described how, after receiving chlorpromazine, initially 'patients spend most of their time in sleep,' and, although this effect lessened as treatment continued, patients remained 'a little sleepy and indifferent' (Delay et al., 1952, pp. 114–5). A subsequent paper contains a lengthy description of the general effects induced by chlorpromazine. In an effort to distinguish the drug from barbiturates, the report minimises the sleep-inducing effects noted in the earlier paper, but it is worth reproducing because it remains one of the most detailed accounts of the effects induced by antipsychotic drugs in the psychiatric literature:

> Seated or lying down, the patient is motionless on his bed, often pale and with lowered eyelids. He remains silent most of the time. If questioned, he responds after a delay, slowly, in an indifferent monotone, expressing himself with few words and quickly becoming mute. Without exception, the response is generally valid and pertinent, showing the subject is capable of attention and of reflection. But he rarely takes the initiative of asking a question; he does not express his preoccupations, desires, or preference. He is usually conscious of the amelioration brought on by treatment, but he does not express euphoria. The apparent indifference, or delay in response to external stimuli, the emotional and affective neutrality, the decrease in both initiative and preoccupation without alteration of conscious awareness or in intellectual faculties constitute the psychic syndrome due to treatment (Delay et al., 1952, pp. 503–4).

Delay and Deniker had recognised that the new drug affected some of the most fundamental human characteristics: emotion, initiative and the ability to respond to the world around us. When the drug was stopped and the effects wore off they noted how the patient regained 'his normal colour, and activity and his normal "spirit"' (Delay et al., 1952, pp. 504).

Other clinicians who used chlorpromazine at this time made similar observations.

Two Parisian neurologists, for example, employed the drug as a painkiller, among other uses, and suggested that 'it had an effect different from other analgesics, producing an indifference to the pain, rather than analgaesia' (Sigwald and Bouttier, 1953, pp. 150–1). From their experience of using the drug in patients with a variety of psychiatric and neurological conditions, they described how it could lessen the' imperative character' of obsessional thoughts and the emotional distress associated with hallucinations and delusions (Sigwald and Bouttier, 1953, pp. 175–6).

At the end of 1952 Rhône-Poulenc decided to market the drug under the name of Largactil. Initially, it was promoted to three groups: surgeons and anaesthetists, obstetricians and gynaecologists, and psychiatrists. The decision to target obstetricians and gynaecologists implies that one of its principle intended uses was for morning sickness, which, before the thalidomide scandal, was a legitimate and potentially lucrative market.

Chlorpromazine Reaches Other Countries

Among the first British psychiatrists to use chlorpromazine was David Anton-Stephens, who worked in Warley hospital in Essex. He described the main effects of chlorpromazine as 'somnolence' and 'psychic indifference,' and, like other investigators, felt its most useful effects were the 'lessening of disturbed behaviour' (Anton-Stephens, 1954, p. 557). Joel and Charmain Elkes from Birmingham conducted what is generally recognised as the first controlled experiment involving the drug. They had been experimenting with other sorts of drugs, and the chlorpromazine study involved 27 patients with chronic psychiatric conditions who all displayed 'over-activity'. The patients were given chlorpromazine for a few weeks, alternating with a placebo. The Elkes judged the trial to have been a success, with 7 of the patients showing 'definite' and 11 showing 'slight' improvement on the drug. According to the Elkes, this improvement consisted of patients becoming 'quieter and more amenable to suggestion by the nursing staff', and the drug did not change basic psychotic phenomena. 'Schizophrenic and paraphrenic patients continued to be subject to delusions and hallucinations' they commented, 'though they appeared to be less disturbed by them' (Elkes and Elkes, 1954, p. 563).

The man credited with first introducing chlorpromazine to North America is Heinz Lehmann, a German Canadian, who was given some chlorpromazine by Rhône-Poulenc, who operated in Canada, as well as France. Lehman soon organised a study of the new drug at the Verdun hospital where he worked in Montreal. Like Delay and Deniker, Lehman considered that the drug was of most value in 'the symptomatic control of almost any kind of severe excitement' (Lehman and Hanrahan, 1954, p. 232), and described results in people classed as having chronic schizophrenia as disappointing. Lehman was also a keen observer of drug-induced effects and reported how the drug made patients lethargic, and how 'patients under treatment display a lack of spontaneous interest in their environment, yet are easily accessible and respond as a rule immediately and relevantly to questions' (Lehamnn and Hanrahan, 1954, p. 230).

Chlorpromazine in the USA

Chlorpromazine was introduced into the USA by the drug company Smith Kline & French, who were approached by Rhône-Poulenc in 1952. The company was initially concerned that American psychiatrists might not give drug treatment the same enthusiastic welcome it was receiving in Europe owing to the influence of psychoanalysis (Swazey, 1974). Sections of US psychiatry, however, had never abandoned the biological approach to understanding and treating mental illness. The principle American psychiatric journal (*The American Journal of Psychiatry*) showed a continual preponderance of articles on biological theories and treatments throughout the mid-twentieth century (Moncrieff, 2008a). On top of this, concern about poor conditions and overcrowding in the state mental hospitals meant that many psychiatrists were desperate to find a simple medical procedure that would help to manage disturbed behaviour and reduce the inpatient population. Moreover, for many psychiatrists, biological interventions and psychotherapeutic approaches could be combined without contradiction. Psychiatrist John Vernon Kinross-Wright, for example, who published the first report of the treatment of hospital patients using chlorpromazine in the USA, expressed how 'for decades psychiatrists have searched for a simple chemical agent with which to treat mental illness, one that would be effective without producing narcosis or coma and at the same time increase the patients capacity to respond to psychotherapy' (Kinross-Wright, 1954, p. 297). N. William Winkelman, Jr, who prescribed chlorpromazine to his outpatients and described the drug's ability to reduce almost any nervous complaint, also warned that 'it should never be given as a substitute for psychoanalytically oriented psychotherapy' (Winkelman, Jr, 1954, p. 21).

Another US psychiatrist, Henry Brill of New York, recalled how he 'was searching for a treatment that was simple to administer and so safe that it could be administered to large numbers of patients' (Brill, cited in Johnson, undated, pp. 7–8, cited in Swazey, 1974, p. 200). After introducing chlorpromazine into his own hospital, he organised a meeting to report on the benefits he had seen to other New York psychiatrists (Healy, 2002). In the late 1950s Brill published a series of papers that documented a decrease in the numbers of mental hospital inpatients and attributed the decline to the introduction of the new 'tranquillisers'. Brill claimed the figures demonstrated that these drugs were producing a 'revolution in the care and treatment of mental patients', enabling even the most chronic patients to be discharged (Brill and Patton, 1957, p. 509). For many decades these papers were cited as demonstrating beyond doubt that the new drugs had emptied the asylums, despite the fact that several other studies contradicted this interpretation (see Chapter 7).

Smith Kline & French's campaign to introduce chlorpromazine into the US was unprecedented at the time. A few days after the company received permission to market the drug in 1954, the president, Francis Boyer, appeared on a national television programme, *The March of Medicine*, to announce the arrival of Thorazine, the company's brand name for chlorpromazine. A Thorazine 'Task Force' worked with state legislatures and the staff of mental hospitals in a programme that was presented not as a marketing campaign, but as a 'true educative effort' intended to highlight the need for more 'intensive treatment' of the mentally ill (Johnson, undated, cited in Swazey, 1974, p. 203). The company organised council meetings at local mental hospitals, provided training for psychiatric administrators on how to obtain state funding for drug treatment, and organised and funded American Psychiatric Association symposia to discuss the use of the drug. The task force also emphasised 'aftercare', or the continuation of drug treatment after discharge. As well as extending the market considerably by promoting the idea of lifelong treatment, the focus on aftercare allowed the task force to deflect criticism that its drug might be increasing discharge rates, but increasing readmission rates, leading to people going in and out of hospital in a 'revolving door' fashion (Swazey, 1974).

The campaign was a huge success and the task force remained in existence for 6 years, indicating the value that chlorpromazine represented for the company. Within 8 months of Thorazine's launch, it had been given to more than 2 million patients (Swazey, 1974). At the time, Brill pointed out that 'no previous method of psychiatric therapy has ever had such rapid and general acceptance' (Brill, 1956, p. 181). Despite the reservations of a few psychoanalytically-minded psychiatrists, he later reflected the use of drugs 'became almost universal. Only a few diehards refused to use them at all' (cited in Johnson, undated, p. 39, cited in Swazey, 1974, p. 196).

Reserpine

More or less concurrent with the introduction of chlorpromazine into psychiatry, a drug with similar properties, originating from a native

Indian plant known as *Rauwolfia serpentina* (named after its use for the treatment of snake bites) was receiving increasing attention. The plant had been used in Indian medicine for centuries to combat fever, sickness, snake bite, insomnia and insanity, and, during the twentieth century, it started to be used to treat high blood pressure. Its potential as an anti-hypertensive attracted the attention of Western drug companies, and, in 1953, researchers at the company Ciba isolated the chief active ingredient of the plant preparation, which they named reserpine.

In the same year *The New York Times* reported on the news that an Indian doctor, Dr R.A. Hakim, had been awarded a gold medal for the presentation of a paper describing his successful treatment of patients with schizophrenia with *Rauwolfia* preparations. The report stimulated the interest of psychiatrist Nathan Kline, recently appointed as research director at Rockland State hospital. This large asylum had become notorious through its portrayal in the highly critical film, *The Snake Pit*, and Kline had set up a research unit to try and improve its image and boost staff morale (Healy, 2002). Kline is an important figure in the story of modern drug treatment because of his domineering influence over American psychiatry. Although he had trained in psychoanalysis, he became an ardent advocate of biological psychiatry in general and drug treatment in particular. He was also known for his blunt manner, and Paul Janssen of Janssen pharmaceuticals, who knew and liked him, nevertheless describes how he ridiculed and intimidated those who challenged him. 'By the end of his life', Janssen recounted, 'he behaved like a kind of Pope ... he had this habit of coming to conferences with a small dog on his lap and patting it all the time and attracting attention whilst smiling to the speaker' (Janssen, 1998, p. 60).

Kline obtained samples of reserpine and started to give it to large numbers of inpatients. In 1954 he published a paper claiming that the drug was responsible for a decline in the number of assaults by patients, and he reported a slight improvement in their condition as rated by nursing staff. He concluded that the drug had 'a definite sedative action', but, in contrast to his later views, he emphasised that there was no evidence that it altered 'the schizophrenic process itself' (Kline, 1954, p. 123). In a paper published the following year, Kline reported how hospital nursing staff were convinced that the drug made 'the patients definitely quieter' with fewer 'assaults, arguments and disturbances in the wards', and he suggested the drug could 'prove a tremendous economy' by reducing disturbed behaviour and enabling patients to be discharged earlier than before (Kline and Stanley, 1955, p. 90).

Other psychiatrists corroborated the behavioural improvements brought about by reserpine, and the economic benefits this promised. Two Canadian psychiatrists reported that the drug produced a 'definite reduction in agitated or overactive behaviour, and made patients less troublesome and easier to manage' (Tyhurst and Richman, 1955, p. 459). Like chlorpromazine, they reported that reserpine produced a 'general decrease in the intensity of the patients' reactions to stimuli, usually associated with somnolence' (p. 459) and that the drug's principle benefit was to reduce the 'emotional disturbance and concern associated with abnormal mental content' (p. 459). Three Californian psychiatrists described how patients underwent a 'metamorphosis from raging, combative, unsociable persons to cooperative, friendly, sociable, relatively quiet persons' who were more amenable to psychotherapy and rehabilitation (Noce et al., 1954, p. 822). Another US psychiatrist commented on the benefits of the drug for ameliorating the 'serious ... national problem' posed by the chronically mentally ill (Naidoo, 1956, p. 12).

The use of reserpine in psychiatry was short-lived, however. It could cause a dangerous lowering of blood pressure, and was associated with a restlessness and agitation in the early days of treatment that was greater than that produced by similar drugs. Given these drawbacks, it was soon swept away by competition from chlorpromazine and other early antipsychotics. Reserpine was important, however, because it was through studying its effects that American Steve Brody started to establish the idea that psychiatric drugs worked through having effects on specific brain chemicals (Healy, 2002).

A New Beginning?

The introduction of drugs like chlorpromazine and reserpine into psychiatry is usually presented as one of the greatest achievements of twentieth-century medicine. Henri Laborit is regarded as one of the principle heroes of this story and shared the Lasker prize for his role in the introduction of chlorpromazine. It is little known that his ideas about the mechanism of surgical shock were based on theories that had already been discredited, and that his techniques for preventing it were dangerous, ineffective and regarded as bizarre by many of his surgical colleagues. Psychiatrists were ready to embrace such unorthodox procedures because they were already conducting their own hazardous treatments, such as insulin coma therapy and lobotomy—therapies which were also based on unfounded theories and a disregard for the safety and dignity of patients. But a simple intervention in the form of a pill was even more appealing and leading European psychiatrists were experimenting with various pharmaceutical candidates. Even in the USA, where psychoanalysis was more influential, many psychiatrists had been longing for an easily administered solution to the problem of mental disturbance, especially one that would ease the problems encountered in the increasingly large and overcrowded mental hospitals. In the event, psychoanalysis never seriously challenged the biological approach to managing mental disturbance and it presented no obstacle to the widespread adoption of the new drug treatments.

Chlorpromazine was not the only drug with antihistamine properties to be found useful in psychiatric patients during the 1950s, but the prestige of Delay and his department combined with the efforts of Rhône-Poulenc and Smith Kline & French helped chlorpromazine to be recognised as the first new and revolutionary drug treatment in psychiatry. A recent revival of interest in the use of promethazine, another early antihistamine, for the emergency treatment of aggression and agitation in psychiatric institutions suggests that other, possibly equally useful candidates, may have been overlooked.

Despite their enthusiasm for the new drugs, in the early days few of the clinicians that prescribed chlorpromazine or reserpine believed that the drugs targeted the underlying psychiatric condition. They thought they were using special sorts of sedative, and, according to this drug-centred understanding of drug action, they were keen observers of the nature of the altered state the drugs produced. After the subsequent transformation of these drugs in the professional and popular imagination into disease-specific treatments charted in the following chapter, this sort of information disappeared from official literature. These early accounts consistently described the state of sedation, detachment and indifference produced by the drugs, and identified its benefits as calming excited or disruptive behaviour, and reducing the intensity of psychotic phenomena and emotional reactions. At this stage the idea that drugs constituted a disease-specific treatment for schizophrenia or psychosis was barely imagined, but the seeds of this view were present in the overwhelming desire that existed in the old institutions to find a proper medical treatment for severe mental disturbance.

3
Magic Bullets: The Development of Ideas on Drug Action[1]

The inscription on the Lasker prize awarded to Deniker, Delay, Laborit and Lehmann in 1957 read 'for the introduction of chlorpromazine into psychiatry and for the demonstration that a medication can *influence the clinical course* of the major psychoses' (Deniker, 1989, p. 253, my emphasis). These words encapsulate the importance that was attributed to finding a physical intervention that was more than just a sticking plaster—to finding something that could change the very nature of psychiatric disorders. Although chlorpromazine and other early anti-psychotics were thought to be uniquely useful, few people believed at this time, however, that they acted on the disease or abnormality that was presumed to give rise to schizophrenia or any other serious mental illness. The disease-centred view of the action of antipsychotics took a while to develop and, in the meantime, the unusual neurological effects the drugs induced were proposed to be the basis of their action, in what was essentially a drug-centred model. But, as the inscription on the Lasker award suggests, psychiatry was already aspiring towards having a drug that would modify the very nature of the problems it was confronted with.

The idea that mental conditions are just the same as any other disease pre-dates the introduction of the early antipsychotics, and, just as this idea generated a story about the effects of insulin coma therapy and electro-convulsive therapy (ECT), it helped to transform the way that drug treatment was understood. In turn, the establishment of a disease-centred view of the nature of psychiatric drug action strengthened and bolstered the medical model of mental disorders, and gave psychiatry the confidence to present itself to the world as a thoroughly medical enterprise, a view that was enshrined in the third edition of the *Diagnostic and Statistical Manual*, the American Psychiatric Association's surprising best-seller (American Psychiatric Association, 1980a). Before this model took hold, however, interest in the nature of the drug-induced state produced by the early antipsychotics revealed the extent of their neurological effects. Plausible, drug-centred explanations of their mechanism of action were proposed, which were subsequently swept away when the disease-centred model took hold.

The Neurological Effects of the New Drugs

In 1954, two separate researchers, Professor Hans Steck of Lausanne, and German psychiatrist Hans Joachim Haase provided the first unambiguous descriptions of a syndrome of abnormally reduced and restricted movement that was associated with chlorpromazine. They both remarked on the similarity between the drug-induced effects—the decreased movement, loss of initiative and muscular rigidity—and the symptoms of Parkinson's disease. They also described the drug-induced agitation known as akathisia (Hasse, 1954; Steck, 1954). Steck compared the Parkinson's disease-like symptoms produced by chlorpromazine to the neurological syndrome seen after the epidemic of encephalitis that hit Europe in the early decades of the twentieth century. This was known as 'encephalitis lethargica', and its consequences are vividly described in Oliver's Sach's famous book *Awakenings* (Sacks, 1990). Steck referred to the drug-induced condition as an 'akinetic picture' (akinetic meaning lack of movement), and noted how, as well as the more obvious signs of slowness and rigidity, the condition was manifested in subtle tendencies, such as walking without swinging the arms, a 'frozen' facial expression and an impaired ability to initiate movement, which are also recognised early features of Parkinson's disease proper. Steck remarked on how the signs of this neurological, drug-induced condition were particularly striking when patients congregated together, conjuring an image of a 'slightly sad procession' (Steck, 1954, p. 739).

Within a couple of years these neurological effects were well recognised and were often referred to as drug-induced 'Parkinsonism'. Other dramatic effects, such as the sudden muscular spasm that usually affects the head and neck muscles, now known as 'acute dystonia', had also been described (Kline, 1956; Hollister, 1957). Collectively, these effects on the body's motor system subsequently came to be referred to as 'extrapyramidal' effects, after the extrapyramidal brain system responsible for the modulation and regulation of movement.[2] The term 'extrapyramidal' effects is also frequently used to refer simply to drug-induced Parkinsonism, however, because this is the most common motor effect encountered.

The Concept of a Neuroleptic

In early attempts to define the nature of drugs like chlorpromazine and reserpine, Delay and Deniker stressed two aspects of the drugs' effects: the peculiar nature of the sedation, which, in contrast to barbiturate-induced sedation, consisted of sleep from which people could be easily roused, and the state of emotional indifference produced by the drugs (Delay and Deniker, 1956; Deniker, 1956). They saw the Parkinson's-like motor effects as incidental to the drugs principle actions, but the sedation and indifference were also regarded as neurological effects by virtue of being induced by drug action on the brain and nervous system. In early papers, following Laborit, they referred to chlorpromazine as a 'neuroplegic' drug (from the Greek to paralyse), and, in 1955, they replaced this term by the term 'neuroleptic' (from the Greek to seize), still emphasising the sedative and emotional effects the drugs produce rather than their motor effects (Delay and Deniker, 1955).

In 1957, Delay and Deniker came across a new drug called prochlorperazine (Stemetil), which was being tested in psychiatric patients in Lyon. Prochlorperazine is a phenothiazine compound like chlorpromazine, but is less sedating in its actions and can produce dramatic neurological reactions that were described at the time as 'excito-motor' effects. These include muscular spasms, severe akathisia and other movement abnormalities, and they were reported to occur both in psychiatric patients and in military personnel who were given the drug to combat sea sickness (Delay et al., 1957; Comite Lyonnais de Recherches Therapeutiques en Psychiatrie, 2000). When Delay and Deniker started using the drug, they witnessed these striking neurological symptoms. Deniker later recalled that the experience of using prochlorperazine persuaded him and Delay that these characteristic effects on movement and muscle tone were an intrinsic part of the neurological state produced by this class of drugs (Deniker, 1989).

Henceforward, the term 'neuroleptic' became associated with the idea that the drugs acted through inducing a neurological syndrome characterised by restricted and abnormal movement, and Deniker, like Steck, started to refer to the distinctive effects of the new drugs as 'akinesia'. Deniker outlined the theory of neuroleptic action most explicitly in a paper published in 1960, entitled 'Experimental Neurological Syndromes and the New Drug Therapies in Psychiatry.' In this paper he suggested that neuroleptics achieve their useful or therapeutic effects by producing a characteristic neurological state akin to post-encephalitis-type Parkinson's disease. As in his other publications, Deniker described in some detail the way the drugs made patients appear and behave. They 'look as if they have been turned to stone' he said and continued 'they are usually indifferent to themselves and their environment, they are stuporous or prostrate, even before the clinical symptom of hypertonia (rigidity) appears' (Deniker, 1960, p. 96). Although Deniker admitted that he had previously found chlorpromazine useful in doses low enough not to cause marked physical effects, he nevertheless suggested here that it was necessary to 'resolutely and systematically aim to produce neurological syndromes to get better results than can be obtained when neuroleptic drugs are given at less effective doses' (Deniker, 1960, p. 100).

The theory propounded in this paper harks back to the idea that mental disorders could be cured by inducing a bodily disease, and Deniker places neuroleptics alongside other examples of treatments inspired by this idea such as ECT and insulin coma therapy. This orientation also explains why he was not ashamed to suggest that the neuroleptic drugs would 'undoubtedly' produce brain damage—irreversible changes in the brain's cellular structure—and why he referred to preliminary animal work demonstrating drug-induced 'lesions' in various parts of the brain as positive evidence of the drugs' effectiveness (Cazzullo and Guareschi, 1954).

In the early days of the 1950s, Delay and Deniker were not the only ones putting forward what amounts to a drug-centred thesis about how the new drugs might work, although Deniker would probably not have seen his ideas as such. Indeed, from time to time, he speculated on how the site of neurological action of the drugs might be involved in the pathology of the psychotic process (Deniker, 1970). German psychiatrist Hans-Joachim Haase also proposed that the therapeutic effects of the new drugs consisted of a mild version of the Parkinson disease-like syndrome they induced (Haase, 1956). In 1961 Haase described the 'handwriting test', which was based on the characteristic shrinking of handwriting that occurs early in Parkinson's disease. In Hasses's test, patients' handwriting was measured each day while they were given gradually increasing doses of the antipsychotic drug haloperidol. Haase suggested that when the handwriting size had decreased by 20%, the 'threshold' dose had been reached. At the threshold dose it was proposed that the early symptoms of Parkinson's disease—the slowed thinking and emotional suppression—would produce therapeutic benefits without producing the more obvious and burdensome physical symptoms, such as slowed movement and muscular rigidity (Haase and Janssen, 1965). The test charts the early signs of Parkinsonism that are produced by the drugs, and the concept of the 'neuroleptic threshold' attained some degree of acceptance.

Similar views were proposed by American psychiatrist, F.A. Freyhan, speaking at a symposium held in Switzerland in 1957 (Freyhan, 1959). He stressed the belief that the effects of the new drugs were not specific to any diagnostic group, but acted on signs of over-arousal, excitement and abnormal preoccupations owing to their ability to reduce movement and initiative, and blunt emotions. Like Deniker and Haase, Freyhan suggested that the drugs' useful or therapeutic effects were on a continuum with their obvious extrapyramidal or Parkinson's-like effects:

> From the beginning it was evident that no lines of demarcation could be drawn between therapeutic degrees of reduced psychomotor activity and early symptoms of Parkinsonism...What we witnessed were gradual transitions from hypermotility to hypomotility, which, in a certain proportion of patients, progressed to the more pronounced degrees of Parkinsonian rigidity. Clinical evidence therefore, indicated that the therapeutic function of chlorpromazine and reserpine could not be separated from their modifying influence on the function of the subcortical motor system in transacting volitional, affective and intentional functions (Freyhan, 1959, p. 10).

Freyhan was still expressing these views in the early 1960s, when the tide was turning against this view of drug treatment, and international meetings were dominated by studies of the biochemical and cellular effects of the new drugs. Instead of trying to identify the specific mechanism for a disease-based action of the drugs, Freyhan called for researchers to abandon the 'arbitrary distinction between main and side effects', and to conduct detailed observations of the 'full range of effects on psychic, vegetative, sensory, motor and other somatic functions' (Freyhan, 1964, p. 561).

Psychiatrists in England and Canada echoed these views (Sarwer-Foner, 1960; Denham, 1965), and there was also support for Deniker's suggestion that producing overt symptoms of Parkinsonism was necessary to achieve the therapeutic benefits of the neuroleptics (Flugel, 1959; Karn, Jr and Kasper, 1959; Denham and Carrick, 1960). The 'drug-centred' viewpoint was summarised by participants at a symposium held in 1955, who concluded that chlorpromazine could be used to 'attain a neuropharmacologic effect, not to "cure" a disease' (Smith Kline & French Laboratories, 1955, p. 158; cited in Whitaker, 2002, p. 146).

The Discovery of Haloperidol

The discovery of haloperidol in 1958 seemed to clinch the theory behind the concept of the neuroleptic, as its therapeutic potency was strongly correlated with its ability to produce Parkinson's disease-like, neurological effects. Ironically, however, as we shall see further in the following chapter, by giving rise to the dopamine hypothesis of schizophrenia, haloperidol hastened the demise of this drug-centred way of understanding the nature of the 'neuroleptic' drugs.

Haloperidol was synthesised by a team led by Belgian researcher Paul Janssen, then director of part of the family pharmaceuticals firm that his father had founded. Janssen's team were working on producing synthetic opiate drugs following the successful development of Palfium (dextromoramide). During this process they attached a molecule known as a 'butyrophenone' group to the compounds they were exploring, and found that, in animal tests, drugs containing this molecule appeared to produce the striking immobility and inertia characteristic of high dose chlorpromazine, a state which had been named 'catalepsy'. Janssen has also described that they tested and were impressed by these drugs' ability to counteract the effects of amphetamines (Granger and Albu, 2005).

The similarity between the observed effects of haloperidol and chlorpromazine suggested the drug might be useful in psychiatric patients, so only 5 weeks after its synthesis in February 1958, Janssen started to give out samples of the drug to psychiatrists he knew. Two psychiatrists at the University of Leige, Paul Divry and Jean Bobon, prescribed the drug to a number of patients with various forms of agitation, and, in line with the first accounts of chlorpromazine, they reported that haloperidol was effective in calming agitated behaviour without inducing irreversible sleep (Divry et al., 1958). They expanded on their observations in a second paper, in which they commented on the facility with which haloperidol produced Parkinson's-like effects: 'here parkinsonism is the norm, not the incident' (Divry et al., 1959).

At this point Janssen gave samples of the drug to investigators in several different European countries, including Delay and Deniker in Paris. In September 1959 he convened a conference at which the investigators reported their findings, documenting the ability of haloperidol to reduce psychotic symptoms, calm agitation, reduce involuntary movements (like tics) and to produce the range of movement abnormalities characteristic of a neuroleptic, including Parkinsonism, acute dystonia and akathisia. A month later, in October 1959, just over 18 months since its synthesis, haloperidol was launched onto the European market (Granger and Albu, 2005).

One of the first patients to be administered haloperidol by Divry and Bobon was a young student, the son of a local doctor, who was admitted to the university hospital at night suffering from paranoid symptoms and agitation. He was given a 10-mg injection of haloperidol, and, by the next morning, he was apparently cured. According to Janssen, who recounted the story to David Healy in the 1990s, following his recovery, the young man was given a low dose (1 mg) of haloperidol every day for the next 7 years, during which time he remained well, completed his studies, worked, married and had children. At first, the drug was given to him surrepticiously in his drinks, but later he took it himself. After 7 years he decided to stop the drug, in conjunction with his doctors, and, after 3 weeks, he apparently became psychotic again, never recovering to the same level as before (Janssen, 1998).

Janssen regarded the outcome as evidence that the young man had genuinely had schizophrenia, which the haloperidol had successfully kept at bay, and the story was interpreted as demonstrating the remarkable benefits of the new drugs. The brevity of the man's symptoms and the lack of any previous psychiatric disturbance make this explanation doubtful, however. An alternative interpretation of events is that the second episode of psychosis was a result of the haloperidol itself, in what may be one of the first recorded cases of 'supersensitivity' or withdrawal-induced psychosis (Moncrieff, 2006). There is now evidence that long-term exposure to antipsychotics may make people vulnerable to experiencing psychotic symptoms when the drugs are withdrawn, even people with no previous history of psychotic problems. The mechanism may be related to the drug-induced changes that cause the abnormal movement disorder known as tardive dyskinesia. These issues are described in further detail in Chapters 5 and 6, but it is interesting to note here that the young man who has been held up as evidence for the benefits of long-term antipsychotic treatment may possibly be one of the first victims of a serious iatrogenic problem.

Paradoxically, although haloperidol had the strongest potential to cause extrapyramidal effects and thus appeared to confirm the neuroleptic theory of antipsychotic action, it also ushered in the dopamine theory of schizophrenia, which, by suggesting that the drugs acted by counteracting an underlying disease, rendered these effects less visible and apparently less significant. Although the dopamine hypothesis was not clearly articulated until the 1970s, its origins lay, as described in the following chapter, in the specific effects of haloperidol on dopamine receptors—effects that were never as clear with broader-acting drugs like chlorpromazine and reserpine. Janssen himself subscribed to a version of the dopamine theory of schizophrenia, believing that the condition was caused by abnormally elevated phenylethylamine levels, an endogenous brain chemical that causes dopamine release (Janssen, 1998).

From Tranquillisers to Antipsychotics

The idea of a neuroleptic was never accepted to the same degree in the USA, where drugs like chlorpromazine and reserpine were referred to as 'tranquillisers'. The term tranquilliser was popularised by the manufacturers of a drug called meprobamate, also known by its brand name, Miltown, who used it to distinguish their drug from the numerous barbiturates on the market at the time (Janssen, 1998). By the 1960s, drugs used in psychosis and schizophrenia started to be referred to as 'major tranquillisers' to distinguish them from sedatives, like meprobamate, and the newly-launched benzodiazepine drugs, including Librium and Valium, which were increasingly referred to as 'minor tranquillisers'. The term 'tranquilliser' was appealing for marketing purposes because its derivation from 'tranquillity' helped to represent the drug-induced state as pleasant and calming, and it also indicated the potentially wide application of such treatments. In the 1950s, for example, reserpine was advertised as having 'a remarkable calming action...capable of wide application in mental illness' (Reserpine advertisement, 1956) (Figure 3.1).

Early advertisements for the drug Melleril (thioridazine), a drug that came to be widely used in psychiatry and general practice, described it as a 'tranquilliser pure and simple', and used the image of a lake to convey its 'specific psychosedative action' (Melleril advertisement, 1960) (Figure 3.2). Other advertisements from the same period recommended many different situations in which the drugs' tranquillising properties could be employed, including anxiety, childhood behaviour problems, and agitation and aggression in the elderly. Dartalan (thiopropazate dihydrochloride), for example, was advertised for use in psychoses, neuroses, geriatrics and general medicine (Dartalan advertisement, 1960).

As early as 1954, however, participants at a psychiatric symposium in Washington, DC, clearly stated they believed chlorpromazine and reserpine were attacking the 'underlying schizophrenic process' (Kinross-Wright, 1956) and exerting a 'specific effect on the basic schizophrenic mechanisms' (Sainz, 1956). A participant, who did not share this view, bemoaned the tendency to jump from the effects of drugs to making generalisations about the genesis of psychotic behaviour (Meyers, 1956). In 1955, the President of the Society of Biological Psychiatry of the United States reflected that the new drugs were of a 'different order'

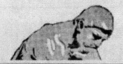

for use in psychiatry

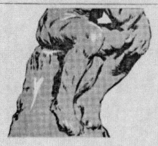

RESERPINE
'SERPILOID' BRAND

Is now available in ampoules, and in tablets of high strengths more suited to administration of the high doses required in the treatment of mental illness.

Tablets of 1 mg. in bottles of 100 and 1,000, tablets of 3 mg. and 5 mg. in bottles of 100, ampoules of 5 mg. in boxes of 6 and 50.

Reserpine, an alkaloid of Rauwolfia serpentina, possesses a remarkable calming and relaxing action, and is capable of wide application in mental illness. Its use is rapidly increasing, and if early reports are confirmed, Reserpine will stand as a very real advance in psychotherapeutics.

"The drug (reserpine) provides a far more rational approach to the treatment of the chronically and acutely disturbed patient than any other method we have used to date."
J. Amer. med. Ass. (1954) 156:821

Reserpine—'Serpiloid' brand is also available in 0.25 mg. and 0.5 mg. tablets in bottles of 100 and 1,000 for those clinicians who prefer a single alkaloid for use in hypertension.

SIDE-EFFECTS

The use of Reserpine in psychiatry is still in the experimental stage, and although no serious side effects have so far been reported, the following conditions may be produced in some patients:

1. Nasal congestion.
2. Weakness and giddiness.
3. A degree of hypotension with bradycardia.
4. A Parkinson-like syndrome following the administration of high doses.

These symptoms will probably disappear in 5/8 days without the need for discontinuing treatment. They will regress if dosage is reduced.

RIKER

'SERPILOID' is a registered trade mark
Regd. Users:

RIKER   LABORATORIES   LIMITED
MORLEY STREET, LOUGHBOROUGH, LEICS

Figure 3.1   Reserpine advertisement
Copyright of 3M, reproduced with permission.

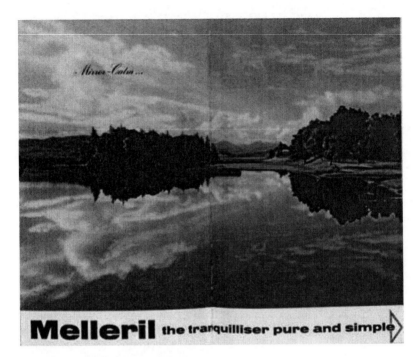

Figure 3.2   Melleril advertisement
Reproduced with kind permission of Novartis.

from previous drugs, and that they could 'wipe out the symptoms of psychotic patients just as internists can use insulin for the elimination of the symptoms of diabetes' (Himwich, 1955).

At the same symposium in 1957 in which Freyhan outlined his drug-centred view of the action of the new tranquillisers, Heinz Lehman set out the first explicit, disease-centred theory of the actions of chlorpromazine and similar drugs (Lehmann, 1959). As well as attempting to classify the new drugs by their physiological effects on the nervous system in a drug-centred manner, he suggested that the effects of drugs could also be divided into those that were 'curative', 'corrective' and 'symptomatic'. Whereas a curative substance was one that reversed the original cause of the disease, like antibiotics, a corrective was one that attacked a 'nucleus of symptoms that is fairly close to the primary disturbance', although the primary cause of the condition need not be known. Examples of correctives in medicine were insulin for diabetes and digitalis for heart disease, and Lehmann identified chlorpromazine and reserpine as 'typical corrective agents in a number of acute and chronic psychotic conditions'

(Lehmann, 1959, p. 22). He contrasted their effects to symptomatic treatments, like morphine for pain, barbiturates for insomnia, and chlorpromazine when it was used for the control of behavioural excitement, which only affected symptoms that were 'rather remote and indirect manifestations' of the disease process (p. 23).

Heinz Lehmann has said that he introduced the term 'antipsychotic' at a Canadian Medical Association meeting in 1956, but that he meant it more metaphorically than literally at this time (Lehmann, 1993). The first paper listed on the medical database Medline using the term 'antipsychotic' was published in 1962, in which two psychiatrists distinguished an 'antipsychotic drug' which 'antagonises major psychotic symptoms' from other tranquillisers, which ameliorate the 'symptom of anxiety' (Mapp and Nodine, 1962, p. 458). Despite this distinction, however, the authors did not attribute 'curative' or 'corrective' properties, in Lehmann's terms, to the drugs they were describing, but expressed confidence that 'more specific agents' would be developed in the future, which would act on the 'etiology of the symptoms rather than the symptoms themselves'. Their longing for such a discovery was conveyed by their dramatically expressed aspiration for a drug which could 'chemically remove' mental symptoms, permitting the patient to 'sever the blocking strings of the past and like some giant Gulliver, step forth as a strong, fully productive adult' (p. 463).

US psychiatrist, Nathan Kline, was one of the most influential proponents of a disease-centred theory of psychiatric drug action. In 1959 Kline described chlorpromazine and reserpine essentially in drug-centred terms, calling them 'ataraxics', a term which, according to Kline, meant a substance that relieved 'turmoil and confusion' (Kline, 1959, p. 398). As well as their ability to 'restrict and inhibit' mental disturbance, however, he believed they could also 'remove or reverse' symptoms, hinting at a putative disease-centred mechanism of action (p. 398). But it was his characterisation of what later came to be known as 'antidepressants' in which Kline expressed the disease-centred view most explicitly. Kline distinguished drugs that he called 'psychic energisers' (later referred to as antidepressants) from stimulants by claiming that they normalised mood in those who were depressed without causing the general arousal and euphoria associated with drugs like amphetamines (Kline, 1959). His assertions were contradicted by data suggesting that the early antidepressants he referred to *did* induce euphoria, and had stimulant effects that were remarkably similar to those of amphetamines (Crane, 1956), but no one pointed this out at the time, and Kline helped to establish the idea that 'antidepressants' worked in a targeted, disease-centred fashion.

In 1964, a well-known study funded by the United States National Institute for Mental Health (NIMH) boldly claimed to have demonstrated the disease-specific action of the new drugs for the treatment of schizophrenia (National Institute of Mental Health Psychopharmacology Service Center Collaborative Study Group, 1964). The trial, which involved chlorpromazine and two other phenothiazine compounds, found that all three drugs improved a range of symptoms greater than the placebo. As these symptoms included not just excitement, agitation and anxiety, but what were regarded as more fundamental schizophrenic symptoms, including incoherence of speech, social withdrawal and apathy, as well as auditory hallucinations and persecutory delusions, the authors concluded that 'the phenothiazines should be considered to be "anti-schizophrenic" in the broad sense. In fact, it is questionable whether the term "tranquiliser" should be retained' (p. 257). They also noted that the drugs tested varied in their proclivity to produce extrapyramidal or Parkinsonian effects, and, yet, because all were equally effective, they suggested that 'the therapeutic properties of these drugs may be quite independent of their tendency to produce side effects' (p. 255).

Sheldon Gelman has described how the report of this trial encapsulated a new psychiatric 'vision', which suggested that drug treatment was effective and specific with relatively trivial adverse effects (Gelman, 1999). Although the results of the study were subsequently cited to justify the disease-centred model of drug action, it appears that the disease-centred view was already assumed in its conception. As the study included no other type of drug, it could not demonstrate that the antipsychotics were superior to other sorts of sedative, nor could it discount the impact of the neurological effects the antipsychotics exerted. Moreover, the neurological or 'extrapyramidal' effects, now referred to as 'side effects,' were already distinguished from the drugs' therapeutic effects and the concept of the 'neuroleptic threshold', which explains that drugs with different propensities to cause extrapyramidal effects can exert therapeutic neurological effects at variable, 'threshold' doses was not considered.

The idea that drugs like chlorpromazine could suppress a range of symptoms does not in itself necessarily imply a disease-centred view of drug action, although, as we shall see in Chapter 6, other studies have not confirmed the NIMH's findings, and have generally found that the principle effects of antipsychotics are on reducing behavioural disturbance and 'positive' psychotic symptoms. The increasing separation and minimisation of neurological 'side effects', however, and the broad endorsement of the drugs suggests that they were in the process of being transformed into drugs that were suitable for a new era in mental health care. Whereas during the early and middle decades of the twentieth century, people felt able to do practically anything to psychiatric patients in the name of therapy, including putting them into dangerous comas for days at a time, by the 1960s times were changing. There was increasing acceptance that treatments should be properly and scientifically evaluated, and along with organised controlled trials came a greater awareness of the ethics of treating people with mental conditions. The idea that psychiatric therapies, including drugs, worked by inducing other diseases, as Deniker had suggested, was no longer an acceptable basis for treatment. Treatment had to be an unqualified good, except, of course, for troublesome, but essentially trivial, side effects.

The Ascendancy of the Disease-Centred Model

The emergence of the disease-centred model of psychiatric drug action was not premised on research findings, however, or on theoretical discussion or debate. Although a few figures like Deniker and Haase continued to reiterate a drug-centred view, in general, what is striking is that this older conception of drug action simply faded away. Descriptions of the neurological and physiological effects induced by antipsychotics and other psychiatric drugs, such as antidepressants, disappeared from the literature (Moncrieff, 2008b). Henceforth they were referred to, if at all, only as 'side effects', which were regarded as an incidental nuisance, rather than an intrinsic part of a drug's action. Almost no papers discussed the relative merits of different theories of drug action or attempted to justify the disease-centred model, and no research was set up to evaluate different models. When textbooks started to present the disease-centred view, there was little acknowledgement that there was an alternative explanation of how antipsychotics might work and there was no discussion of any evidence to support the disease-centred view of drug action, with the exception of some oblique references to the NIMH study.

Textbooks tentatively started to convey a disease-centred view of the nature of neuroleptic or antipsychotic drugs from the 1960s, with suggestions that 'they appear to do more than tranquilise' (Henderson and Gillespie, 1962, p. 350) and 'penetrate much closer to the site of mechanism of the disease itself than any other procedure applied hitherto' (Mayer-Gross et al., 1960, p. 386). Most descriptions of drug treatment remained only implicitly disease-centred at this period, however, linking

52

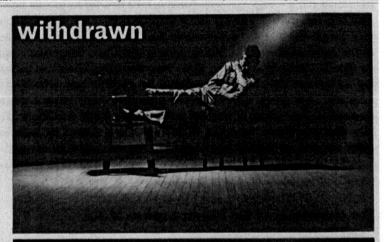

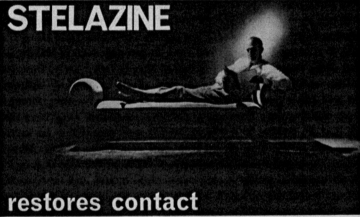

Figure 3.3   Stelazine advertisement
Reproduced with kind permission of GlaxoSmithKline.

particular drugs with particular conditions, omitting any description of their psychoactive or drug-induced effects, and conceptually separating therapeutic effects from 'side' effects, but without any discussion about how the drugs might affect possible disease mechanisms (Hoch, 1959; Malitz and Hoch, 1966).

Hints of a disease-centred view also started to appear in advertisements of the 1960s, where the neuroleptics or major tranquillisers were increasingly associated with the treatment of schizophrenia. Largactil (chlorpromazine) was said to act as a 'psychocorrective' in this situation, for example (Largactil or chlorpormazine; Largactil advertisement, 1965), and Serenace (haloperidol) was said to have a 'profound' action (Serenace or haloperidol) (Serenace advertisement, 1965a). A 1965 advertisement for Stelazine, which depicts a young man looking comfortable and relaxed below a troubled-looking older man, seems to illustrate the idea that drug treatment could restore someone to normal and prevent them deteriorating into a state of chronic patienthood (Stelazine advertisement, 1965a) (Figure 3.3).

By 1970, the majority of advertisements were aimed at people diagnosed with schizophrenia. The Melleril (thioridazine) advertisement from this year, which consisted of two colour pages, described the action of the drug in explicitly disease-centred terms (Figure 3.4). Melleril 'strikes promptly at the target symptoms', the advertisement claimed, and the drug was referred to as an 'anti-psychotic'. The effect on 'target' or psychotic symptoms, which was said to occur after 7 days, was also distinguished from the immediate sedative or 'tranquillising effect' of the drug (Melleril advertisement, 1970).

During the 1970s, the consolidation of the dopamine hypothesis of schizophrenia introduced a new confidence to assertions about the nature of drug treatment for schizophrenia. Commitment to the disease-centred view of drug action was expressed in the belief that clarifying the drugs' mechanism of action would reveal the underlying basis of schizophrenia.

The *Companion to Psychiatric Studies*, one of the most respected British textbooks of psychiatry for many decades, first published in 1973, presented what is probably the last mainstream, drug-centred account of antipsychotic action, alongside the disease-centred view. The general chapter on pharmacology suggested that the drugs damp down responses to stimuli and reduce spontaneity, and, following Delay and Deniker, suggested their unique quality was their ability to induce sedation without sleep (Roberts, 1973). The chapter on the treatment of schizophrenia, however, written by a different author, assumed the drugs

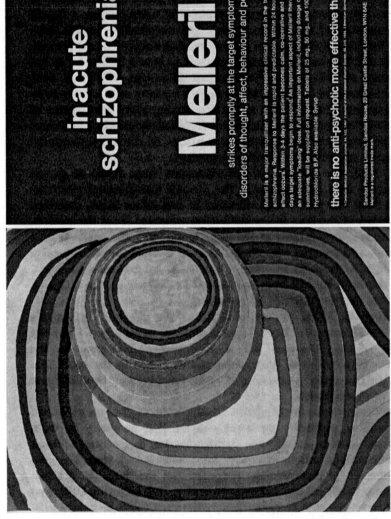

Figure 3.4 Melleril advertisement
Reproduced with kind permission of Novartis.

acted in a disease-centred manner. In this chapter the drugs were referred to as 'anti-schizophrenic' and it was asserted that they exert 'a specific therapeutic effect in schizophrenia, and that the term "tranquiliser" is a misnomer' (Smythies, 1973, pp. 281–2). Serotonin and dopamine were discussed as possible candidates for the underlying basis of drug action and clarification of this, it was suggested, would reveal the 'biochemical lesion of schizophrenia' (Smythies, 1973, p. 282).

The second edition of the *American Handbook of Psychiatry*, the largest American textbook of the mid-twentieth century also claimed that 'specific pharmacological treatments for the major psycho-pathological states have become available' and that these agents were able to elucidate the biochemical origins of these disorders (Maas & Garver, 1975, p. 427). The chapter on 'Antipsychotic Drugs', written by Jonathan Cole, the lead researcher on the NIMH study, and John Davis, another well-known academic, speculated that the drugs may exert their effects by reducing dopamine activity (Davis et al., 1975, p. 446).

By 1980, the first edition of what has subsequently become the major American textbook of psychiatry unequivocally asserted the disease-centred position. The section on antipsychotic drugs, written by John Davis, stated 'antipsychotic drugs have a *normalising* effect. They lessen the typical schizophrenic symptoms, such as hallucinations and delusions. They also normalise various other abnormal behaviours'. Davis also stressed that 'there is a clear cut difference between their sedative and antipsychotic properties' (Davis, 1980, p. 2260, my emphasis). The author of the general section on psychopharmacology, Solomon Snyder, whom we shall meet in the next chapter through his work on dopamine receptors, asserted that the drugs 'exert a selective anti-schizophrenia action' and then provided a detailed description of their actions on the dopamine system (Snyder, 1980, p. 161).

By the mid-1970s advertisements for neuroleptic drugs no longer mentioned their psychoactive properties, and almost all were targeted at the treatment of people diagnosed with schizophrenia. In June 1975 a new drug called Redeptin was advertised for the first time, which was said to have an 'antipsychotic action' that was achieved through its 'specific action on dopamine receptors' (Redeptin advertisement, 1975).

Influences and Motivations

A rare discussion of alternative understandings of drug action by Nathan Kline in 1969 reveals how much was felt to be at stake by acknowledging the drug-centred point of view by this time. In his 1959 paper, Kline rejected the concept of a 'neuroleptic' on the not unreasonable basis that the mode of action the term suggested was unproven. Ten years later, he angrily dismissed a World Health Organization report on psychopharmacology that had accepted the concept, presumably under Deniker's influence. He described the report as being 'deGaulling' in its 'capitulation' to the French point of view, and as using a 'weasling excuse' to defend its position, language far removed from the sober and restrained expression that usually characterises academic writing (Kline, 1969).

Although typical of Kline's forthright personality (Healy, 2002), his fury at the implications of the drug-centred view illustrates the strength of professional interests that were at stake in the transformation of views about the nature of psychiatric drug treatment. Ever since the medical superintendents of the lunatic asylums identified themselves as a profession, they had been on the defensive about the role of medicine in caring for people deemed at that time to be 'insane' (Scull, 1993; Rogers and Pilgrim, 2001). After decades of impotence, as they perceived it, physical treatments like insulin coma therapy, ECT and lobotomy had helped psychiatrists to present a medical face to the world (Moncrieff and Crawford, 2001). From the 1940s, however, with the introduction of penicillin and an array of other drugs, medicine came to be identified more than anything with drug treatment. Thus, the new drugs helped bring psychiatry further into line with existing medical practice, and contemporaries expressed their delight that the drugs made 'the mental hospital a medical institution in the minds of the public' (Overholser, 1956). Deniker, too, described approvingly how the new drugs had strengthened the medical and scientific approach in psychiatry (Deniker, 1970).

The drug-centred view of how psychiatric drugs might work was not, however, a model that could be easily married with the increasingly specific nature of other medical treatments. Medicine in the twentieth century was increasingly identified with the notion of treatment that worked by targeting an underlying disease. 'Cure by specific therapy' had become 'the only really proper sphere for the physician' (Pellegrino, 1979, p. 255). Suppressing symptoms by drugging people, even if the characteristics of the drug-induced state were uniquely useful, as Deniker and others argued, was not a model that could be married with the mechanisms of antibiotics, hormones or other emerging medical therapies. So psychiatrists borrowed the notion of specificity from their medical colleagues and soon forgot that there was any other way to conceive of the effects of the drugs that they used.

A parallel process occurred during this period with other types of drugs, and a belief developed that most of the major classes of drugs used in psychiatry represented specific treatments that worked by targeting the biological processes underlying particular mental conditions. As this way of understanding drug treatment coalesced, the psychoactive and physical effects the drugs produced gradually became invisible. Taking attention away from the mind-altering properties of psychiatric drugs helped to distance the use of drugs that were prescribed as medicines from the rapidly expanding recreational drug scene (DeGrandpre, 2006). In this way, the disease-centred model of drug action helped to preserve psychiatry's respectability at a time when levels of barbiturate and stimulant prescribing were causing concern and when stimulant drugs were still being promoted for the treatment of depression and fatigue (Hammond, 1964; Ritalin advertisement, 1964). Even the benzodiazepine drugs like Valium, with their obvious and appealing sedative-psychoactive effects, were presented as a targeted treatment for the 'disease' of anxiety, despite their prolific use for numerous situations across a range of diagnoses.

The consolidation of the idea that psychiatric drugs constituted disease-specific treatments formed an important building block for the project that has sometimes been referred to as the 'remedicalisation' of psychiatry, which took place during the 1970s, culminating in the publication of the third edition of the *Diagnostic and Statistical Manual of Mental Disorders* (*DSM*) in 1980. The *DSM-3* expunged the influence of psychoanalysis and social psychiatry that had infiltrated twentieth century psychiatry—quite illegitimately in the opinion of its authors— and helped to present psychiatric practice as a thoroughly medical process in which discrete disease entities could be identified, labelled and treated with specially targeted interventions (Wilson, 1993). Without being able to predict treatment, psychiatric diagnosis was an easy target, and hence the claim that psychiatric treatments act on underlying processes was a prerequisite for the consolidation and acceptance of the philosophy that underpinned the *DSM-3*.

Professional interests were not the only drivers of the change in understandings of psychiatric drug action, however. The disease-centred model seemed to promise that the use of properly targeted medical treatment could resolve the age-old problem of what to do with people who became mentally disturbed. Instead of having to be contained and cared for, this new orientation suggested that people with psychiatric problems could be 'cured' and returned to society to resume a normal life. It was a view that was enormously appealing to politicians and policy makers, who could now regard a complex problem of social control and welfare as a simple situation requiring only the correct technical intervention. Moreover, the idea that people could be cured provided a way of conceptualising mental health care that was in tune with the liberal and progressive ideals of the post-war world, and, co-incidentally, afforded the justification to run down the expensive mental hospitals and replace them with cheaper 'care in the community'. The attempt to reframe madness as a medical problem that started in the nineteenth century was finally cemented by the disease-centred view of the new tranquillisers.

By 1970 the disease-centred model was so well accepted that Deniker was forced to admit that his views were controversial, acknowledging how unpalatable it was to many psychiatrists to define a group of drugs by their adverse effects (Deniker, 1970, 1983). Although he continued to stress that the 'therapeutic effects of the neuroleptics are inseparable from the psychomotor, neurological and vegetative modifications which they produce' (Deniker, 1983), he recanted on the idea that advanced symptoms of Parkinsonism were required for the best therapeutic effects (Deniker, 1970). He was sceptical of the dopamine hypothesis of schizophrenia, however, and maintained that 'neuroleptics diminish the phenomena of schizophrenia, but do not pretend to be an etiological treatment of these psychoses' (Deniker, 1989). Also interesting from a drug-centred perspective is that Deniker was one of the first people to comment on how the 'neurovegetative' effects of clozapine, which he acknowledged were different from those induced by other, more 'typical' antipsychotics, were likely to mediate its therapeutic effects (Deniker, 1989). We shall see how this idea is confirmed by other accounts in Chapter 7.

When dopamine receptor blockade was demonstrated to be the principle mechanism of both the therapeutic action of most early antipsychotics and their propensity to induce neurological or extrapyramidal effects, it might have seemed as though mainstream psychiatry would have to acknowledge the truth of Deniker's position. In the 1990s it was established that the level of dopamine receptor blockade required to produce therapeutic effects (65–80%) was only slightly lower than the level found to produce overt evidence of drug-induced Parkinsonism (above 80%), in a pattern reminiscent of Haase's concept of the 'neuroleptic threshold' (Farde et al., 1992; Nyberg et al., 1995). Somehow, psychiatry managed to maintain the distinction between the therapeutic effects and the neurological effects of antipsychotics, however, and the idea that these were one and the same started to become unthinkable as the disease-centred view gained wider acceptance. The development of the dopamine hypothesis of schizophrenia played a crucial part in this evasion. By focusing attention on the biological nature of the underlying disorder, and suggesting a mechanism whereby drugs *might* reverse a proposed abnormality, the theory consigned the drug-centred understanding of the new drugs to history. The neurological alterations produced by antipsychotics and described so vividly by Deniker and others, along with the theories they inspired, slipped quietly, but thoroughly, out of view.

4
Building a House of Cards: The Dopamine Theory of Schizophrenia and Drug Action

By presenting a theory of schizophrenia suggesting that some or all of its symptoms are caused by a biochemical abnormality that antipsychotics happen to reverse, the dopamine hypothesis of schizophrenia is a key part of the story of how the group of drugs we are considering came to be understood as 'miracle cures'—as drugs that target the basis of schizophrenia or psychosis. Although the inadequacy and inconsistency of the theory have been acknowledged ever since it was articulated, the dopamine hypothesis of schizophrenia has occupied research activity for decades and consumed vast amounts of funding. In fact, for many academics and practising clinicians, it has long moved beyond hypothesis into the realm of fact.

The original hypothesis proposed that schizophrenia is caused by over-activity of the brain chemical, dopamine. The theory has existed in many different versions, however, over the course of its life. Stephen Stahl, author of many best-selling textbooks on psychopharmacology, presents an elaborate version of the hypothesis in his 2008 book *Antipsychotics and Mood Stabilisers*. Backed up by numerous scientific-looking illustrations of brain circuits and neurons, he suggests that schizophrenia is caused by simultaneous over-activity of dopamine in one part of the brain, the limbic system, and under-activity in another, the cortex. Furthermore, he postulates that atypical antipsychotics simultaneously correct these opposing defects. No conflicting evidence is mentioned, and there is no acknowledgement of the implausibility of a situation involving opposing biochemical states co-existing in different, but inter-related, brain regions, or of the idea that one drug can simultaneously act in different ways in different areas (Stahl, 2008).

'The history of schizophrenia research', said pharmacologist Les Iverson in an interview with psychiatrist and academic David Healy, 'is littered with the skeletons of chemical hypotheses' (Iversen, 1998, p. 345). Before the dopamine hypothesis there was a thyroid hormone hypothesis of schizophrenia, a sex hormone hypothesis, the transmethylation and serotonin hypotheses, and many others. Since the 1990s glutamate has come into fashion, and interest in serotonin has been revived. The dopamine hypothesis seems to be the most persistent, however, but, in order to survive, it has had to absorb, transform or expel many awkward pieces of evidence. The popularity and longevity of the theory tells us something important about the vision psychiatry wishes to promote of itself and its treatments. The dopamine hypothesis of schizophrenia suggests, as many psychiatrists have wanted to believe for a long time, that psychiatric conditions are real diseases with tangible and specific biological origins, and that antipsychotic drugs constitute a genuine and innocuous medical treatment, which counteract the underlying defect in a highly targeted manner.

In fact, however, the dopamine theory was elaborated on the *assumption* that antipsychotic drugs act in a disease-specific way on the underlying pathology of schizophrenia or its symptoms. Because this view of antipsychotic action was already unquestioned, it was presumed that the origins of schizophrenia or psychosis could be deduced to be the opposite state from that produced by the drugs. So, according to a recent textbook of psychiatry, 'the fact that every effective antipsychotic drug blocks dopamine D_2 receptors is powerful evidence of the importance of dopamine in the pathogenesis of schizophrenia' (Wright et al., 2012, p. 272). Even in the early days of the dopamine hypothesis, few of its proponents seemed aware that they were making an assumption of this sort. The dopamine hypothesis of schizophrenia is a consequence of the fact that the disease-centred model had already eclipsed other ways of understanding drug action by the time the hypothesis was elaborated in the 1970s.

This chapter will demonstrate that decades of research have failed to provide evidence that the symptoms of either schizophrenia or psychosis result from an underlying abnormality of dopamine activity. What research has clearly demonstrated, in contrast, is that antipsychotic drugs disturb dopamine function to a greater or lesser extent, and that their action on the dopamine system is responsible for many of the characteristic neurological disturbances they produce. The dopamine theory of schizophrenia has, however, helped to ensure that such effects are decisively relegated to the place of second fiddle behind the drugs' proposed ability to rectify the underlying disease. In this way, the dopamine hypothesis provided an important bulwark against the potential threat posed to the modern vision of drug treatment by the emergence of tardive dyskinesia. Moreover, as we shall see in the next chapter, an adapted version of the dopamine hypothesis was an important tool in the early marketing of the atypical antipsychotics.

Origins of the Dopamine Hypothesis

The activity of dopamine as a neurotransmitter, or chemical messenger, was discovered by the Nobel prize-winning Swedish pharmacologist Arvid Carlsson, while he was investigating the chemical basis of the action of reserpine. In the 1950s the newly described effects of the drug lysergic acid diethylamide (LSD) made some people speculate that schizophrenia was due to abnormalities of the serotonin system (Woolley and Shaw, 1954). Bernard 'Steve' Brodie, the leading scientist at the National Institute of Mental Health (NIMH) in the USA, under whom Carlsson worked for a period in the mid-1950s, showed that reserpine reduced brain serotonin levels when given to rabbits (Pletscher et al., 1955). Carlsson's later work showed that reserpine depleted not just serotonin but dopamine and noradrenaline as well, and that dopamine and not serotonin was responsible for the slowing and lethargy caused by reserpine (Carlsson et al., 1957, 1959). The similarity between the state of reduced movement induced by reserpine and Parkinson's disease lead Carlsson to speculate that the latter might involve the dopamine system, and this was confirmed in the 1960s (Ehringer and Hornykiewicz, 1960).

So, the discovery of the activity of dopamine in the brain was a consequence of the investigation of the abnormal state of reduced movement produced by reserpine. In other words, it proceeded according to a drug-centred model of drug action. As the neuroleptics were transformed into 'antipsychotics', this research metamorphosed into something quite different. The drug-induced abnormalities that had been observed were inverted and the research became focused on the origins of schizophrenia itself. From this point on, the perturbations induced by drugs were only interesting in so far as they indicated something about the pathology of the disease that was presumed to lie behind the symptoms of schizophrenia, and there was little interest in the effects of the drugs for their own sake.

Although reserpine had been shown to deplete dopamine stores, the mechanism of action of the other antipsychotics remained uncertain, as they could not be shown to have the same depleting action. A Dutch researcher, Jacques van Rossum showed that haloperidol, and a related drug, spiramide, reversed the effects of dopamine on blood pressure in cats, confirming his hypothesis that 'dopamine receptor blockade is an important factor in the mode of action of neuroleptic drugs' (van Rossum, 1966a, p. 492). In a book published the same year he briefly speculated that the discovery might have 'fargoing consequences for the pathophysiology of schizophrenia. Overstimulation of dopamine receptors could then be part of the aetiology' (van Rossum , 1966b, p. 327).

The dopamine hypothesis of schizophrenia was not clearly expounded in the scientific literature until the 1970s, however, although there are indications that it was already influential by this time. By 1974, for example, it was claimed to be a central theme in psychopharmacology, which was 'shared by many investigators' and was said to exert 'a substantial influence on the design of experiments' (Matthysse, 1974a, p. 107). In spite of its increasing importance, other theories continued to be put forward, however, particularly variants of the serotonin hypothesis of schizophrenia, the 'transmethylation' hypothesis and a phenylalanine hypothesis (Faurbye, 1968; Fischer, 1970). A deficit of noradrenline, another neurotransmitter, was proposed to be the origin of schizophrenia (Wise et al., 1974), and research continued into the role of noradrenaline in the effects of stimulants and antipsychotics (Bartholini et al., 1972). As late as 1973, in one of the first reviews of research pertaining to a possible dopamine theory of schizophrenia, Steven Matthysse, professor of psychobiology at Harvard, argued 'this simple hypothesis is by no means the only possible interpretation [of the research data]. It is not even the most plausible'(Matthysse, 1973).

Three international conferences on dopamine and noradrenaline, also known collectively as 'catecholamines', had been organised by 1973. At the third meeting, Steven Mattysse proposed a further meeting, which took place the following year, on the role of these chemicals in the 'neuropathology of schizophrenia,' in order, as he said, to assemble the world's most 'critical and productive investigators in the field' (Matthysse, 1974b, p. xiii). The two main strands of evidence that were cited as the basis for a dopamine theory of schizophrenia in the collection of conference papers published in 1974 were the effects of antipsychotic drugs, and the ability of the drug amphetamine to induce psychotic symptoms. Many of the authors highlighted the contradictory nature of the evidence, however, and few were confident that the origin of schizophrenia or its symptoms had been uncovered. As Mattysse pointed out in the epilogue to the volume, the state of the evidence allowed only limited conclusions. These were simply, he thought, that antipsychotic drugs block dopamine activity and that amphetamines can cause psychosis. In Matthysse's view, it had not even been established that dopamine was involved in the therapeutic effects of antipsychotics or the psychosis-inducing effect of amphetamines (Matthysse, 1974b).

These modest and uncontested claims jar with the space devoted to speculation about the role of dopamine in schizophrenia and the enthusiasm expressed about the potential of the research being conducted. Leading psychiatric geneticist Seymore Kety summed up the atmosphere of the conference by noting how the area was creating 'considerable ferment throughout the world'. There was a feeling, he suggested, that the 'psychobiological substrates' underpinning schizophrenia were, at last, being laid bare (Kety, 1974, p. x). Despite his cautious assessment of the existing evidence, Mattysse himself declared that the research being conducted would eventually make a substantial contribution to the 'matrix of scientific knowledge' on the biological nature of schizophrenia (Matthysse, 1974b, p. xvi).

Antipsychotic Action and the Dopamine Hypothesis

Matthysse noted that most of the contributors to the 1974 conference took as 'axiomatic' the idea that antipsychotics exerted their therapeutic effects in people diagnosed with schizophrenia by acting on the abnormalities that gave rise to the condition. The only contributor who acknowledged that this view required justification was Solomon Snyder, a scientist already renowned for his work on identifying and locating opiate receptors. Snyder subsequently identified the first dopamine receptors and became one of the principle proponents of both the dopamine hypothesis of antipsychotic action, and the dopamine hypothesis of schizophrenia. Snyder's main line of research into dopamine concerned the actions of amphetamine, but, in his contribution to the 1974 conference, he also claimed emphatically that antipsychotic drugs had been shown to be specifically 'antischizophrenic', referring to the NIMH study and the claim by its authors that the drugs affected all the 'fundamental' symptoms of schizophrenia (Snyder, 1974). As we have seen, however, the study was already influenced by a disease-specific view of antipsychotic action and, moreover, was contradicted by other studies on the effects of antipsychotics.

Having supposedly established the disease specificity of antipsychotic action, and although he admitted that the drugs 'produce biochemical effects on almost every system that has been examined', Snyder concluded that the therapeutic effects of antipsychotics were achieved through their effects on the dopamine system on the basis of studies showing correlations between the dose range of various antipsychotics and their effects on dopamine receptors (Snyder, 1974; Snyder et al., 1974, p. 1246). Drugs with stronger actions on these receptors were active at lower doses than those with weaker actions, and this finding has been cited many times since to support the dopamine hypothesis of drug action and of schizophrenia. David Healy suggested it was 'among the most clear-cut findings in psychopharmacology' (Healy, 2002, p. 214).

The relationship between dopamine blockade and therapeutic activity is not as strong or as simple as is often suggested, however. It was already apparent in the 1970s that some drugs, such as clozapine and thioridazine (Melleril), which had relatively weak dopamine-blocking properties, were as effective as other antipsychotics. Several of the presenters at the 1974 conference pointed out this discrepancy, including Matthysse (Crow and Gillbe, 1974; Matthysse 1974a). Snyder himself acknowledged another inconsistency: that the dopamine-blocking properties of the antipsychotics were more strongly correlated with their propensity to induce Parkinson's-like or 'extrapyramidal' neurological effects, than their therapeutic efficacy (Snyder, 1974). Evidence suggested there was a 'dissociation between dopaminergic blockade and antipsychotic activity' (Stawarz et al., 1975).

The discrepancy problem was largely ignored, however, until the re-introduction of clozapine in the early 1990s. At that time, receptor binding studies carried out with the new technology of radio-actively labelling chemicals that bind to receptors in living subjects confirmed that clozapine, at clinically effective doses, occupied a lower proportion of the now identified dopamine D_2 receptors, compared with most conventional antipsychotics. Moreover, occupancy rates were closely associated with the presence of Parkinsonism, which clozapine does not produce to the same degree as other antipsychotics (Farde et al., 1992; Nyberg et al., 1995). A more recent meta-analysis of dopamine receptor studies failed to find a statistically significant correlation between D_2 receptor occupancy levels and clinical response. Excluding studies involving clozapine and quetipine (another antipsychotic with low dopamine receptor blocking properties) still did not produce evidence of a correlation between receptor occupancy and clinical response. Excluding one other study, on the basis that it had overly high dopamine receptor occupancy levels, did, finally, produce a statistically significant result. The authors had to conclude, however, that 'D_2 receptor occupancy is only part of the story regarding antipsychotic medication response' (Yilmaz et al., 2012, p. 216). By implication, therefore, drug action on dopamine receptors cannot be presumed to reveal the underlying pathology of schizophrenia or psychosis.

Another explanation offered for the problem of clozapine is the suggestion that clozapine and some other antipsychotics block dopamine receptors, but then rapidly detach themselves again (Kapur and Seeman, 2001). Somehow, this transient attachment is proposed to facilitate antipsychotic effects, but prevent the occurrence of drug-induced, extrapyramidal effects. It seems more likely that the failure to produce these neurological signs indicates that no clinically significant dopamine blockade is occurring, and that the drugs' much stronger effects on other neurotransmitter systems account for their psychoactive effects and their impact on psychotic symptoms.

Amphetamine-Induced Psychosis and the Dopamine Hypothesis

Snyder and others had been conducting research to elucidate the mechanism of action of the stimulant drug amphetamine since the 1960s, and several authors, including Snyder, drew on this line of evidence for the dopamine hypothesis in their 1974 conference papers. Amphetamine psychosis was first described in the scientific literature in 1938 (Young and Scoville, 1938). Although it is often indistinguishable from an unexplained psychotic episode in a particular individual, as a group people with stimulant-induced psychosis exhibit a slightly different range of symptoms, as Snyder himself pointed out in 1972 (Snyder, 1972). Amphetamine psychosis is primarily a paranoid state; therefore, although there is clearly overlap with the paranoid delusions that characterise some episodes of schizophrenia, other sorts of symptoms that occur in acute episodes of schizophrenic-type psychosis, such as the verbal ramblings known as 'thought disorder', delusions of being controlled, and inappropriate or flattened emotional responses, are rarely seen in the drug-induced state. The latter is more often characterised by heightened anxiety, and visual or tactile (sensations of touch) hallucinations may be present, which are uncommon in episodes of schizophrenia. Some authors have pointed out, however, that stimulant-induced psychosis can occasionally produce symptoms more usually associated with schizophrenia, including bizarre delusions, third person hallucinations, social withdrawal and apathy (Harris and Batki, 2000; Batki and Harris, 2004). It seems possible to conclude both that the psychotic state induced by amphetamines and other stimulants is somewhat distinctive, and that it shares some features with spontaneous psychotic or schizophrenic episodes.

For researchers in the 1960s, however, the fact that psychosis could be produced by chemical means seemed highly significant, and unlocking the key to this experience appeared to promise the explanation of mental disturbance more generally (Randrup and Munkvad, 1972). Amphetamine affects many neurochemical systems, however, including noradrenaline, and serotonin, as well as dopamine, and, initially, interest focused on its effects on noradrenaline (Brodie et al. 1959; van Rossum et al., 1962). Indeed, amphetamine increases the release of noradrenaline more potently than it releases dopamine or serotonin (Rothman et al., 2001). In the 1960s a group of Danish researchers, lead by Axel Randrup, described how rats treated with high doses of amphetamine developed abnormal, repetitive, 'stereotyped' movements, which they called 'stereotypies'. These consisted of licking, sniffing, and biting their cage or themselves. These stereotyped behaviours could be distinguished from the general hyperactivity that was produced at lower doses of amphetamine (Randrup et al., 1963). Later, abnormally obsessive and repetitive behaviours, sometimes referred to as 'punding', were noticed to occur in humans after prolonged exposure to stimulant drugs, including amphetamine. Men were reported to tinker with mechanical equipment, such as car engines and clocks, and women repetitively sorted through handbags, or engaged in compulsive tidying or grooming. Humans also develop involuntary movements, including twitches and tics, when taking stimulant drugs (Costall and Naylor, 1975). Randrup proposed that these stereotypies were attributable to amphetamine's effects on the dopamine system because they were modified by antipsychotic drugs, but not by barbiturates (Randrup et al., 1963; Randrup and Munkvad, 1967).

The proposed association between stereotypies, dopamine and the effects of antipsychotics led to the suggestion that stimulant-induced stereotypy was a 'model' for psychosis, in other words that it constituted an animal equivalent of a psychotic state. The ability of drugs to counteract the motor effects of stimulants, particularly amphetamine, was widely adopted as a method of evaluating the potential antipsychotic activity of a chemical substance, and Janssen Laboratories, for example, was said to be using this screening test from the early 1960s (Baumeister and Francis, 2002).

Stereotypies are clearly not the same thing as psychotic experiences, however, and they occur in people on amphetamine in the absence of psychotic symptoms. Equally, drug-induced psychosis is not necessarily accompanied by stereotypical behaviours. Moreover, the idea that the motor effects of amphetamines in general, or stereotypies in particular, were mediated purely by dopamine was not firmly established, and some research suggested that noradrenaline was also involved in stimulant-induced hyperactivity and stereotypies (Herman, 1970; Mogilnicka and Braestrup, 1976; Borison and Diamond, 1978). It is also becoming clear that it is difficult to map any complex behaviour to a single neurotransmitter system, and it is likely that both noradrenaline and dopamine, and possibly other systems, are involved in most aspects of amphetamine's effects (Berridge, 2006).

In the 1970s, Snyder attempted to demonstrate that dopamine was the chemical involved in the psychosis-inducing effects of amphetamine through studying the effects of the two different chemical forms or 'isomers' of the drug. Snyder suggested that the positive isomer of amphetamine, (+)-amphetamine, had been found to have stronger noradrenaline-enhancing activity than the negative, (−)-amphetamine isomer, whereas the two isomers had more equal dopamine-stimulating activity as measured by their ability to provoke stereotypies in animals. As the two isomers were equal in their ability to precipitate psychotic symptoms in humans, Snyder concluded that dopamine must be responsible for this effect (Snyder, 1974). However, he admitted that other studies had produced conflicting evidence, and Matthysse, in his main contribution to the 1974 conference report, listed numerous studies that contradicted Snyder's findings on the relative effects of the different isomers (Matthysse, 1974a). Another group of researchers, based on their own studies of amphetamine isomers, came to the opposite conclusion that noradrenaline and not dopamine was the system involved in the psychotic state induced by amphetamines (Bunney et al., 1975).

In a comprehensive overview of the evidence for the dopamine hypothesis published in 1976, the only evidence cited to support the idea that amphetamine psychosis is mediated by dopamine was the effectiveness of antipsychotic drugs in reducing its symptoms (Meltzer and Stahl, 1976). In other words, the pharmacology of amphetamine played no independent role in establishing the dopamine hypothesis by this time, and the evidence came back, once again, to the assumption that the antipsychotics act in a disease-centred manner.

Further difficulties for the dopamine hypothesis of schizophrenia or psychosis are presented by the fact that other drugs that increase dopamine activity do not produce the same sort of schizophrenia-like psychosis as amphetamine and other recreationally used stimulant drugs like cocaine. L-dopa, for example, the chemical precursor of dopamine used for the treatment of Parkinson's disease, can induce psychotic symptoms in patients with Parkinson's disease, but, as Snyder recognised, these are usually part of a toxic confusional state, and not the lucid, paranoid-type symptoms seen most commonly with amphetamine (Snyder, 1972). The drug apomorphine, which has specific dopamine-stimulating effects and can induce stereotypies, produces some psychotic symptoms when used in the treatment of Parkinson's disease, but it has not been noted to produce a psychotic state in the thousands of people in whom it has been used for other problems, such as alcoholism, and it does not reliably provoke or worsen psychotic symptoms in people diagnosed with schizophrenia (Depatie and Lal, 2001).

Cannabis also presents a difficulty for the dopamine hypothesis of schizophrenia and psychosis. It is well known that heavy and prolonged use of cannabis can induce a psychotic state, involving paranoid delusions, that resembles both stimulant-induced psychosis and schizophrenia. Cannabis, however, does not elevate dopamine to the same degree as stimulant drugs and does not produce stereotypies.

Despite the folklore, therefore, the occurrence of psychosis following the ingestion of amphetamine or other stimulants has not been demonstrated to be attributable to the effects of these drugs on dopamine. The ambiguous nature of the evidence was forgotten, however, and what passed down into psychiatric thinking was the idea that the effects of amphetamine *in general* are attributable principally to the drug's effects on dopamine. This view was stated repeatedly in authoritative reviews and textbooks over subsequent decades, and the fact that the drug had profound effects on a whole range of other brain chemicals just stopped being mentioned (Crow, 1987; Lieberman et al., 1990; Wright et al., 2012).

The Mirage of Dopamine Receptors

Efforts went on throughout the 1970s and 1980s to demonstrate abnormalities of dopamine activity in people diagnosed with schizophrenia. Dopamine can only be measured directly after death, so dopamine concentrations in post-mortem brain specimens were sampled, levels of dopamine metabolites in blood, urine and cerebro-spinal fluid were measured, and studies were conducted to assess the status of the hormones that are related to dopamine activity—growth hormone and prolactin. Although some early studies reported differences between people diagnosed with schizophrenia and 'healthy' controls, these were not confirmed in further studies, and, in the end, none of these areas yielded evidence that suggested there were any abnormalities of dopamine activity in people with schizophrenia (the evidence is well reviewed in Kendler and Schaffner, 2011).

In the same period, post-mortem studies suggested that dopamine receptors might be over-abundant, or overly sensitive, to dopamine in people considered to have schizophrenia, sparking renewed optimism that a link between dopamine and schizophrenia might yet be found (Owen et al., 1978; Lee and Seeman, 1980). Animal studies were simultaneously demonstrating, however, that antipsychotic treatment caused the brain to produce more dopamine receptors and resulted in existing receptors becoming more sensitive (Burt et al., 1977; Muller and Seeman, 1978; Clow et al., 1980). The fact that the post-mortem studies included brains from a few patients who either had no exposure to antipsychotic drugs or were drug-free when they died was suggested to confirm that the effect was intrinsic to schizophrenia, and not simply an artefact of drug treatment (Owen et al., 1978). Other research failed to confirm these findings in larger groups of non-medicated patients, however, and concluded that the increased D_2 receptor density and sensitivity detected in people diagnosed with schizophrenia was attributable to antipsychotic treatment (Reynolds et al., 1981; Mackay et al., 1982).

The debate replayed in a similar form in the late 1980s and 1990s when it became possible to visualise dopamine receptors in the living brain using positron emission tomography (PET) scans.[1] In 1986 a study published in *Science* reported that ten young people with schizophrenia who had received no drug treatment showed higher D_2 receptor density then a control group of people of similar age and gender without schizophrenia (Wong et al., 1986). The analysis involved various complex and unreliable assumptions, however, and, as Barry Zeeberg and colleagues from Washington DC demonstrated, the data were compatible with a number of different conclusions, including that there was no difference or even decreased density of dopamine receptors in the group with schizophrenia (Zeeberg et al., 1988). In any case, several subsequent studies showed no difference in dopamine receptor density in untreated people with a diagnosis of schizophrenia compared with controls (Farde et al, 1987; Martinot et al., 1990; Pilowsky et al., 1994).

Just as the link between amphetamine psychosis and dopamine survived contradictory data, psychiatrists found it hard to give up on the only demonstrable abnormality of dopamine that had so far conclusively been shown in people with schizophrenia, and showed a tendency to minimise, or even ignore, the evidence that the finding was attributable to antipsychotic treatment. Thus, two meta-analyses concluded that elevated dopamine receptors in people diagnosed with schizophrenia indicated an underlying disease process, despite demonstrating a statistically significant relationship between antipsychotic drug exposure and receptor density (Zakzanis and Hansen, 1998; Kestler et al., 2001). Only when other evidence was acquired that was thought to support the dopamine hypothesis did it start to be widely acknowledged that changes in dopamine receptors are accounted for entirely by prior drug treatment (Guillin et al, 2007; Howes et al., 2012).

The Revival

Although it was never completely abandoned, by the 1990s the dopamine hypothesis looked increasingly tenuous. None of the many areas of research that had attempted to detect dopamine abnormalities in people with schizophrenia had yielded any confirmatory data, and the reintroduction of clozapine was a stark reminder of the limitations of conventional, dopamine-blocking antipsychotic drugs. They were often ineffective, and even when they helped reduce 'positive' psychotic symptoms, many people continued to show considerable impairments.

In this context, Kenneth Davis and colleagues tried to rescue the hypothesis by outlining a version in which positive symptoms were said to originate from *increased* dopamine in the brain stem area and negative symptoms from *reduced* dopamine activity in the frontal lobe of the brain (Davis et al., 1991). The theory was founded on studies that demonstrated that the frontal lobes of the brains of patients with chronic schizophrenia showed lower levels of activity than those of healthy controls (as measured by blood flow and energy consumption) (Franzen and Ingvar, 1975; Jacquy et al., 1976). This research was claimed to indicate that 'hypofrontality' was a characteristic of schizophrenia. Most of the studies, however, involved patients who had been medicated for many years, and antipsychotic drugs have been shown to reduce activity in the frontal lobe, as well as other areas (Ngan et al., 2002; Lane et al., 2004). Moreover, studies with unmedicated patients did not detect the same abnormalities (Volkow et al., 1986). This new version of the dopamine hypothesis proposed the unusual and biologically improbable situation that the condition of schizophrenia arises from the development of simultaneous, opposing biochemical deviations in different brain regions. Despite its implausibility, it remains a popular conception and continues to be promulgated by textbooks of psychopharmacology, such as those of Stephen Stahl (Stahl, 2008).

Other attempts to rescue the dopamine hypothesis involved combining it with a serotonin and later a glutamate hypothesis of schizophrenia, as other brain chemicals went in and out of fashion (Huttunen,

1995; Meltzer, 1995; Carlsson, 2006; Winterer, 2006). Then, in the 1990s, a group of researchers based in Columbia University headed by Professor Marc Laruelle started giving amphetamine to people with schizophrenia and indirectly measuring the dopamine that was subsequently released using single photon emission computed tomography (SPECT) scans. The group reported that people with schizophrenia released more dopamine than the control sample, including the small number of people, seven in total, who had had no previous antipsychotic treatment (Laruelle et al., 1999). Starting around the same time, studies were conducted that looked at the rate at which a radioactively-labelled preparation of L-dopa (the chemical from which dopamine is synthesised), was taken up into various brain regions by people diagnosed with schizophrenia. Some, but not all, of these studies indicated increased uptake of L-dopa in some parts of the brain, suggesting that synthesis of dopamine was accelerated. The results for different brain regions were highly inconsistent across individual studies, however (Moncrieff, 2009). The study reporting the largest effects was conducted exclusively with patients who were taking antipsychotics (McGowan et al, 2004), and the largest study of drug-naive subjects (14 in total) found no effect (Nozaki et al., 2009). Moreover, a study of healthy volunteers confirmed that treatment with haloperidol enhances L-dopa-uptake (Vernaleken et al., 2006), indicating that, as with other attempts to identify dopamine abnormalities in people with schizophrenia, current studies probably reflect changes induced by drug treatment.

However, many factors other than prior drug treatment might influence the results of the L-dopa uptake and amphetamine challenge studies. To interpret the differences between people diagnosed with schizophrenia and controls properly, we need to understand something of the various functions of dopamine. These have not been fully mapped out, but numerous human and animal studies suggest that dopamine is involved in motor activity, attention and arousal, and that it is released in response to various stressful stimuli, such as pain, hypoglycaemia and examination stress (Frankenhaeuser et al., 1986; Breier, 1989; Rauste-von Wright and Frankenhaeuser, 1989; Finlay and Zigmond, 1997; Adler et al., 2000; Goerendt et al., 2003; Nieoullon and Coquerel, 2003; Sawamoto et al., 2005; Berridge, 2006). One study of a milder stressor—mental arithmetic—did not show increased dopamine activity, however (Montgomery et al., 2006). As we saw in Chapter 3, we know from observations of the dopamine deficiency state seen in drug-induced and normal Parkinson's disease that dopamine is involved in movement, speed of thinking and mood (Laruelle et al., 1997; Verhoeff et al., 2001; Voruganti and Awad, 2006). There is also some evidence that dopamine is affected by smoking, including one study that showed increased uptake of L-dopa in smokers compared with non-smokers (Salokangas et al., 2000). People diagnosed with psychosis or schizophrenia, especially those who are acutely psychotic, are likely to differ from controls in many of these factors. They may be agitated and therefore be more physically active; they may be in a state of heightened arousal; they may be overly attentive to their delusional ideas or hallucinations; they are more likely to be long-term smokers; and research indicates that people in an acute psychotic state are more stressed than controls (Tandon et al., 1991; Pariante et al., 2004).

It was pointed out in the 1970s that increased dopamine activity in psychosis may reflect increased movement rather than anything specific about psychosis (Van Praag and Korf, 1975), but there has been little consideration of the non-specific factors that might influence measures of dopamine action in the amphetamine-induced dopamine release and L-dopa uptake studies (Moncrieff, 2009). Nevertheless, they are now considered to constitute 'compelling' evidence of a dopamine abnormality in the latest version of the dopamine hypothesis of schizophrenia (Kapur, 2003, p. 14). This new version, first proposed in 2003 by psychiatric researcher Shitij Kapur, proposes that dopamine is responsible for the 'salience' of events—the degree to which events appear as personally significant and important—and that psychosis is a state of abnormally increased salience caused by a defect of the dopamine system. Kapur's argument was once again built up from the effects of antipsychotic drugs, assuming that they act in a disease-centred manner. He cited the older literature on the psychoactive effects of antipsychotics—the first time in many years that these descriptions had appeared in the pages of an academic journal—to illustrate how the drugs reduce the salience of events, which he attributed to their ability to block the effects of dopamine. He concluded from this that psychosis must represent the opposite state of heightened salience and increased dopamine activity (Kapur, 2003).

The new version of the dopamine hypothesis represents a restatement of the early position, except that it links dopamine only with positive psychotic symptoms. In more recent accounts a complex array of chemical and environmental pathways and interactions is postulated which eventually converge to produce 'dopamine hyperfunction', which produces psychotic symptoms (Howes and Kapur, 2009, p. 556).

Kapur's ideas captured the psychiatric imagination and sparked another revival of interest in the dopamine theory of schizophrenia.

In 2006 a large international conference organised at the Institute of Psychiatry in London had the dramatic title 'Dopamine – Tempter and Tormenter of the Soul', and presentations included one entitled 'Why dopamine is psychiatry's favourite transmitter'! In 2009 leading British psychiatrist Robin Murray described the latest version of the dopamine hypothesis in a keynote address to an audience of thousands at the conference of the World Psychiatric Association in Italy. Decades of contradictory findings notwithstanding, the hypothesis remains at the heart of the psychiatric conception of schizophrenia and antipsychotic action.

A Smokescreen

Although its proponents admire the ability of the dopamine hypothesis to 'evolve' (Howes and Kapur, 2009, p. 549), others have commented that the contortions and transformations the theory has undergone to accommodate or side-line contradictory evidence makes it look very much like the philosopher Karl Popper's idea of a pseudoscience (Kendler et al., 2011). For Popper, a pseudoscience, like psychoanalysis in his view, was a theory that could not be refuted because it could explain everything—but to explain everything is, in fact, to explain nothing. In view of the considerable evidence that the only dopamine abnormalities in people with schizophrenia are caused by antipsychotic treatment, it is hard to think what evidence could convince the promoters of the dopamine theory of schizophrenia or psychosis that the theory is mistaken.

The particular tenacity of the dopamine hypothesis can be explained by the way that it appears to validate a disease-centred model of drug action. Despite the fact that the hypothesis was premised on the assumption that the drugs act in a disease-centred manner, the theory has itself become a crucial plank of support for the idea that psychiatric drugs in general, and antipsychotics in particular, represent a targeted treatment for a particular disease process. The longevity of the dopamine theory in the face of decades of contradictory and conflicting evidence testifies to the importance of keeping this belief afloat. Other theories in biological psychiatry come and go, but theories that present psychiatric treatment as a medical enterprise, and clearly distinguish it from the physical and chemical restraint that took place in earlier periods, cannot be easily abandoned without risking the whole intellectual framework within which psychiatric care and 'treatment' now takes place.

By focusing on the basis of the disease the drugs were presumed to treat, the dopamine hypothesis also conveniently diverted attention away from the effects of the drugs themselves. As David Healy has suggested, the hypothesis blurred the boundaries between the 'illness and the effects of the treatments given for it' (Healy, 2002, p. 218). In this way the dopamine hypothesis played its part in mitigating the consequences of the emerging evidence that antipsychotic drugs cause permanent brain damage. The story of tardive dyskinesia, as we shall see in the next chapter, illustrates how the dopamine hypothesis kept the antipsychotic bandwagon afloat.

5
The Phoenix Rises: From Tardive Dyskinesia to the Introduction of the 'Atypicals'[1]

By the 1970s the rose-tinted spectacles were securely in place. The new tranquillisers, now increasingly referred to as 'antipsychotics', were widely believed to be the first truly specific treatment for schizophrenia—a view that appeared to be confirmed by the emergence of the dopamine hypothesis. By this time public mental health systems had become dependent on the widespread use of these drugs both within hospitals and after discharge. Psychiatrist George Crane, whom we shall meet shortly, commented that the trend towards the management of more and more patients in the community had 'generated the feeling that drug therapy is indispensable'. The primary purpose of community psychiatric services had become to dispense and administer medication, and almost everyone diagnosed with severe mental illness was taking antipsychotics (Crane, 1973, p. 125).

As their use became the norm, and as they came to be seen as targeting an underlying disease, the wide range of serious adverse effects induced by antipsychotic drugs were sapped of their significance and relegated to the status of relatively trivial 'side effects'. A new 'vision' of drug treatment was cemented, as described by author Sheldon Gelman, exemplified by the National Institute of Mental Health study report, which proclaimed the 'anti-schizophrenic' properties of the drugs, while declaring that unwanted effects were 'generally mild or infrequent' (National Institute of Mental Health Psychopharmacology Service Center Collaborative Study Group, 1964, p. 255; Gelman, 1999). These conclusions threw a veil over previous observations of the neurological impairment the drugs produced, and evidence of other harmful effects. The emergence of enduring involuntary movements in people on long-term treatment was more difficult to ignore, however. The gradual recognition of what came to be known as tardive dyskinesia[2] threatened to destroy the 'study vision', thrusting the dangerous nature of the drugs back into public view. The anxiety it provoked laid the foundations for the introduction of the atypical antipsychotics.

As we saw in Chapter 3, movement disorders that arise immediately or shortly after starting treatment with antipsychotics, including Parkinsonism and acute dystonia, had been identified soon after chlorpromazine was first introduced into psychiatric practice. Then, in 1956 and 1957, two German papers described the occurrence of distinctive mouth and facial movements that began a few weeks after the start of antipsychotic treatment (Kulenkampff and Tarnow, 1956; Schoenecker, 1957). One of these papers described abnormal movements in three women, which persisted for several weeks after the drug was discontinued (Schoenecker, 1957). In 1959, Sigwald, the French neurologist, described involuntary movements of the tongue, lips, jaw and facial muscles in four women aged 54–69 years who had been treated with antipsychotics for between 3 and 18 months. The movements persisted for more than 2 years after the drug was stopped in one patient, and for 6 months or more in the others (Sigwald et al., 1959).

In 1960 two Danish psychiatrists described 29 patients with abnormal involuntary movements of the mouth muscles, which were associated, in some severe cases, with abnormal twisting and rocking movements of the body and restless, akathisia-like movements of the feet. The movements persisted in most patients in whom the medication was stopped, and in some cases the movements started only after medication was withdrawn, a phenomenon known as 'unmasking' (Uhrbrand and Faurbye, 1960).

In 1964 the Danish group proposed the term 'tardive dyskinesia' to denote the characteristic abnormal, involuntary movements that occurred after a period of antipsychotic therapy, and the syndrome was reported by clinicians in the USA and the UK in the first half of the 1960s (Kruse, 1960; Druckman et al., 1962; Faurbye et al., 1964; Hunter et al., 1964a). Despite the fact that the disorder was reported in younger people, and in people who were prescribed the drugs as outpatients for depression, anxiety and pain (Sigwald et al., 1959; Evans, 1965), the view emerged that the condition was uncommon and restricted to elderly people with pre-existing brain disease. Nevertheless, the syndrome was recognised as a form of brain damage in its own right and a British psychiatrist suggested it should be regarded as a chemical form of 'encephalitis' (Hunter et al., 1964b). It was American psychiatrist George Crane who eventually changed perceptions about the disorder, however, establishing and publicising its frequency and significance, although not without considerable resistance from much of the rest of the psychiatric world (Gelman, 1999).

The story of tardive dyskinesia reveals the psychiatric profession in a state of denial about the effects of its treatments. Leading psychiatrists argued that the condition was infrequent and unimportant. They suggested the movements were a pre-existing feature of schizophrenia, and nothing or little to do with antipsychotic medication, even though the syndrome had been clearly recognisable to those who first observed it as something distinct and new. Finally, the full nature of tardive dyskinesia has never been properly acknowledged, particularly the fact that the condition is characterised by intellectual decline, as well as abnormal movements. Although some early reports referred to tardive dyskinesia as 'brain damage' (Anonymous, 1965; Schmidt and Jarcho, 1966), to this day it continues to be understood as a usually trivial disorder limited to the presence of involuntary movements

Minimising the Problem

In 1967 and 1968 George Crane published papers suggesting that up to a quarter of patients in psychiatric hospitals suffered from tardive dyskinesia, that antipsychotic drugs were most probably its cause and that it was frequently irreversible. He described the abnormal movements of tardive dyskinesia in considerable detail in order to distinguish them from other types of unusual movements occasionally seen in long-term psychiatric patients (Crane, 1967, 1968). Crane was immediately criticised by Nathan Kline, among others, who challenged Crane's claims about the frequency and persistence of the condition, and asserted that the majority of cases occurred in people with pre-existing brain damage. Despite Crane's meticulous observations, Kline also suggested that Crane had mistaken movements that were inherent in schizophrenia itself for drug-induced movements and he concluded that tardive dyskinesia was 'not of great clinical significance' (Kline, 1968, p. 51). The dispute became personal with Kline accusing Crane of causing 'another epidemic of side effects' without solid scientific evidence (N. Kline, cited in Crane, 1967, p. 218). Another American psychiatrist accused Crane of making 'sweeping, generalised conclusions that would undo the past 15 years of work' and also called for 'sober, unemotional, objective and unbiased observations', implying that Crane's work was none of these things (H. Denber cited in Crane, 1967, p. 218).

At the time that Kline and others were decrying Crane's findings other psychiatrists and neurologists, who believed the link with antipsychotic drugs was well established, were surprised that a contrary 'consensus' had survived 'despite many observations that contradict it' (Schmidt and Jarcho, 1966, p. 373). An editorial in no lesser place than the *Journal of the American Medical Association* warned that a reappraisal of the benefits and indications of antipsychotic drugs was necessary (Anonymous, 1965).

In 1973, the first of three US 'Task Forces' on tardive dyskinesia gave the official stamp of approval to the condition's existence. However, the Task Force report asserted, without citing any studies, that prevalence rates were low, at between 3 and 6%, and concluded that, generally, the drugs could be 'used with confidence' and should continue to be prescribed for most people with schizophrenia (Freedman, 1973, p. 463). The report referred to tardive dyskinesia as the 'unavoidable price to be paid for the benefits of prolonged neuroleptic therapy' (p. 464). Crane was a member of the Task Force, but in a paper published around the same time as the report, he argued much more forcefully that the benefits of antipsychotics had been overstated, that they were given indiscriminately to far too many people and he referred to how 'permanent neurological disorders have become very common among patients treated with neuroleptics' (Crane, 1973, p. 127). He criticised the psychiatric community which was, in his opinion, 'completely unconcerned' about the problem, and he expressed his anxiety about the situation in which the public mental health system of the USA had come to depend on widespread, long-term drug treatment to the detriment of patients' welfare.

A few years later the general attitude towards tardive dyskinesia was said to have 'shifted from curiosity and mild concern to panic' in the face of rising litigation (Gardos and Cole, 1980, p. 776). In 1974 Smith Kline & French settled a claim for chlorpromazine-induced tardive dyskinesia for $1 million, and more cases followed (Healy, 2002). Often, it was shown that the treating psychiatrists had not noticed or had ignored the symptoms (Gelman, 1999). A second Task Force was set up in 1980, under the auspices of the American Psychiatric Association, which estimated from existing prevalence studies that around 20% of adults might develop tardive dyskinesia, rising to 40% or more in the elderly. Reviewing the evidence on the reversibility or otherwise of the condition, the Task Force concluded that in people who had been on long-term medication, symptoms persisted after drug withdrawal in two thirds of cases. The Task Force produced sensible guidelines for minimising the occurrence of tardive dyskinesia, including careful consideration of whether long-term drug treatment was really justified, the use of minimally effective doses, constant monitoring and attempts to withdraw medication in long-term hospital patients who were clinically stable. It stopped short of recommending this course of action for patients in the community, however, because of the 'ubiquitous and critical shortage of aftercare systems' (American Psychiatric Association, 1980b, p. 170).

Despite concern over litigation, increasing publicity and the American Psychiatric Association's exhortations, antipsychotics continued to be prescribed to ever increasing numbers at increasingly high doses throughout the 1980s. In 1986, two leading psychiatrists concluded that the Task Force recommendations about careful and cautious prescribing had been 'honored more in the breach than in the keeping' (Gualtieri et al., 1986, p. 206). The increasing popularity of antipsychotic use seemed unstoppable, even in the face of almost certain drug-induced brain damage.

Blaming Schizophrenia

When prevalence rates could not be ignored, another tactic of denial was adopted that helped to defuse the tardive dyskinesia time bomb. Suggestions that the abnormal movements, now labelled as tardive dyskinesia, pre-dated the use of antipsychotic drugs and were a feature of schizophrenia, had been made by Kline in the 1960s, and periodically thereafter. Reference was frequently made to the observations of Kraepelin and other early psychiatrists that patients with 'dementia praecox' or schizophrenia showed abnormal movements long before the introduction of antipsychotic drugs. These claims were revived and widely publicised in a paper by a group of researchers based at Northwick Park hospital on the outskirts of London.

In 1982, psychiatrist David Cunningham Owens and colleagues reported on rates of abnormal movements in a group of long-term hospital patients. What was novel about the study was that 47 out of the 411 patients studied had never been exposed to antipsychotic drugs. These patients had been resident in a 'therapeutic community' within the hospital, where the emphasis was on psychotherapy and family therapy, and drugs and physical treatments were avoided, although several of the patients were said to have had electro-convulsive therapy (ECT), insulin coma therapy or a lobotomy in the past (Owens et al., 1982).

The study reported that rates of abnormal movements were just as high among the non-drug treated group as among those who had received drug treatment, and, based on these results, the researchers questioned whether tardive dyskinesia existed at all (Crow et al., 1983).

Little attempt was made to differentiate the movements that characterise tardive dyskinesia from other sorts of movements, however. In
fact, the paper revealed that more patients on drugs had the specific
movements suggestive of tardive dyskinesia, such as grimacing and
tongue movements, whereas movements that are not a feature of tardive dyskinesia, like head-nodding, were found to be more common in
those who were not on medication. The drug-naive patients were also
10 years older than the drug-treated patients, and the rate of spontaneously developing movement disorders is known to increase with age.

In 1985 Owens modified his conclusion, suggesting that antipsychotic medication did increase rates of abnormal movements, but that
it did this by revealing an underlying tendency inherent in the condition and, in this sense, the drugs could not be held to cause the disorder
directly (Owens, 1985).

Owens' claims were revived in the 1990s by a group of US researchers,
including psychiatrist Richard Wyatt, who went on to develop influential theories about schizophrenia causing progressive brain damage (see
Chapter 11). First, Wyatt published a review of studies such as Owens',
concluding that many cases of tardive dyskinesia were a result of the
underlying mental illness rather than drug treatment (Khot and Wyatt,
1991). Second, the group conducted a retrospective study of the case
notes of patients who had been admitted to Chestnut Lodge, a psychiatric therapeutic community hospital, who, like Owens' sub-sample, had
not received antipsychotics. Twenty-three per cent of the patients were
reported to have shown abnormal movements of some sort, with 15%
showing abnormal mouth or face movements considered to be equivalent to tardive dyskinesia (Fenton et al., 1997). However, the majority of
patients had received ECT and insulin coma therapy, which have been
found to be associated with higher rates of tardive dyskinesia in some
studies (although not this one). Moreover, a selection of excerpts from
the case notes indicates that few of the abnormal movements resembled tardive dyskinesia and that the majority of patients were highly
psychotic at the time the movements were noted (Fenton et al., 1994).
Tardive dyskinesia, in contrast, is most clearly observable in patients
who are mentally stable. Overall, therefore, it appears that this study
identified the many bizarre mannerisms and movements that people
can demonstrate when they are severely mentally disturbed, which are
quite different from the involuntary twitching or writhing character of
tardive dyskinesia (Paulson, 2005).

Animal studies and evidence from populations of patients without schizophrenia have confirmed that antipsychotics cause tardive

dyskinesia. Although rats and mice do not show exactly the same picture as humans, antipsychotic treatment can produce pointless or 'vacuous' and repetitive chewing movements, tongue protrusions and facial twitches similar in nature to tardive dyskinesia (Kulkarni and Dhir, 2011). Studies conducted in the 1970s revealed that primates and monkeys develop signs of tardive dyskinesia indistinguishable from those shown in humans when given antipsychotics on a long-term basis (Gunne and Barany, 1976; Barany et al., 1979; Domino, 1985). Many studies have shown that people with mental handicap or learning disability, and people diagnosed with mood disorders, like depression and manic depression, develop tardive dyskinesia when treated with long-term antipsychotics just as commonly as people diagnosed with schizophrenia (Wolf et al., 1983; Youssef and Waddington, 1988).

The idea that tardive dyskinesia might be part of the underlying mental condition of schizophrenia was enormously appealing to a profession that was finding that its central and most celebrated form of treatment caused brain damage. A final Task Force on tardive dyskinesia, which reported in 1992 and confirmed that the disorder developed in around 15–20% of long-term antipsychotic users, placed great emphasis on the Northwick Park study (Gelman, 1999). The findings were described in detail and the report repeated Owens' later conclusion that antipsychotics might bring out an inherent vulnerability to abnormal movements latent in some people with schizophrenia. The very suggestion that the drugs might not be responsible for tardive dyskinesia, however tenuous, allowed psychiatrists to continue to go about their business, without having to fully confront the now long-buried facts that the drugs they used were neurological poisons.

Ignoring Mental Impairment

The most persistent and effective strategy to deflect attention from the importance of tardive dyskinesia has been the neglect of its 'cognitive' or mental component. In mainstream psychiatric literature, tardive dyskinesia is described simply as a movement disorder, and although it is sometimes acknowledged to represent a form of brain damage or malfunction, the full consequences of that damage are rarely explicated. Coupled with the evidence that many patients are unaware of the abnormal movements, it is easy to see how the condition could be regarded as inconsequential. Of course, some patients do care about the disfiguring nature of the movements, which immediately mark them out, but there is a more worrying aspect to tardive dyskinesia.

Numerous studies show that people who develop the condition have lowered intellectual capacity, suggesting that mental impairment may be a feature of tardive dyskinesia. This should not be surprising, given the interconnectedness of different areas of the brain, and several commentators have drawn attention to the similarities between tardive dyskinesia and other forms of generalised brain disease like lethargic encephalitis and Huntingdon's chorea (Wade et al., 1987; DeWolfe et al., 1988; Breggin, 1990).

An early study found that patients with tardive dyskinesia also had 'dementia' (Hunter et al., 1964b) and subsequent research supported the view that tardive dyskinesia is only one aspect of a wider 'chronic neuroleptic-induced neurotoxic process' (Wade et al., 1987, p. 395). Mainstream psychiatric literature explained the association between tardive dyskinesia and mental impairment by adopting Kline's explanation, however. Tardive dyskinesia was said to occur more frequently in those with 'vulnerable' brains—people who had pre-existing brain damage or intellectual impairment—and nothing was said about the possibility that the condition itself might compromise mental ability. Current psychiatric textbooks reiterate this position (Wright et al., 2012), although research has been inconsistent, with by far the largest study finding no association between prior mental capacity and subsequent development of tardive dyskinesia (Jeste et al., 1995).

In the 1990s a group of researchers from Ireland reviewed 29 studies on tardive dyskinesia and found that 23 of these found an association between tardive dyskinesia and mental dysfunction of some sort. The studies used different tests and measures, and found different sorts of impairments, including deficiencies in memory, executive function (planning and organisational abilities) and abstraction (Waddington et al., 1993). Another review found a similar picture with 24 out of 31 studies finding an association (Paulsen et al., 1994). The Irish group also followed a cohort of 64 patients over a period of 5 years to explore changes in their mental or cognitive function. They found a correlation between intellectual deterioration and the onset of tardive dyskinesia, especially that affecting the face and mouth, and they concluded that mental impairment is an intrinsic part of tardive dyskinesia (Waddington et al., 1990).

In the 1980s and early 1990s several authors suggested that tardive dyskinesia could also be associated with the sort of personality changes that can occur following a severe brain injury, which typically include unstable mood, loud speech, tension, aggression and elation (Wilson et al., 1983; Mukherjee, 1984; Jones, 1985; Goldberg, 1985;

Myslobodsky, 1993). Peter Breggin has also drawn attention to the parallel between the lack of awareness of movements in tardive dyskinesia and the denial of disability in other brain disease, like stroke, and more generalised conditions, such as neurosyphilis (Breggin, 1993b).

Despite these indications that long-term antipsychotic treatment leads not only to a persistent movement disorder, but also to intellectual impairment and personality changes characteristic of widespread brain damage, the subject has since disappeared from the research agenda and the scientific literature. Even the Irish researchers switched their interest to movement disorders in untreated schizophrenia (Whitty et al., 2009). Although studies continued to examine the mechanism of tardive dyskinesia, its prevalence and treatment, no research programme was set up to elucidate the overall nature of the brain impairments caused by antipsychotics. We remain uncertain about the full consequences of long-term antipsychotic treatment, especially to what extent and how commonly the drugs impair mental functioning.

Although research has continued to demonstrate that tardive dyskinesia is linked with deteriorating mental function (Byne et al., 1998), the psychiatric establishment continues to be reluctant to acknowledge the problem. The Clinical Antipsychotic Trials of Intervention Effectiveness (CATIE) study, for example, a large and well known randomised comparison of various antipsychotics, revealed a strong association between mental impairment and tardive dyskinesia, but what was reported were the results of a complex statistical analysis in which the association had disappeared. The analysis included several variables, such as the length of antipsychotic treatment, which should not have been included because they are part of the putative causal mechanism. This basic statistical error, which is likely to have wiped out the association between tardive dyskinesia and reduced intellectual performance, apparently passed unnoticed through this high-powered journal's refereeing process (Miller et al., 2005).

By the twenty-first century, when the CATIE study reported its results, psychiatry did not want to be reminded of the evidence that antipsychotics cause generalised brain dysfunction. The introduction of the atypical antipsychotics had thrown a welcome veil over the powerful neurological effects the drugs produce and helped to reinforce what had looked like an increasingly vulnerable view of these drugs as disease-targeting treatments. The ascendance of the atypicals closed down an opportunity to develop a proper understanding of the nature of antipsychotic drugs and the consequences of long-term use, and returned psychiatric research to its preoccupation with locating the pathology underlying schizophrenia. Moreover, as we shall see in subsequent chapters, the atypicals reinvigorated the quest to expand the use of antipsychotics far beyond what had been achieved with the older antipsychotic drugs.

The Introduction of 'Atypical' Antipsychotics

Antipsychotic drug development ground to a halt in the 1980s in the face of increasing lawsuits concerning tardive dyskinesia (Healy, 2002). Revival of interest in clozapine in the late 1980s, however, suggested that it might be possible to produce drugs with greater efficacy and lower rates of neurological side effects, and this provided the stimulus for the pharmaceutical industry to develop other drugs for the antipsychotic market—drugs that are often referred to as 'atypical' antipsychotics.

The term 'atypical' has been used in a bewildering variety of ways over the last two decades. It is commonly used to describe drugs that are useful for the treatment of psychosis but induce lower levels of extrapyramidal effects than older, standard antipsychotics, but it is also used to refer to drugs that have particular chemical properties, such as combining serotonin and dopamine receptor blockade. It has also been suggested that the term was little more than a marketing device, deployed to convince prescribers that the drugs were distinctive and superior (Tyrer and Kendall, 2009).

The name 'atypical' is first used in a paper listed on the electronic index Medline in 1975 to describe the properties of clozapine and two other older antipsychotics, sulpiride and thioridazine (Melleril). Early papers on the atypical qualities of these drugs noted that their effects on stimulant-induced movement disorders like hyperactivity and stereotypies were weaker than the effects of the other, more 'typical' antipsychotics (Costall and Naylor, 1975). There were also reports that they caused lower rates of adverse neurological or extrapyramidal effects in humans, including tardive dyskinesia (Borison and Diamond, 1986).

Clozapine

Clozapine was synthesised in 1958, as part of a group of compounds that were based on the chemical structure of the drug imipramine. Imipramine was initially proposed as a treatment for schizophrenia and, like imipramine, clozapine was found to have similar properties to chlorpromazine in laboratory studies (Crilley, 2007). Whereas imipramine, through the efforts of Swiss psychiatrist Roland Kuhn, came to be regarded as an 'antidepressant' (although it is doubtful that it, or any other drug, has specific antidepressant properties, see Moncrieff and Cohen, 2006; Moncrieff, 2008b), clozapine continued to be investigated as a treatment for people with schizophrenia. German psychiatrist Hans Hippius conducted several clinical studies, concluding that clozapine was an effective antipsychotic with a lower propensity to induce extrapyramidal movement disorders than other antipsychotics (Hippius, 1999). In the early 1970s a patented version of clozapine, named Leponex, was launched in several European countries, including Germany and Finland, and the manufacturer, Sandoz, began to plan research in the USA (Crilley, 2007).

In 1975, however, a report in *The Lancet* announced that 18 patients in Finland had developed severe blood disorders shortly after starting clozapine, nine of whom had died (Idanpaan-Heikkila et al., 1975). Most of the blood disorders consisted of 'agranulocytosis', a condition in which the white blood cells known as granulocytes, which fight infection, are suppressed. The Finnish government ordered clozapine to be withdrawn immediately and other European countries followed suit. Sandoz suggested that the drug could be used safely as long as frequent blood tests were carried out to monitor blood cell numbers, but, in 1976, Sandoz called a halt to its clozapine research programme (Crilley, 2007).

Clozapine continued to be used in some parts of the world, however, and in the mid-1980s the tardive dyskinesia epidemic, combined with rising doubts about the efficacy of the antipsychotics in use at the time, re-ignited interest in the drug. Sandoz applied for a licence in the USA in 1983, but the Food and Drug Administration (FDA) insisted that the drug should be aimed at people who had failed to respond well to other drugs because only in this population were the benefits thought to outweigh the risks (Crilley, 2007). In 1988 a randomised trial funded by Sandoz was published showing that clozapine produced a greater reduction in symptoms than chlorpromazine in people with 'treatment resistant schizophrenia' (Kane et al., 1988). In the same year, the company was granted a licence to market clozapine in the USA under the trade name Clozaril.

The re-launch of clozapine revived interest in developing new antipsychotic drugs and suggested the possibility of finding drugs with greater efficacy than the early antipsychotics. The 'antidepressant' drug Prozac was launched in 1989 and it's phenomenal success confirmed that it was possible to make a great deal of money from drugs for mental disorders. Prozac, or fluoxetine, was one result of a renewed interest in the neurotransmitter called serotonion, or 5 hydroxy-tryptamine (5-HT), which started in the 1970s. Since the 1960s, it had been suggested that serotonin might be involved in the genesis of schizophrenia owing to the structural similarities between serotonin and lysergic acid diethylamide (LSD), a drug which could produce hallucinations and sensory distortions. It had been shown in the 1960s that LSD had some similar actions to endogenous serotonin, although it also had some opposing actions (Woolley and Campbell, 1962b). Originally, it was thought that schizophrenia might represent a deficiency of serotonin (Gaddum and Hameed, 1954; Woolley and Shaw, 1954), but it was later proposed that schizophrenia could be due to over-activity of serotonin (Woolley and Campbell, 1962a). Interest in serotonin continued during the 1970s, when its role in other physiological functions was investigated, including its effects on sleep. Paul Janssen became interested in this area, and set out to synthesise a serotonin antagonist. At first he produced a drug called ritanserin which, among other actions, reduced transmission at one of the serotonin receptors thought to be influential in the actions of LSD, the 5-HT$_{2A}$ receptor.

Janssen was particularly interested in serotonin's ability to reduce and disrupt sleep, and speculated that serotonin-blocking drugs might therefore be useful in conditions in which sleep is disrupted, such as chronic depression (Janssen, 1998). During the 1980s, interest also developed in the interaction between serotonin and dopamine, with suggestions that drugs that reduce serotonin release might inhibit the extrapyramidal neurological effects produced by anti-dopaminergic drugs, such as haloperidol (Waldmeier and Delini-Stula, 1979; Gerlach, 1985). Janssen and others started to conduct studies using ritanserin added to conventional antipsychotics, speculating that the combination would improve clinical outcome and reduce drug-induced movement disorders (Janssen, 1998). At the same time Janssen set out to develop a drug that would simultaneously inhibit the activity of dopamine and serotonin. Risperidone was synthesised in 1983, and in 1988 Janssen suggested that risperidone's actions on these two systems could combine antipsychotic activity with beneficial effects on mood and negative symptoms, and lower levels of extrapyramidal effects (Janssen et al., 1988). The theory that serotonin blockade might improve mood went against the emerging serotonin hypothesis of depression, but this inconsistency was never pointed out. Risperidone was not launched until 1993, by which time the combined fortunes of clozapine and Prozac made a new antipsychotic a viable and attractive proposition.

Marketing 'Atypicality'

The launch of risperidone and clozapine ushered in a new phase in the story of antipsychotic drugs. The idea that they did not induce extra-pyramidal symptoms, later shown to be incorrect in the case of risperidone, conveniently diverted attention from the neurological effects of antipsychotics, including tardive dyskinesia. Moreover, the credibility of the disease-centred theory of drug action was revived by renewed speculations about the biochemical basis of schizophrenia and the mechanism of drug treatment. Some claimed the 'atypical' antipsychotics had ushered in a whole new era in psychiatry (Meltzer, 1995), one in which the drug-centred model could finally be consigned to oblivion and psychiatry could get on with the business of applying specific medical treatments to real underlying diseases. To support such claims, an apparently coherent concept of 'atypical' action was moulded out of still uncertain and inconsistent evidence, which enabled the new antipsychotics to be presented as something quite distinct from their older counterparts.

Although it is now only one of many theories about the mode of action of atypical antipsychotics, in the early days the idea that they achieved their effects through blockading serotonin, as well as dopamine receptors, predominated, and they were frequently referred to as 'serotonin–dopamine antagonists' in the scientific literature and advertisements of the time. This proposed action simultaneously rescued the dopamine hypothesis of schizophrenia, while presenting the atypical antipsychotics as novel and unique. US psychiatrist Herbert Meltzer, an enthusiastic advocate of clozapine in particular, was a strong proponent of the serotonin–dopamine antagonism hypothesis, claiming that the additional effects of serotonin antagonism made the new antipsychotics more effective and less toxic than their predecessors (Meltzer, 1994). Later, claims that they enhanced cognitive function or halted the decline in mental functioning associated with a diagnosis of schizophrenia were added, and alongside these claims came a resurgence of interest in the role of serotonin in the aetiology of schizophrenia. A burgeoning literature on schizophrenia and serotonin receptors appeared, and research to develop new drugs with anti-serotonin activity flourished (Breier, 1995; Brunello et al., 1995; Remington, 2008).

As before, however, there was a disjunction between the representation of the atypical antipsychotics and the science behind them. Although interest in the effects of the serotonin system survives, it is now acknowledged that the relationship between drug action and clinical effects is more complex than early accounts allowed (Remington, 2008). In 1995, psychiatrist William Carpenter pointed out that if serotonin antagonism counteracted dopamine blockade, and dopamine blockade was still believed to be necessary for reducing positive psychotic symptoms, then drugs with anti-serotonin action would be expected to be less effective, not more effective, than other antipsychotics (Carpenter Jr, 1995). Moreover, it is not even clear whether blocking serotonin receptors reduces extrapyramidal effects, as claimed, as animal studies with the drug ritanserin have yielded conflicting findings (Remington, 2008). Among atypical antipsychotics, the proposed correlation between anti-serotonin effects and the liability to induce extrapyrdamidal adverse effects has not been borne out. It was clear from the time of its introduction, as Janssen himself acknowledged (Janssen, 1998), that despite its anti-serotonergic action, risperidone causes extrapyramidal effects at higher doses in the same fashion as the older antipsychotics (Chouinard et al., 1993; Marder and Meibach, 1994; Kapur et al., 1995). Moreover, the proposed benefits of the atypical antipsychotics on negative symptoms of schizophrenia have been suggested to be a consequence of the unduly high doses of older drugs used in comparative studies (Carpenter Jr, 1995; Geddes et al., 2000), and the much-hyped improvement in cognitive symptoms has not materialised in well-designed studies (Green et al., 2002; Keefe et al., 2007).

As further atypical antipsychotics appeared, other theories were concocted, like Stephen Stahl's idea that the drugs somehow block the effects of dopamine in one area of the brain, the limbic system, but not in another area, the basal ganglia (Stahl, 2008).[3] The fact that most of these drugs induce neurological movement disorders, at least at higher doses, suggests that they do affect the basal ganglia, however, where these abnormalities originate. Moreover, no explanation was ever satisfactorily offered for how such selective effects could come about. It was also suggested that other dopamine receptors might be involved in atypical antipsychotic action, such as the D_1 receptor or subtypes of the D_2 receptor (Meltzer, 1991). Little attention was paid to the profound effects of clozapine and some other atypical antipsychotics on other neurochemical systems in the brain, however, such as those involving histamine, acetylcholine and noradrenaline.

As with the first generation of antipsychotic drugs, the fact that the proposed mechanism of action lacked coherence and was not supported by firm evidence did not matter. The assumption that the drugs worked on the underlying disease was already in place, and speculation about novel actions was all that was needed to convince disappointed clinicians that a new miracle cure was about to arrive. Over the last few years, however, it has become clear that the original hopes and claims for these medications have not been fulfilled. Prominent psychiatrists, including David Cunningham Owens (whose research had been used to argue that tardive dyskinesia was part of schizophrenia, but who, in later years, has become more critical of drug treatment), have started to suggest that the story of atypical antipsychotics as a group of compounds with unique therapeutic properties is a myth, largely constructed by the pharmaceutical industry, and swallowed hook, line and sinker by the psychiatric profession (Owens, 2008; Tyrer and Kendall, 2009; Kendall, 2011).

As well as its yearning for new and effective medical treatments, the profession was won over by the results of the first clinical trials of the atypical antipsychotics, which were rapidly set up by the pharmaceutical companies in the USA in the 1990s. We shall look in more detail at some of these trials in the next chapter because it is now apparent that they were hopelessly flawed. Journalist and author of *Mad in America* Robert Whitaker goes further: 'Behind the public façade of medical achievement', he cautions, 'is a story of science marred by greed, deaths and the deliberate deception of the American public' (Whitaker, 2002, p. 254.) But most of the psychiatric community was happily oblivious to the machinations that propelled the atypical antipsychotics into the limelight, and within a few years they were widely recommended as the first-line treatment for someone diagnosed with schizophrenia (National Institute for Health and Clinical Excellence, 2002).

6
Looking Where the Light is: Randomised Controlled Trials of Antipsychotics

This chapter reviews some of the reams of evidence that has been collected on the effects of antipsychotics in people diagnosed with schizophrenia or psychosis, focusing on randomised controlled trials, especially those that have compared an antipsychotic drug with a placebo. It is important to review this data because randomised controlled trials are universally regarded as the proper scientific method for evaluating the effects of an intervention. They are applied throughout medicine, they are required by drug licensing authorities and no new medical therapy would be accepted nowadays without having passed through this testing procedure. And yet the placebo-controlled trials of antipsychotics, both those conducted shortly after their introduction and more recent studies, are severely limited. They provide little information about how the drugs might impact on the experiences we call mental disorders and whether taking them is ultimately better than not taking them.

As we saw in Chapter 4, by the time the first large-scale, systematic studies of antipsychotics were published in the early 1960s, there was already a consensus developing that they constituted a disease-centred form of treatment. The results of these studies, particularly the National Institute of Mental Health (NIMH) study, further cemented this view, but they were also a product of it. Instead of trying to understand *how* the drugs affected the brain and behaviour, the increasing assumption that the drugs had disease-specific effects encouraged research that simply aimed to establish whether or not the drugs reduced symptoms. Randomised controlled trials came to dominate research on psychiatric drug treatment and soon they were almost the only means available with which to assess the usefulness and safety of psychiatric medications. They continue to be regarded today as the only credible and relevant evidence as far as drug treatment is concerned. Although well-conducted randomised controlled trials have an important part to play in evaluating psychiatric medications, and are certainly preferable to anecdotal claims of miraculous recoveries, the inadequacies of existing studies have not been properly appreciated. Moreover, as they proliferated they eclipsed other important information on the nature of the mental and physical alterations the drugs produce and the consequences of long-term use.

Jonathan Cole, the psychiatrist who became head of the Psychopharmacology Service centre at the NIMH, and conducted the NIMH antipsychotic study, was one of the leading figures in advocating the use of randomised trials of psychiatric treatments. Apart from a few small randomised studies that took place in Europe, such as the Elke trial in Birmingham, the first large-scale trials of the new drugs were conducted in the USA. By the mid-1950s United States Congress had already earmarked $2 million for research into new drug treatments in psychiatry, testifying to the confidence that already existed in the potential of drugs to treat mental disorders (Cole, 1996, p. 242).

The Limitations of Randomised Trials of Antipsychotics

Before we look in more detail at some of the hundreds of trials of antipsychotics that have been conducted over the last 60 years, we need to consider some theoretical and technical problems involved in conducting such trials. From a conceptual point of view, it is important to recognise that measuring and categorising behavioural and emotional difficulties is an imprecise and subjective affair. The changing ways that mental disorders have been classified over the last century, as well as the jostling and wrangling that occurs in the production of a system like the *Diagnostic and Statistical Manual of Mental Health* (*DSM*), testifies to the difficulty in achieving consensus about how such difficulties should be understood. Supposedly homogenous conditions like 'schizophrenia' and 'depression' involve numerous and diverse experiences, follow varied patterns, have unpredictable outcomes, their manifestations and consequences are difficult to quantify, and they impact in different ways on different parties. So quite apart from the issue of whether or not schizophrenia is a valid and useful label, interpreting results of studies that involve people labelled as having schizophrenia is far from straightforward.

Randomised trials of antipsychotics measure the effects of the drugs using rating scales, for example, that consist of collections of more or less randomly collated symptoms and include many factors like anxiety, irritability and hostility that are not specific to a psychotic syndrome or schizophrenia. Improvements in scores do not necessarily tally with functional improvement and it is easy for scores to improve quite a lot if someone is more subdued, and expressing their abnormal ideas less frequently, but they might, nonetheless, remain profoundly impaired. Occasionally, measures of social functioning are employed to address this problem, but they, too, consist of subjective evaluations about what constitutes normal activity in particular areas. Moreover, what counts as improvement varies according to the perspective of the person making the rating. In a German study of definitions of 'remission', for instance, it was found that patients, their relatives and psychiatrists only agreed in 18% of cases (Karow et al, 2012).

Technical problems are numerous, and have been well reviewed by other authors (Leucht et al., 2008). 'Double-blind' studies, in which those involved are meant to be ignorant of who receives the drug and who receives placebo, are likely to be 'unblinded' by the fact that antipsychotics produce obvious physical and mental alterations, for example. In other words, both participants and researchers are likely to be able to detect who is receiving the drugs and who is on placebo, and non-blinded studies produce larger differences between groups than those that are conducted double blind (Leucht et al., 2012b). Furthermore, large numbers of people drop out of antipsychotic trials before the end of the study, and the way this missing data is dealt with can have an impact on study results, while many other factors can also distort results and the way these are presented. Recent exposés have shown how the pharmaceutical industry can cherry-pick positive findings and neglect to mention, or fail to publish, results that do not show their drug in the best possible light (Melander et al., 2003; Jureidini et al., 2008).

Withdrawal Effects

It is the variety of effects that can occur after stopping antipsychotic drugs that present the greatest impediment to accepting the results of randomised controlled trials at face value, however. Because antipsychotics came into widespread use so early after their introduction, even the earliest clinical trials mostly involved people who were already taking the drugs on a long-term basis before the trial began. At the start of the study, therefore, participants would have to be taken off their previous medication, and those who were allocated to the drug being tested would have it replaced by the new drug, but those allocated to placebo would have nothing to replace it. By the 1960s there were already descriptions of the withdrawal effects that occurred when people discontinued antipsychotics after taking them for some time. These are known to include agitation, anxiety, insomnia, restlessness and irritability (Brooks, 1959; Judah et al., 1961; Lacoursiere, 1976). All these experiences can be mistaken for signs of the underlying condition, especially if rating scales are used that contain items referring to these behaviours, as they mostly do, and if the people making the ratings have no awareness of the possibility that the placebo-treated subjects might be experiencing withdrawal effects.

Occasionally, the withdrawal of antipsychotics can itself produce psychotic symptoms that had not been present before drug treatment started. This phenomenon was first recorded in the 1950s, but the implications were ignored until Canadian psychiatrist Guy Chouinard proposed the idea of 'supersensitivity' psychosis in the 1980s. The term 'supersensitivity' psychosis refers to the idea that long-term antipsychotic treatment could make people more vulnerable to psychotic symptoms by increasing the sensitivity of dopamine receptors, in a mechanism analogous to that which was proposed (although not proven) to cause tardive dyskinesia. Just as tardive dyskinesia could appear either during treatment or after drug treatment was stopped, so Chouniard proposed that supersensitivity psychosis could occur after drug withdrawal, or during on-going treatment, with pre-existing psychotic symptoms re-emerging after being dormant, and new ones developing (Chouinard and Jones, 1980).

Despite Chouinard's work and several other reports documenting the emergence or deterioration of psychotic symptoms after antipsychotic discontinuation (these are described in detail in Moncrieff, 2006), there was little interest in the area, but by the 2000s it was becoming clear that people could become extremely psychotic when they stopped clozapine. Moreover, several studies showed that symptoms were worse after stopping clozapine than they had been before starting it (Diamond and Borison, 1986; Borison et al., 1988; Apud et al., 2003). In 2002, a paper from Hong Kong reported that two elderly men with no previous psychiatric problems had developed a short-lived psychotic state after stopping metaclopramide, a dopamine-blocking drug used for nausea, similar to the antipsychotic drug sulpiride. Their symptoms rapidly subsided when they were treated with risperidone, which was then gradually withdrawn without further problems (Lu et al., 2002). Combining all the descriptions of withdrawal-induced psychosis suggests that its symptoms have a slightly different profile from a typical episode of spontaneous psychosis or schizophrenia, and are more reminiscent of those provoked by heavy use of amphetamines or other stimulants. Paranoid ideas, hostility and aggression are common, and although people experience auditory hallucinations, common in schizophrenia, some also report visual hallucinations, which are not. It seems, therefore, that stopping antipsychotics can sometimes provoke a psychotic episode, even in someone who does not have a history of schizophrenia or psychosis (Moncrieff, 2006).

The chemical mechanism of withdrawal-induced psychosis is unclear, and the role of supersensitive dopamine receptors has not been confirmed. As we saw in Chapter 5 there is, in any case, much more to the biochemistry of antipsychotics than dopamine, and the fact that clozapine, which has relatively weak D_2 receptor-blocking properties, is one of the most likely candidates to provoke withdrawal psychosis, suggests that dopamine may not be the only, or even the most important, brain chemical to be involved. The symptom profile suggests that the mechanism may be similar to the still unknown process by which stimulant drugs, like amphetamine, induce psychotic symptoms.

In the 1990s another potential problem of withdrawal from psychiatric drugs was described. A group led by psychiatrist Ross Baldessarini at Harvard medical school produced several studies that suggested that stopping long-term psychiatric drug treatment of various sorts may precipitate a recurrence or deterioration of the underlying condition. In other words, stopping medication may, in itself, be a risk factor for relapse. This effect was shown convincingly in the case of lithium treatment for 'bipolar disorder' or manic depression. When an individual stops long-term lithium treatment, the risk of that person having a relapse of manic depression is higher than it was before they started lithium (Cundall et al., 1972; Suppes et al., 1991; Baldessarini et al., 1999). The group's work suggested that a similar effect might occur in people treated with antipsychotics for schizophrenia or psychotic disorders, and part of the evidence for this proposal was that withdrawal studies show that relapses cluster soon after the point of withdrawal. In one analysis, for example, 50% of relapses occurred within 3 months of the discontinuation of the antipsychotic (Baldessarini and Viguera, 1995). This observation suggests, however, that in many cases 'relapse' may have consisted of antipsychotic withdrawal symptoms, especially in studies where relapse was defined as a small increase in score on a rating scale.

The fact that the withdrawal of antipsychotic medication can produce mental and behavioural difficulties, whether or not this involves the precipitation of relapse, potentially undermines all studies that have involved the discontinuation of previous antipsychotic treatment in people on placebo, and this includes almost all the placebo-controlled studies that have ever been conducted. Although Baldessarini and his group recognised the profound implications of withdrawal effects back in 1995 (Baldessarini and Viguera, 1995), drug trials and reviews of research have continued more or less as if they did not exist.

Treatment of an Acute Psychotic Episode

Despite the hundreds of randomised trials of antipsychotics conducted with people with schizophrenia and psychosis, evidence on the effects of drugs in people experiencing a recent, 'acute' episode is surprisingly sparse. This is unfortunate because studies involving people who are experiencing a new episode are more likely to entail the actual initiation of drug treatment than studies with people with a chronic condition, although in some cases the acute episode may have been precipitated by the patient previously discontinuing long-term medication.

Table 6.1 lists randomised trials of treatment of an acute episode of psychosis or schizophrenia that have compared antipsychotics with a placebo, another sort of sedative drug or other sorts of treatment.

The first study of the use of antipsychotics for acute treatment was not the NIMH study discussed in Chapter 3, but an earlier study conducted in the late 1950s in the Veterans Affairs (VA) hospitals in the USA, the system of hospitals reserved for veterans of the US armed forces. Multi-site studies of anti-tuberculous drugs and of lobotomy had already been conducted in the VA hospitals, and early attempts to create psychiatric rating scales were made by those who were studying the effects of lobotomy (Cole, 1996). Two studies involving a number of early antipsychotic drugs were conducted in the VA hospitals in the 1950s involving 37 hospitals and a total of 1445 male veterans. One of them investigated the treatment of an acute episode and one primarily involved long-term hospital patients (Casey et al., 1960a, 1960b).

The acute treatment study enrolled 640 'newly admitted schizo-phrenic men' and is one of the largest studies of antipsychotic drugs ever conducted, but it is little known in comparison with the NIMH study. The control, or comparison, group took phenobarbital, the stand-ard barbiturate of the time, not an inert placebo as would become the norm later (Casey et al., 1960a). At the time the study was designed, it seems it was deemed necessary not just to show that the drugs did something rather than nothing, but to demonstrate that they were

Table 6.1 Randomised trials of antipsychotic treatment of an acute psychotic episode

Study	Number of patients enrolled	Duration of randomised treatment	Treatments compared	Previous treatment	Global results	Effects on different symptoms
VA study (Casey et al., 1960a)	640	12 weeks	Chlorpromazine, prochlorperazine, perphenazine, triflupromazine, mepazine, phenobarbital	56% had had past treatment with antipsychotics, 82% had had previous admissions	A 10–15 point difference between antipsychotics, excepting mepazine, and phenobarbital in scores on a 140-point symptom scale	Symptoms that showed greatest responsiveness to antipsychotics included 'resistiveness', 'belligerence', paranoid ideas, hallucinations, participation in activities
NIMH study (National Institute of Mental Health Psychopharmacology Service Center Collaborative Study Group, 1964)	463	6 weeks	Chlorpromazine, fluphenazine, thioridazine, placebo	50% had previous admissions	1.1-point difference between drug- and placebo-treated patients on a 7-point scale of improvement; 40% of drug-treated patients rated as 'much improved' vs 30% of placebo-treated patients	13 of 21 symptoms of all types showed more improvement with drugs than placebo
May (1968)	247 (good and poor prognosis patients excluded)	1 year	Antipsychotic alone, psychotherapy alone, psychotherapy plus antipsychotic, ECT, 'milieu' therapy	First admission— no details on previous treatment	Rates of discharge from hospital within 1 year: 96% for drug-treated patients, 96% drug plus psychotherapy, 79% ECT, 65% psychotherapy alone, 58% milieu therapy	—
Johnstone et al. (1978)	45	4 weeks	Flupentixol, beta-isomer flupenthixol, placebo	No details	Flupenthixol-treated patients improved by 8 points on a 15-point scale; placebo patients by 5 points	'Positive' symptoms responded better than 'negative' ones

(continued)

Table 6.1 Continued

Study	Number of patients enrolled	Duration of randomised treatment	Treatments compared	Previous treatment	Global results	Effects on different symptoms
Braden et al. (1982)	78	3 weeks	Chlorpromazine, lithium	55% had previous hospital admissions	Diagnosis did not affect response to either drug	No difference in psychotic or schizophrenic symptoms; over-activity improved more with chlorpromazine
Johnstone et al. (1988)	120	4 weeks	Pimozide, lithium, placebo	No details	Diagnosis did not affect response to either drug	Positive symptoms said to respond better to pimozide

ECT: electro-convulsive therapy; NIMH: National Institute for Mental Health; VA: Veterans Affairs.

superior to a commonly used alternative sedative, indicating the continuing influence of the drug-centred model at the time the study was planned. In this sense, the trial can be seen as an attempt to quantify the descriptive comparisons made by the likes of Deniker and others between the drug-induced state produced by antipsychotics and that produced by barbiturates.

All studies involving people with an acute episode found that antipsychotics were superior to other treatments in terms of symptom improvement, but often by only a modest margin. In the VA study and the NIMH study, however, a substantial number of patients dropped out of the placebo or phenobarbital group because they were not improving, so, in this respect, results are likely to underestimate the effects of the antipsychotics used. On the other hand, even in the earliest study, many participants had received antipsychotics in the past, introducing the possibility of withdrawal-related effects adversely affecting outcome in the control groups. Moreover, the double-blind design was likely to have been compromised in all studies involving a placebo. In 1956 Jonathan Cole, presiding over a conference on methods of evaluating the new drugs, commented at length on the problem that the 'side effects' of the new drugs would immediately reveal to everyone involved in a trial which participants were taking active drugs and which were on placebo (Cole, 1959, p. 97). The fact that the study he set up a few years later, the NIMH study, took no account of this problem is an indication of the growing influence of the disease-centred model.

The only study that lasted for longer than 12 weeks was the comparison of drug treatment and psychotherapy conducted by the Californian-based British psychiatrist Philip May in the 1960s. This study involved people admitted to hospital with a first episode of 'schizophrenia' and compared treatment with antipsychotics, electro-convulsive therapy (ECT), psychoanalytic psychotherapy and milieu therapy. The latter consisted of all the usual activities available in the hospital at the time, including occupational therapy and 'industrial therapy', and doctors were also permitted to prescribe barbiturates and hydrotherapy.[1] The principle outcome was discharge from hospital, and the group who received drug treatment had a clear advantage in this respect. Patients who had ECT also fared well, and the majority of patients in all groups were discharged from the hospital within a year. It is important to note that the trial excluded people who were thought to have a good chance of recovery without drug treatment, as well as those who were thought to be too chronic to benefit from it. Therefore, the trial population probably represents patients who obtain the most benefit from drug therapy, and not the general run of people who experience a first episode of psychosis (May, 1968).

Whereas the NIMH study found that antipsychotics reduced a wide range of symptoms, prompting the study authors to comment that 'the characterisation of these phenothiazines as agents which calm and tranquilize excited or boisterous patients is a greatly oversimplified one' (National Institute of Mental Health Psychopharmacology Service Center Collaborative Study Group, 1964, p. 254), other studies found that it was mostly 'positive' symptoms and behavioural disturbance that showed a specific response to antipsychotics, although the VA hospital study also indicated signs of improved social functioning (Table 6.1).

In the 1980s two studies compared the effects of antipsychotics and lithium in people with different types of acute psychosis, including those with a diagnosis of schizophrenia, mania, psychotic depression and those with mixed features, usually given the catch-all label of 'schizoaffective' disorder. Both studies clearly demonstrated that diagnosis did not predict response to treatment. In other words, people diagnosed with a schizophrenic or schizoaffective episode, according to a range of diagnostic criteria, responded equally well to lithium as to antipsychotic treatment. In one study, lithium was found to be less effective for controlling over-activity, but the authors noted that 'the presence of schizophrenic symptoms did not predict a poor response to lithium' (Braden et al., 1982). In the other study, after dividing the sample up into small groups and applying a complex statistical analysis, the authors claimed to show that there were differences in the response of some symptoms and that 'positive symptoms' responded better to the antipsychotic drug pimozide. Differences were not striking, however, and no direct comparison data were provided (Johnstone et al., 1988).

A small number of studies have compared the effects of antipsychotics and benzodiazepines. These studies are old, mostly small and publications provide few details about their methodology, but they do not provide convincing evidence of the superiority of antipsychotics. Among seven comparisons, described in a review published in 1990, three found no difference between the antipsychotic and the benzodiazepine, three found the benzodiazepine to be superior and two found that the antipsychotic was more effective. Several trials also reported that the benzodiazepine reduced psychotic symptoms, alongside the more familiar sedative effects of these drugs (Wolkowitz and Pickar, 1991).

Overall, therefore, studies of the treatment of people with a recent acute episode of psychosis or schizophrenia show that the use of antipsychotics leads to more improvement than a placebo, a barbiturate, psychotherapy or milieu therapy, but in some studies people allocated to placebo or other treatments also improved to a considerable extent. The NIMH study showed a superior effect on a wide range of symptoms, but other studies suggest that it is the positive 'symptoms,' particularly hallucinations and delusions, that respond most to the drugs (National Institute of Mental Health Psychopharmacology Service Center Collaborative Study Group, 1964). In contrast, a later study comparing clozapine and chlorpromazine for 31 'acutely schizophrenic' patients reported that although clozapine reduced typical psychotic symptoms, chlorpromazine did not, and the authors concluded that it had 'little impact on the acute schizophrenic process in the group of patients examined' (Shopsin et al., 1979, p. 659). This study was conducted when clozapine was new and exciting, and chlorpromazine was old and uninteresting, suggesting that the effects reported in earlier studies might, at least partly, reflect investigators' enthusiasm for new treatments.

Two of the studies of short-term treatment followed up participants after the trial had ended to ascertain whether there were any lasting effects. One year after the NIMH study people randomised to placebo were no different from people who had been treated with antipsychotics in terms of symptoms and level of functioning, except that they had a *lower* chance of being readmitted to hospital (Schooler et al., 1967). Participants in Philip May's study were followed up for between two and five years after the end of the study, and there was found to be 'no startling difference in follow-up outcome between the five original treatment groups' (May et al., 1981, p. 781). On the overall measure of outcome used, people who had had ECT performed best, and there was almost no difference between those who had received 'milieu therapy' and those who had been allocated to antipsychotics. As treatment was not controlled after the initial admission, many participants in all groups received antipsychotics at some point during the follow-up period, although, impressively, 51% of people originally allocated to ECT did not use them at all, as well as 40% and 38% of those in the psychotherapy and milieu therapy groups respectively (May et al., 1981).

So, although studies of antipsychotic drug treatment for an acute psychotic episode suggest that people who receive drug treatment fare better than those who do not in the short-term, there is little evidence that these benefits are sustained. Comparative studies, although few in number, suggest that antipsychotics are superior to barbiturates, but they are not differentiated from other sedative drugs like lithium

and benzodiazepines in studies conducted to date. It is also important to note, given the emphasis now put on starting drug treatment
early in people experiencing a first episode of psychosis, that no
placebo-controlled studies of the treatment of a first episode of psychosis have ever been conducted. May's comparison of antipsychotics
and other types of intervention suggested that antipsychotic treatment
helped people to improve more rapidly in the short-term, although,
interestingly, people who received ECT also fared well in this respect.
In the long-term, however, those who had not received drug treatment
initially improved to around the same level and many were never subsequently exposed to antipsychotic treatment.

Long-Term Treatment

Studies of long-term treatment have two possible objectives—they can
assess the effects of drugs in people with on-going, chronic symptoms
or they can evaluate whether drug treatment helps prevent recurrence
in people who have had a discrete episode of psychosis from which
they have recovered. Unfortunately, these two situations have not been
clearly distinguished in the many hundreds of research studies that
have been conducted in this area. Although studies often purport to
measure 'relapse' this is often defined, if at all, as an exacerbation of
symptoms and does not necessarily indicate that the individual had
previously recovered completely.

The idea that antipsychotics should be continued on a long-term
basis appears to have been established early in the history of their
use. Members of the Thorazine Task Force reminisced to Judith Swazey
that the continuation of drug treatment after discharge was the norm,
but there was concern that doses might be lowered, leading to relapse
or readmission (Swazey, 1974). Smith Kline & French quickly realised that 'aftercare' was a potentially profitable area, and it became a
principle component of the Thorazine marketing campaign. The task
force funded regional aftercare clinics to monitor and prescribe for
recently discharged patients, forging links between hospital and community services, and ensuring that hospital treatment was extended
beyond its walls. The task force also sponsored symposia held by
the American Psychiatric Association on caring for patients after discharge, and it worked with the American Academy of General Practice
and with individual general practitioners and private psychiatrists to
encourage on-going prescribing. The fact that 56% of the newly admitted patients in the VA hospitals' acute treatment study were already

taking antipsychotics at the time of admission suggests the policy of extending drug treatment to the community had been widely adopted by the late 1950s.

Subsequent attempts to test whether or not long-term continuation of treatment with antipsychotics prevents relapse or rehospitalisation were therefore confounded by the fact that most people were already taking the drugs. In other words, the studies could not test the effects of starting out on long-term treatment; they could only assess the effects of stopping it.

A recent meta-analysis of 65 randomised withdrawal studies conducted since 1960 found that 64% of people who were withdrawn from antipsychotics met study criteria for relapse within 1 year compared with 27% who continued the treatment. Only 26% and 10% of patients from each group, respectively, were admitted to hospital, however. No difference in relapse rates was detected between studies in which patients were withdrawn from antipsychotics overnight and studies in which withdrawal was conducted more gradually, although the average period for gradual withdrawal was only 28 days. Moreover, in contrast to previous findings, the risk of relapse did not appear to abate with time, except in some longer studies. People who had not relapsed after 6 or 9 months still had higher relapse rates if they were randomised to take placebo than if they continued on drug treatment. Studies that lasted longer than a year, however, found that rates of relapse in people who continued on drug treatment started to catch up with those who had come off it. The review also revealed that studies that were conducted double blind found smaller effects than ones that were not (Leucht et al., 2012a, 2012b).

In contrast to the situation of acute treatment, there is a small number of studies of the value of maintenance antipsychotic treatment involving patients with a first episode of psychosis or schizophrenia. As these patients are likely to have received antipsychotic treatment for shorter periods of time than patients with a long history of psychiatric problems, and would therefore be expected to experience less severe withdrawal effects, these studies might provide more reliable evidence about the real effects of taking antipsychotics on a long-term basis. Leucht et al. identified seven placebo-controlled trials and found that overall relapse rates in people with a first episode of psychosis or schizophrenia were similar to those reported in other studies of maintenance treatment (Leucht et al., 2012b). This may suggest that withdrawal-related adverse effects do not contribute to relapse rates, but, even in these studies, patients had been taking antipsychotic medication for up to a year after recovering from their initial episode.

The only sizeable study conducted until recent years was published in 1986 and conducted at Northwick Park hospital. One hundred and twenty patients who had recovered from their first episode of psychosis and been stable for 1 month were randomised to continue antipsychotic medication, or have it withdrawn over a month and replaced by placebo. They were followed up for 2 years, and, by the end of the study, 54% of patients who continued on their antipsychotic medication experienced a relapse, defined by requiring additional treatment or hospital admission, which was only slightly less than the 62% of people who relapsed while allocated to placebo. Most patients who relapsed were said to have psychotic symptoms, but not all. Looking at the pattern of relapses (Figure 6.1) suggests a withdrawal effect may have been present in this study despite the fact that it only involved people with a first episode of psychosis. The majority of relapses among the placebo-treated group occurred within the first year, whereas drug-treated patients continued to relapse during the second year (Crow et al., 1986). A more recent comparison of risperidone and haloperidol in people with a first episode of psychosis found similarly high rates of relapse in both groups of drug-treated patients, with 41% of those allocated to risperidone and 48% allocated to haloperidol relapsing within two years (Schooler et al., 2005).

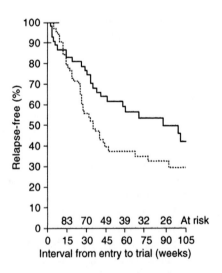

Figure 6.1 Northwick Park first episode study: patients remaining relapse-free on drug and placebo (reproduced with kind permission of the Royal College of Psychiatrists)

In more recent years, three studies have been conducted using open, non-blinded designs, and one large placebo-controlled trial has been carried out, funded by the makers of quetiapine, GlaxoSmithKline (Table 6.2). They all reported higher rates of relapse in people who were withdrawn from antipsychotic medication, but results varied according to the way 'relapse' was defined and on the strategies employed to manage withdrawal-related deterioration. In a study conducted in Germany some of the patients withdrawn from antipsychotic medication were given intermittent drug treatment if they exhibited symptoms suggestive of possible impending relapse, such as insomnia, restlessness, poor concentration and nervousness—symptoms which might equally have been indicative of antipsychotic withdrawal. These first episode patients were only slightly more likely to relapse than those who took antipsychotic medication continuously (36% vs 28%). Patients who did not receive this early or 'prodromal' treatment relapsed at a higher rate of 55%, but even in this group almost half the patients did not relapse after medication withdrawal (Gaebel et al., 2002). Another German study, which used a stringent definition of relapse involving a substantial increase in symptoms, found that only a minority of patients withdrawn from antipsychotics had a full relapse, although 57% showed some clinical deterioration. Even so, 38% of patients were able to withdraw from medication successfully (Gaebel et al., 2011). In contrast, only 20% of the patients in a Dutch study were successfully withdrawn from medication without subsequent relapse, but criteria for relapse were more inclusive (Wunderink et al., 2007). Sixty-three per cent of patients in the placebo-controlled trial of quetiapine were classified as having 'relapsed' using broad criteria, but only 16% were hospitalised, which was only 10% more than the proportion in the drug-treated group (Chen et al., 2010).

Again, few studies have assessed the effects of maintenance treatment with antipsychotics compared with other sorts of sedatives. The second VA study, which involved people with chronic symptoms, included a group who took a barbiturate, and found that this group fared no better than placebo (Casey, 1960b). Another study compared the effects of the benzodiazepine drug diazepam (Valium) with the antipsychotic drug fluphenazine for the treatment of signs of 'exacerbation' in 53 patients diagnosed with schizophrenia who had been withdrawn from their previous antipsychotic regime. In contrast to the VA study, diazepam was as effective as fluphenazine and superior to placebo in preventing a full-blown relapse (Carpenter, Jr, et al., 1999). Similarly, in one of the German studies short-term treatment of deterioration subsequent to

Table 6.2 Recent randomised trials of antipsychotic discontinuation

Study	Number of patients enrolled	Treatment strategies	Duration of follow up	Definition of relapse	Results
Gaebel et al. (2002)	115 with first episode	Patients 'stabilised' on antipsychotic medication for at least 3 months after acute episode, then randomised to be openly withdrawn from antipsychotics within 6 months or continued	2 years	'psychotic deterioration… usually demanding hospitalisation'	28% relapsed with continued drug treatment vs 36–55% in withdrawal group
Wunderink et al. (2007)	131	All patients continued drug treatment for 6 months after 'remission' of an episode, then randomly assigned to open gradual withdrawal over a year or more, or continuation	18 months	Clinical deterioration of at least 1 weeks' duration, with at least one 'moderately severe' positive symptom*	21% relapsed in drug continuation group, vs 43% in withdrawal group; 14 patients (22%) in withdrawal group successfully stopped drug treatment
Chen et al. (2010)	178	Patients had received antipsychotics for an average of almost 2 years before entering the study (618 days)	12 months	Emergence of 'definite psychotic symptom'* plus CGI score >3	30% relapse in drug-treated group vs 63% in placebo group; hospitalisation rates were 6% vs 16%
Gaebel et al. (2011)	44	Antipsychotic treatment continued for 1 year after remission, then randomly assigned to open withdrawal over 3 months or continuation	1 year	Increase of PANSS positive score >10, CGI change >6, decrease in GAF score >20	None of the continuation group relapsed versus 4 patients (19%) in withdrawal group 8 (38%) patients in withdrawal group remained in the study and off anti-psychotic medication

*As measured by PANSS positive symptom subscale.
CGI: Clinical Global Improvement scale; GAF: Global Assessment of Functioning scale; PANSS: Positive and Negative Symptoms of Schizophrenia scale.

antipsychotic withdrawal with a benzodiazepine was just as effective as using an antipsychotic (Gaebel et al., 2011).

Putting aside methodological reservations, the figures of Leucht et al. indicate that 36% of people who stop antipsychotic medication in randomised trials do not relapse in the following year (Leucht et al., 2012a). Some studies with people who have only experienced one episode of psychosis or schizophrenia suggest that 40% or more may remain well after stopping their antipsychotic. Although we remain uncertain about the precise impact of antipsychotic discontinuation, it seems probable that at least some of the events that are classified as 'relapse' in these studies represent the effects of withdrawing from long-term medication, and a gradual reduction that took place over months, rather than weeks, might increase the proportion of patients who could do well without long-term antipsychotic medication. Moreover, the majority of people who experience a relapse after discontinuing antipsychotics can be treated without recourse to hospital admission, and a short course of a benzodiazepines has found to be as effective as antipsychotics for treating early signs of relapse or antipsychotic withdrawal. As we shall see in the next chapter, evidence from other sorts of studies does not support the notion that long-term antipsychotic treatment substantially improves the outlook of everyone diagnosed with schizophrenia, and, even if it did, a reduction in the risk of having a relapse would have to be balanced against the serious consequences of taking these toxic substances over many years.

Trials of Atypical Antipsychotics

As the atypical antipsychotics rapidly came to replace the use of the older drugs for the treatment of people diagnosed with schizophrenia or any 'psychotic' disorder, it is worth looking in more detail at some of the research that forms the basis of their adoption as the principle form of treatment for this situation. After the re-introduction of clozapine in the early 1990s, interest in other 'atypical' antipsychotics accelerated. In the US the Food and Drug Administration (FDA) requires that at least two placebo-controlled trials are conducted to establish the efficacy of a new drug and gain a licence for its use, and approval in many other countries is based on evidence submitted to the FDA. Trials of atypical antipsychotics were submitted rapidly after their development, and could only have been produced so quickly by involving long-term patients on long-term medication.

Robert Whitaker has described in detail the commercial structure behind these studies, and how they were conducted by newly emerging private research companies that tendered their services out to the pharmaceutical companies wanting to test the new drugs. As the research companies were paid per patient they recruited, there was an incentive to be flexible with the eligibility criteria in order to recruit as many patients as possible. The wealth that could be accrued through running these trials and the methods used to entice patients into studies was revealed in enquiries into the practice of two psychiatrists, Richard Borison and Bruce Diamond, who were involved in some of the early studies of atypical antipsychotics, including those that formed the basis of the FDA's approval of risperidone. Employing aggressive selling tactics to recruit large numbers of patients, the business netted Borison and Diamond millions of dollars, which they used to fund extravagant lifestyles. They were finally tried and convicted of the criminal offence of defrauding the Medical College of Georgia, the university where they worked, to which the profits from any trials were meant to have been paid. Richard Borison was sentenced to 15 years in prison and Diamond to 5 years (Whitaker, 2002).

You would think that the imprisonment of two of the principle researchers involved in the introduction of a range of new and widely promoted pharmaceuticals would be big news, opening up questions about the nature of the research they had conducted and the value of the products they had tested. The medical press remained mum on the subject, however, and, until recently, no one questioned the research base for the new drugs.

Looking in detail at the placebo-controlled trials that were meant to have established the efficacy of the atypical antipsychotics confirms that they were, indeed, withdrawal studies, involving people with long-standing difficulties, who had been taking some sort of antipsychotic drugs on a long-term basis prior to the study. In some studies patients were described as experiencing an 'acute exacerbation', but this was never defined clearly and appeared to refer to anyone who reached a certain level of symptom severity (Leucht et al., 2008). Despite this, differences between atypical antipsychotics and placebo were modest, and generally not large enough to indicate that the drugs had clinically meaningful effects in real-life settings.

Stefan Leucht and colleagues explored the clinical significance of changes in psychosis rating scales. They defined a significant clinical effect as one that corresponds to a minimal degree of improvement, as assessed by the Clinical Global Improvement scale (Guy, 1976). They estimated that for the commonly used Positive and Negative Syndrome Scale (PANSS), which rates 30 different items and has a maximum score of 210, a change of 15 points or more would be required to indicate a minimally significant clinical effect. For the Brief Psychiatric Rating Scale (BPRS), whose maximum score is 96, they suggested that a change of 10 points would be equivalent to a minimal level of improvement (Leucht et al., 2006).

The first large study of risperidone was set up in the USA and Canada, and involved a comparison between various doses of risperidone, placebo and haloperidol—the latter prescribed at a fixed dose of 20 mg per day. Like many other atypical studies, it was designed to show risperidone in the best possible light since use of this relatively high dose of haloperidol was bound to cause substantial rates of obvious, unwanted 'extrapyramidal' effects. The Canadian part of the study, which was published in 1993, involved 135 participants who were described as having 'chronic schizophrenia', and had been taking quite high doses of antipsychotics (an average of 753 mg of chlorpromazine or equivalent doses of other antipsychotics) prior to entering the study. No details were provided about how this prior medication was withdrawn (Chouinard et al., 1993).

Despite the fact that many placebo-treated patients were almost certain to have suffered from antipsychotic withdrawal symptoms, and that 48% of participants dropped out before the end of the study, which makes the results difficult to interpret, only the group taking 6 mg of risperidone showed a moderate decrease in symptoms—26 points on the PANSS. People on other doses of ripseridone (2 mg, 10 mg and 16 mg), or haloperidol, showed symptom reductions of less than 15 points. The US arm of the study was conducted with 388 patients, including a mixture of long-term hospital patients and those who had been recently admitted. Most participants, however, had been diagnosed many years before and most were likely to have been on medication prior to study entry as in the Canadian study, although the published report did not mention previous medication. Again, only the group taking 6 mg of risperidone qualified as showing just a minimal degree of improvement in this part of the study, with a reduction in PANSS score of just 16 points. People on other doses of risperidone and those taking haloperidol did not fare markedly better than those on placebo, whose symptoms worsened somewhat in this arm of the study (Marder et al., 1994).

Olanzapine was licensed for use in the USA in 1996 on the basis of two studies, both of which were funded by Eli Lilly and involved people whose condition had a 'chronic course'. The first trial involved a comparison of olanzapine at various doses, haloperidol (10–20 mg per day) and placebo, and lasted for 6 weeks. Three hundred and thirty-five patients were involved and they had been diagnosed with schizophrenia for around 15 years on average, with numerous previous episodes. They were said to be suffering from an 'exacerbation' of symptoms that had lasted around 2 to 5 months before the study started. After medication was withdrawn abruptly over 2 days, patients entered a 'placebo lead-in phase' of 4–7 days. During this time patients were given a placebo, and those who responded well were excluded from randomisation. This technique has been rightly criticised for biasing trials against placebo, but it also demonstrates that the patients entered into the trial were almost certainly suffering from rapidly-occurring withdrawal symptoms, as signs of the underlying condition would be expected to take longer to reappear. After randomisation more than 50% of patients dropped out of the study, including 50–60% of those allocated to olanzapine.

Despite the placebo run-in bias, the drop-out rate and the fact that patients had been withdrawn from previous medication, the difference in improvement between people on placebo and people taking olanzapine only just reached criteria for clinical significance in the group taking the highest dose, where it was 12.1 points on the BPRS. People on other doses of olanzapine and those treated with haloperidol showed an improvement that was less than 10 points different from that shown by the placebo-treated patients. Moreover, there was no difference between the groups in the amount of additional medication used (lorezepam, a benzodiazepine drug, was allowed) (Beasley, Jr, et al., 1996b).

The other trial consisted of a simple comparison between placebo and olanzapine at two different fixed doses: 1 mg and 10 mg. It involved 152 inpatients who had been diagnosed with mental health problems for around 15 years. Sixty-five per cent were said to be experiencing an acute exacerbation and 78% had been taking antipsychotics in the week prior to the study. A quarter of the patients had been on clozapine before entering the study and, given clozapine's potential to provoke withdrawal-related psychotic symptoms, it is highly likely that some patients in the placebo group would have been in a state of antipsychotic withdrawal. This may have contributed to the fact that a phenomenal 80% of the placebo group and 38% of the olanzapine group dropped out of the study early. Like the previous study, this one started with a placebo lead-in phase of 4–7 days and the double blind treatment phase lasted 4 weeks. Again, the results are remarkable for the small difference between olanzapine and placebo, with the group taking 10 mg of olanzapine showing a 7.7-point improvement in its BPRS rating compared with a 0.2-point improvement in the group on placebo (Beasley, Jr, et al., 1996a).

Both studies reported similar rates of sedation in people on olanzapine and placebo, which is hardly credible and may be accounted for by the fact that researchers relied on spontaneous reporting by participants, rather than asking about adverse effects in a systematic manner. Weight gain, however, showed clear differences from placebo, with people on the highest doses of olanzapine gaining an average of 3.5 kg in just 6 weeks in the first study (Beasley, Jr, et al., 1996b).

More recent trials have produced even smaller differences between atypical antipsychotics and placebo. The difference in PANSS scores between drug-treated and placebo-treated patients in trials conducted between 1999 and 2008 was only 6 points, for example (Khin et al., 2012), far below the threshold for clinical significance proposed by Leucht et al. (2006). A meta-analysis conducted by Leucht and colleagues of studies of nine atypical antipsychotics published since 1992 found that the difference between the improvement on the antipsychotic compared with placebo was only 10 points on the PANSS and 9 points on the BPRS. Only 18% more patients taking atypicals showed a 'response' to the drugs than to placebo, although response in these studies was liberally defined as a 20–30% reduction in symptom scores, rather than the 50% reduction that is usually regarded as representing a clinically meaningful change (Leucht et al., 2009). The review also found evidence suggesting the existence of unpublished negative studies and unblinding, and the high levels of drop-out that occurred are likely to further skew the results (Hutton et al., 2012).

Unanswered Questions

The official evidence base for the use of antipsychotics begs more questions than it answers. We know that these drugs improve psychotic symptoms to a greater extent than a placebo, but not how they compare with other sedative drugs, except, perhaps, the barbiturates. In many studies, however, the difference between antipsychotics and placebo is not substantial, and we do not know whether suppressing symptoms with drugs in this way helps more people to make an eventual recovery. Research suggesting that long-term treatment with antipsychotics makes people vulnerable to various withdrawal-induced effects when they discontinue the drugs has not been developed, and it remains possible that such effects fundamentally undermine the results of studies that purport to establish the value of long-term treatment.

The principle problem with antipsychotic trials is that the drugs were already in use before they took place. By the 1960s most patients had been taking these drugs for months or even years before they entered the randomised trials that were supposed to establish whether the drugs worked. Researchers were unaware or unconcerned about the problem this poses, however, despite the fact that withdrawal symptoms had been clearly described by the 1960s. It is difficult not to conclude that leading psychiatrists and researchers did not want to think too deeply about the methodology of their studies because the antipsychotics had already become an indispensable part of psychiatric practice and central to the image that psychiatry was constructing of itself as a bona fide medical speciality.

It is particularly noticeable, in these days when special services have been set up for people experiencing a 'first episode of psychosis', that there are no placebo-controlled trials of acute treatment in people undergoing a first psychotic breakdown, and only a few studies of maintenance treatment in this group. After more than half a century of research into the effects of antipsychotics, and despite the fact that extended use of these drugs is universally recommended, we cannot yet say whether taking antipsychotics in the first place is ultimately better than not taking them or whether starting 'maintenance' treatment offers any real advantages. We know at least that not everyone benefits from taking antipsychotics on a long-term basis, but we need to look elsewhere for evidence about what these drugs actually do that can help us weigh up the pros and cons of taking them in different circumstances.

7
The Patient's Dilemma: Other Evidence on the Effects of Antipsychotics

By the beginning of the 1980s the data from randomised controlled trials and the dopamine hypothesis of schizophrenia had come together to form the foundations of a view that antipsychotic drugs were effective and specific treatments for schizophrenia. Tardive dyskinesia and other 'side effects' were considered, in most cases, a price worth paying for a treatment that was assumed to work on the biochemical mechanism that constituted the condition itself, whether this was the abnormality suggested by the dopamine hypothesis, or a more complex situation involving other neurotransmitters. The drug-centred understanding of the nature and action of these drugs had been well and truly buried, and descriptions of the mental and physical alterations they produced disappeared from the literature. The very idea that psychiatric drugs, like recreational drugs, exert psychoactive effects—alter mental functioning and the nature of consciousness—was banished from mainstream thinking. Research was dominated by the view that these drug-induced alterations were incidental and therefore essentially uninteresting, and could be readily distinguished from the really significant effects of the drugs on the underlying disease. The dopamine hypothesis of schizophrenia ensured that the majority of attention focused on how the drugs reversed this presumed disease, and not how they modified normal brain function.

A countervailing view did emerge in the 1980s, however, which reiterated and restated the drug-centred account, and forced the drug-induced effects of the antipsychotics back into the public domain. American psychiatrist Peter Breggin published his first book *Hazards to the Brain* in 1983, and his best-selling book *Toxic Psychiatry* came out in 1990. Breggin had started to worry about the nature of psychiatric treatments while he was a college student working as a volunteer at a local asylum

(International Center for the Study of Psychiatry and Psychology, 2009). He went on to formulate a comprehensive account of what he called the 'brain disabling' effects of all sorts of psychiatric interventions, including electro-convulsive therapy (ECT), lobotomy and antipsychotics, and he became a vociferous critic of what he believed to be the 'abusive practices' prevalent in mainstream psychiatry (Breggin, 1993a, p. 507).

Breggin put together scattered data from animal research, volunteer studies, the early observations of Deniker and others, and patients' accounts of the experience of taking antipsychotic drugs to construct a drug-centred account of the drugs' effects on mental activity and behaviour. He used the term 'behavioural deactivation' to summarise the characteristics of the state produced by ingesting antipsychotics, an expression intended to capture the generalised restriction of all aspects of activity, from physical movement to intellectual capacity and emotional responses. Like the theory of 'neuroleptic action', this view suggests that, at lower doses, the drug-induced state is mainly manifest in the slowing of intellectual functioning and flattening out of emotions, but at higher doses the classical physical symptoms of Parkinson's disease, such as increased muscle tone and restricted movement, become more apparent. What was most controversial about Breggin's ideas, however, was that he resurrected the views expressed in the 1950s that far from being unwanted 'side effects', it was through these effects that the intended consequences of drug treatment occurred. Breggin linked all physical psychiatric treatments, from lobotomy to Prozac, by suggesting that their purpose was to obliterate troubling behaviours by producing states of reduced brain activity. Antipsychotic drugs, like insulin coma therapy, ECT and lobotomy before them 'exert their primary or intended effect by disabling normal brain function' (Breggin, 1993a, p. 72). Treatment is deemed successful, he explained, when someone, although not necessarily the patient, prefers the 'state of diminished brain function with its narrowed range of mental capacity and emotional expression' (Breggin, 1997, p. 4).

With typical frankness, Breggin pointed out the parallels between the antipsychotic-induced state of deactivation and the effects produced by surgical lobotomy. By severing connections to the frontal lobes, the brain area responsible for characteristics such as spontaneity and motivation, and sometimes referred to as the 'seat of personality', lobotomy results in a state of apathy, emotional disinterest and cognitive impairment. Clinicians and researchers in the 1950s had also made the analogy between the effects of antipsychotics and lobotomy (Lehmann, 1955), but the two states are not quite the same. Lobotomy frequently produces disinhibited and child-like behaviour, which is not characteristic of the antipsychotic-induced state. Like Steck and Deniker, Breggin also compared the effects of the drugs with those of the devastating infectious disease that hit Europe in the early twentieth century, encephalitis lethargica. This neurological disease, which was presumed to be caused by a virus, produced the same range of neurological abnormalities produced by the antipsychotics. Most commonly it involved mental and physical changes that resembled Parkinson's disease, but it could produce other neurological reactions like akathisia, dystonia and a tardive dyskinesia-like condition (Breggin, 1993b).

Breggin attributed the state of deactivation to the dopamine blockade caused by antipsychotic drugs, but even the purest anti-dopaminergic antipsychotics affect other neurochemical systems in complex, interacting and often unmapped ways. Chlorpromazine was given its European brand name Largactil after its 'large action', but even haloperidol and Stelazine, supposedly more specific dopamine blockers, affect numerous other systems, and drugs like clozapine, as already noted, have relatively weak actions on dopamine and stronger effects on other neurotransmitters. The atypical antipsychotics consist of a diverse group of drugs, some of which are similar in nature to some of the older drugs, and some of which appear to have a variety of different types of action. Risperidone, for example, is chemically related to the older drug sulpiride, and exerts a similar range of characteristic effects, whereas olanzapine, quetiapine and aripriprazole, as we shall see, all produce their own subtly distinctive drug-induced state. Although we may be able to map some aspects of the alterations produced by antipsychotics to particular chemical mechanisms, like the induction of 'Parkinsonism' by dopamine receptor blockade, it is rarely possible to find the origin of a complex subjective state in a single biochemical aberration. As philosopher of science Isabelle Stengers suggests, 'between the richness of the psychic effects of a drug and the hypothesis that it disturbs the effects of a type of neurotransmitter, there exists a gulf that no contemporary theory can cross' (Stengers, 1995, p. 134–135, cited in Kirk et al., 2013).

The Subjective Effects of Antipsychotics

In order to understand the nature of a psychoactive drug, whether the drug is used for recreational purposes or prescribed to treat a condition, we have to start with the phenomenology of the drug-induced state. We need to know what sort of physical and mental alterations different drugs produce in people who take them, and how these alterations might vary over the course of longer periods of use. Fortunately, although mainstream psychiatry lost interest in the nature of the drugs it was using, some independent-minded psychiatrists bucked this trend, and patients also continued to speak of the effects the drugs exerted on them. They complained to their psychiatrists in large numbers, they demonstrated their feelings by refusing to take the drugs and some put their experiences down in writing. Put together this information provides an insight into how the state of deactivation Breggin proposed feels from the inside—from the perspective of the person taking the drug. Accounts by people with mental health difficulties also convey how the drug- induced state can suppress a range of unwanted mental experiences and disruptive or unusual behaviours, including the symptoms associated with psychosis or schizophrenia.

Although all drugs have to be tested in 'healthy volunteers' before they come to market, most published volunteer studies provide only brief data on selected physiological parameters or psychological tests, and do not describe the nature of the drug-induced state. Nevertheless, the data indicate that antipsychotic drugs reduce or impair almost all psychological and motor functions that can be measured, and that volunteers find the drug-induced state to be highly unpleasant (Heninger et al., 1965; McClelland et al., 1990; Fagan et al., 1991; Rammsayer and Gallhofer, 1995; Peretti et al, 1997; Ramaekers et al., 1999).

A more informative study was conducted by psychiatrist David Healy in the hospital where he worked in north Wales. In this study staff from the hospital, including nurses, doctors and psychologists, were randomised to receive 5 mg of droperidol (a haloperidol-like antipsychotic), diazepam (Valium) or placebo in a double-blind fashion, and they were required to perform various psychological tests under the influence of the drug. The results of the study, which was only published in a minor pharmacology journal, indicated that almost all of the 20 participants who took droperidol felt heavily sedated, with a feeling that physical and mental activity required greater effort than usual. Concentrating on even simple tasks was difficult and one participant, who happened to be the psychologist and author Richard Bentall, found that obtaining a sandwich from a sandwich machine was just too complicated. All those who took droperidol described feeling 'disengaged' from events around them and found it difficult to motivate themselves to perform the tests they were set. The drug produced feelings of restlessness, anxiety and impatience in all 20 participants, and some felt irritable and uncharacteristically belligerent. Most people found the experience of taking droperidol unpleasant to some degree, in contrast with those who took diazepam who found it either neutral or pleasant. The increased effort required to do anything, the akathisia and the anxiety that the experience would be prolonged all contributed to these negative feelings, and several subjects felt so distressed they entertained suicidal feelings (Healy and Farquhar, 1998).

One of the most interesting aspects of the experiment was that many participants did not recognise the altered state they were in while they were under the influence of the drug. Only two reported feelings of restlessness during the test session, even though many more were observably restless and distressed. Others reported that although they were vaguely aware of being in an altered state, they had an inability or unwillingness to admit to it, in part because they found it difficult to identify and describe its features while under the influence of the drug. Breggin has also highlighted how people's ability to make judgements about their behaviour may be impaired while they are under the influence of a psychoactive substance, an effect he has termed 'spell-binding' (Breggin, 2006).

The Patients' Perspective

Despite the problem of spell-binding, and concerns that people diagnosed with mental disorders might not be able to differentiate between their own difficulties and the effects of drugs, patients' accounts of taking antipsychotics closely mirror those of non-patients. As Marjorie Wallace, founder of the British mental health charity SANE, commented, even people with severe symptoms remain 'extraordinarily articulate and lucid on the subject of their medication' (Wallace, 1994, p. 35).

A survey conducted by SANE provided one glimpse of patients' views prior to the era of the Internet. Most people, Wallace reported, disliked their drugs, whose negative effects were often experienced as 'worse than the illness itself'. Like Healy's volunteers, the respondents felt disengaged from the world around them, as if they were separated from it by a 'glass screen'. They described how 'their senses were numbed, their willpower drained and their lives meaningless', and they often summed up the experience as feeling like a 'zombie' (Wallace, 1994, p. 34, 35). Another account of treatment with antipsychotics describes the adverse impact on imagination and creativity. Peter Wescott, who had suffered from episodes of extreme paranoia and psychosis, felt that his antipsychotic treatment, although effectively suppressing his psychotic symptoms, had fundamentally changed his personality. 'Whereas once I lived in a fascinating ocean of imagination, I now exist in a mere puddle of it', he recounted. 'I used to write poetry and prose because it released and satisfied something deep inside myself; now I find reading and writing an effort and my world inside is a desert' (Wescott, 1979, p. 990).

The Internet has revolutionised possibilities for understanding people's experiences of medical care and prescription drugs. www.askapatient.com, created by a librarian in the USA, is one of several sites that allows users to provide their own perspective on the use of all sorts of medicines, including those prescribed for psychiatric problems. These data are particularly useful for evaluating the subjective effects of the atypical antipsychotics, since there are no descriptions of these in mainstream literature. Table 7.1 lists accounts written on www.askapatient.com by people who had taken some older antipsychotics, as well as the newer drugs risperidone and olanzapine. Comments are artificially separated into different categories of effect, like sedation and emotional effects, but it should be appreciated that what people generally described was a global, drug-induced state, which had both physical and mental aspects (Moncrieff et al., 2009).

Consistent with previous reports, people taking the older drugs chlorpromazine, trifluoperazine (Stelazine) and haloperidol described feeling heavily sedated, and physically and mentally slowed or inhibited. They also depicted the deadening effect on emotions and, like Wescott, reported feelings of having lost important aspects of their personality such as their creativity and humour. Although many disliked these experiences, some people acknowledged that these same effects had led to improvements in mental symptoms. A man diagnosed with bipolar disorder, for example, described how he thought haloperidol had 'decreased brain activity, slowed down racing thoughts'. A woman who had taken haloperidol for psychotic symptoms, including hallucinations, described the suppression of interest caused by the drug, referring to the benefits of this state, as well as a sense of loss:

> Although I felt very well, I felt as if I had absolutely nothing to talk about. I kept wondering about whatever [it] was that had been so interesting during most of my life that I had suddenly lost... But I was very much in contact with reality and for that I was thankful.

Other respondents were also grateful for the effects of the drugs. One suggested that receiving haloperidol for a few days for a manic attack had been life-saving, for example. In contrast, many described the experience as highly unpleasant. One man referred to haloperidol as 'the worst [drug] I have been exposed to' and chlorpromazine was said to be 'horrible stuff'.

Table 7.1 Verbatim descriptions of subjective effects of antipsychotics from www.askapatient.com (from Moncrieff et al., 2009)

Effect	Typical comments
Sedative effects	'I'm still fatigued in the morning and can barely get out of bed some days' (trifluoperazine) 'I feel tired all the time. Too tired to be depressed' (risperidone) 'I was sleeping over 14 hours a night and was so hung over during the day I could hardly go about my normal routines. I couldn't even get myself dressed to go out to the store' (olanzapine)
Cognitive effects	'low ability to make decisions' (trifluoperazine) 'no thoughts or inner world' (risperidone) 'mental fogginess all the time' (risperidone) 'altered mental state, cannot focus. Impaired judgement and thinking' (risperidone) 'blank mind' (olanzapine) 'sluggish thinking' (olanzapine) 'loss of wits' (olanzapine)
Emotional effects	'I feel absolutely nothing!! No sadness, no joy, NOTHING' (haloperidol) 'emotionally empty, dead inside...took away my sense of humour' (trifluoperazine) 'oblivious to my surrounds...all creativity was squashed' (trifluoperazine) 'no emotions, only a weird, spacey, empty feeling, no arousal, no excitement, no joy, nothing' (risperidone) 'total shut down of my outgoing personality' (risperidone) 'emotionless zombie' (risperidone) 'lack of interest in life, no will to carry on living' (risperidone) 'too zoned, too robotic, emotion dead' (olanzapine) 'lost of emotions and general feeling that everything doesn't matter at all' (olanzapine) 'personality is dampened' (olanzapine) 'general lack of interest in anything' (olanzapine)
Parkinsonian effects	'...extremely hard to move, think, talk' (haloperidol) 'I feel like a zombie, I can't think clear and my movement is slow' (haloperidol) 'heavy mental and physical stagnance...retarded feeling' (haloperidol) 'I felt like I was in slow motion' (risperidone) 'I am not able to think properly and am experiencing the world at about half the normal pace...Can't keep my mind focused and my eyes are slow' (olanzapine) 'mild inhibited feeling' (olanzapine)

(continued)

Table 7.1   Continued

Effect	Typical comments
Akathisia	'horrible restlessness' (haloperidol) '...extreme physical agitation combined with a zombielike mind state' (chlorpromazine) 'I felt like scratching my eyes out and my skin off and running into the walls' (risperidone) 'ineffable anxiety, which was sort of like restless leg syndrome' (risperidone) 'restlessness, the kind where you wanna kill yourself' (olanzapine)
Sexual effects	'I lost my ability to feel emotions, I lost my libido, I lost my drives, I lost my ability to get an erection' (risperidone) 'Low motivation, narrow emotional range, can't get excited about things, libido and drive have been obliterated' (risperidone) 'Even at 2.5mg, I still have no interest in sex' (olanzapine) 'Reduction in sex drive' (olanzapine) 'Lowered libido' (chlorpromazine)
Metabolic effects	'ravenous, rapacious hunger that never quit' (olanzapine) 'I feel numb, like I've been brainwashed. There is more to life than eating and sleeping' (olanzapine) 'I was a humongous zombie on Zyprexa' (olanzapine) 'I keep eating and eating and sleeping and sleeping and sometimes I manage to do both at the same time' (olanzapine)

People who had taken risperidone described a similar state, but movement disorder was mentioned less frequently and sexual difficulties, including loss of libido and impotence, more frequently. The latter were often linked with the emotional flattening produced by the drug, suggesting that its effects can be understood as a global reduction of arousal that encompasses all aspects of motivation and desire. Again, people described how these same effects had helped reduce troubling thoughts and disabling anxiety. A man with a diagnosis of paranoid schizophrenia described how risperidone had 'numbed my brain from psychotic thoughts, flattened most of my emotions'. Another respondent with anxiety and 'paranoia' described how it 'stops my negative thoughts and feeling being amplified and overwhelming me', and several more commented on how the drug had produced feelings of 'calm' or relief from anxiety. A woman with depression noted how she now felt 'too tired to be depressed'.

As with the older antipsychotics, some people had extremely negative reactions to the effects of risperidone. One recipient described taking it as a 'living hell'. Another warned: 'BEWARE, BEWARE, BEWARE!!! This medication is Satan in a flipping pill'.

People commenting on olanzapine described an altered state consisting of profound sedation accompanied by emotional flattening and indifference, in association with a markedly increased appetite for food. Slow or restricted movement did not appear to be a common feature of the drug-induced experience, in contrast to the older drugs. The following comment by a person diagnosed with bipolar disorder typifies many, and illustrates the close relation between the drug's psychoactive and metabolic effects:

> I've never been able to eat as much as I did when I was on Zyprexa. I gained 40 lbs in no time and my mind was in a constant fog of lethargy and indifference. I didn't care about anything. I just wanted to sit around and eat.

The lethargy was not always experienced as unpleasant, and several respondents described how olanzapine had helped reduce anxiety, irritability and even suicidal thoughts. 'It has a wonderful calming effect' was how one man, with a diagnosis of bipolar disorder, described it. 'The drug saved my life' commented one woman, 'by getting me sleep so my nervous system could rest'. Several mentioned that the drug had stopped or reduced psychotic symptoms. It 'stopped the psychosis and thoughts coming into my head', commented a man diagnosed with schizoaffective disorder. As with the other drugs, some respondents disliked the effects intensely. An older man with anxiety said 'This is the most horrible drug I've ever used', and a woman commented 'if you would not willingly undergo a lobotomy, then do not take this drug'. Some people found the effects unpleasant, but had, nevertheless, found the drug useful: 'Despite its extremely negative side effects' said one respondent, 'this medication does wonders for paranoia and delusional thinking ... the anxiety is non existent now, I am able to function as a normal human being'. A woman with psychosis commented 'It makes me feel like a veggie, but that was better than what I was going through and it kept me out of the hospital'.

Clozapine, now reserved for people who do not improve on treatment with other antipsychotics because of its dangerous effects on the immune system, was also described as producing heavy or 'extreme' sedation, lethargy, weight gain and increased appetite. In keeping with comparative clinical trials, which show that it can reduce positive psychotic symptoms like delusions and hallucinations better than other sorts of antipsychotics, at least in the short term (Moncrieff, 2003), many respondents with a diagnosis of schizophrenia felt the drug had been beneficial. 'It saved my mind', said a 32-year-old woman who had been taking it for 10 years, and a 37-year-old woman, who had been on the drug for 6 years, described how it had helped her relate and 'connect' to people, which she had previously found difficult. Others commented on how the sedating effects were useful for inducing sleep and reducing anxiety. In contrast, several respondents had found the effects frightening and unpleasant, and felt that the drug had changed their personalities in subtle ways which, like the participants in Healy's study, they were not always aware of when under its influence. A 41-year-old woman diagnosed with depression and bipolar disorder described how she lost her 'personality and became like a zombie', but only realised the effect the drug was having when she stopped taking it and the 'sedation wore off'. Another woman described clozapine as the 'most EVIL med I have ever taken' (original emphasis), describing how it made her feel '100% zoned out'.

The comments on www.askapatient.com are consistent with a large interview study conducted in Germany involving 80 patients with a diagnosis of schizophrenia. Around a third of these patients felt that clozapine had been helpful to them, but the most commonly cited benefits were its ability to improve sleep and produce sensations of calmness. The authors concluded that 'a significant proportion of the patients viewed clozapine more as a tranquilliser or a sleeping pill than an antipsychotic drug'. Some patients complained of feelings of demotivation, lethargy and a lack of interest and enthusiasm, which they attributed to the drug. When asked how they thought the drug worked the patients reported that it had made their voices fainter, or less frequent, or that they had disappeared completely. Two described its effects as 'shielding' them from stress and 'irritations'. Some patients imagined that the drug suppressed the actions of the brain and nervous system. One described how it seemed as if the drug 'makes the nerves work more slowly' and another that it caused a 'blockage of brain functions'. Like the www.askapatient.com respondents, some patients reported that the drug had improved their ability to function in the world (Angermeyer et al., 2001, pp. 512, 515).

Trials that demonstrate clozapine's facility to reduce aggressive impulses and behaviour illustrate the unusual state of placidity this particular drug can produce (Spivak et al., 1997b; Volavka et al., 2004; Krakowski et al., 2006). Unlike the older drugs, where the emotional restriction appears to be part of an overall state of physical and mental inhibition, the emotional state produced by clozapine involves a more subtle change in emotional tenor and personality, which people may not find so unpleasant at the time of taking the drug, but which in retrospect might seem even more frightening.

Quetiapine, better known by its brand name Seroquel, has become one of the best-selling drugs in its class since its release in 1997. It shares an intense sedating effect with clozapine and olanzapine, but its effects on weight and metabolism appear to be weaker, although they are by no means insignificant. It is frequently prescribed for insomnia and is said to have a modest street value as a 'downer', where it is know by the slang term 'Suzy Q' (Wen, 2009). Respondents on www.askapatient. com, many of whom said they were taking it for insomnia, as well as bipolar disorder, anxiety, depression and schizophrenia, described it as sapping motivation and sex drive, causing extreme sedation and lethargy, and sometimes increasing appetite and producing weight gain. People reported feeling 'drugged up', and having feelings of 'passivity and 'zombie-like periods' while taking it, but many people commented on its ability to induce and improve sleep.

Aripiprazole (trade name Abilify), has been widely marketed with the curious suggestion that it has the simultaneous ability to stimulate and block dopamine receptors. The rationale for the benefits of this action is said to be reduced neurological adverse effects like Parkinsonism, but why other dopamine-blocking drugs could not just be given at reduced doses is never explained. Judging from clinical experience and comments on www.askapatient.com, the subjective experience of taking the drug suggests it is less sedative than other antipsychotics, and it frequently produces an unpleasant state of insomnia, restlessness and agitation. People also report experiences of the sort of flattened emotions and demotivation associated with the other antipsychotics, however.

Are Antipsychotics Useful?

Patients, volunteers and observers concur that ingesting antipsychotic drugs produces a state of sedation, lethargy, flattening of emotional responses, indifference and feelings of impaired mental functioning sometimes accompanied, depending on the drug to some extent, by the unpleasant agitation known as akathisia. The exact quality of these effects varies between the different drugs, as do the physical effects that accompany these mental changes. So whereas the psychoactive effects of the older drugs are closely associated with their ability to slow and restrict movement, the placidity and indifference produced by some of the newer antipsychotics, notably clozapine and olanzapine, appear to be part of a global state characterised by a striking metabolic disturbance, but less profound effects on movement. The types of mental suppression produced by quetiapine and aripriprazole are subtly different again, but whatever the drug, the physical effects appear to have an intrinsic relation to the mental effects, suggesting they are, in fact, different facets of the same basic physiological process.

It is not difficult to imagine how these drug-induced effects might impact on symptoms of psychosis, schizophrenia and other mental health problems, and patients describe this process from their own perspective. The physical and mental slowing induced by the drugs reduces agitation and helps to calm people who are highly aroused, possibly as a consequence of hearing voices or other disturbing mental phenomena. The mental clouding produced by the drugs may also reduce the intensity of psychotic symptoms, but it is the distinctive ability of the drugs to dampen emotional responses that marks them out from most other sedative, psychoactive substances. The emotional restriction and loss of interest and motivation that the drugs produce can reduce people's preoccupation with intrusive ideas and experiences, and thus also the excitation, anxiety or aggression that such experiences might provoke. The psychotic phenomena seem to fade into the background; they no longer demand so much attention and levels of distress can markedly diminish. With drug treatment people are able to ignore their psychotic symptoms, and although they will still talk about them when asked, the symptoms no longer appear to be at the forefront of their thought. Sometimes the abnormal ideas and experiences might disappear altogether as people simply lose interest in them. Deniker recognised this effect in 1960 when he suggested that the improvement that could occur in an individual's 'previously rigid system of delusions...is really the patient's increasing lack of interest and his loss of feeling for his delusional fantasies' (Deniker, 1960, p. 99).

Although the drugs suppress mental activity indiscriminately—not just aberrant thoughts and feelings—in cases where someone's mental life is dominated by psychotic processes, the dampening down and slowing up of thinking may, by reducing the strength of the troubling thoughts, release the affected person from their internal psychotic world, and enable them to interact more normally with the world

Table 7.2 Changes in dimensions of psychosis after antipsychotic treatment (data from Mizrahi et al., 2006)

Dimension of psychotic experience	Reduction in dimension after 6 weeks of antipsychotic treatment (%)
Behavioural impact	64
Cognitive preoccupation	51
Emotional involvement	56
Conviction	25
External perspective	0

around them. Thus, people who are extremely psychotic may show improved social functioning while taking the drugs, despite also exhibiting signs of drug-induced suppression.

More recently, two studies led by members of a respected research group based in Toronto have confirmed this pattern. One study investigated patients' views on how antipsychotics impacted on their psychotic symptoms, and found that patients described that drug treatment produced a state of detachment from their symptoms, rather than eradicating them. The study included eight patients who had never taken antipsychotics before. Initially, these individuals expected the drugs to eliminate their symptoms, but after receiving the drugs they changed their minds and felt the drugs merely made the symptoms less intense and troublesome (Mizrahi et al., 2005). The second study investigated changes in five dimensions of the psychotic experience in 17 people experiencing a psychotic episode who were starting on antipsychotics, mostly for the first time. The dimension that showed the most change after 6 weeks of drug treatment was the 'behavioural impact' of the symptoms, which referred to whether the symptoms influenced patients' behaviour (Table 7.2). Preoccupation with symptoms also reduced substantially, along with patients 'emotional involvement' with their symptoms. In contrast, belief in the reality of the symptoms (which the researchers referred to as 'conviction') diminished little, and patients' 'external perspective', or understanding of the unusual nature of their experiences, did not change at all (Mizrahi et al., 2006).

Long-Term Effects

The ability of antipsychotics to suppress psychotic symptoms does not necessarily translate into a useful and lasting effect, however. Although many psychiatrists believe that the introduction of these drugs transformed the outlook for people with severe mental disorders dramatically, data from research are more ambiguous. Figures on declining hospital populations, for example, originally interpreted as indicating that the introduction of antipsychotics had enabled people to be discharged from psychiatric institutions more frequently than before, actually showed that in countries like the UK and the USA, rates of discharge started increasing prior to the introduction of antipsychotics (Shepherd et al., 1961; Gronfein, 1985; Grob, 1994). In other places, like France and Norway, discharge rates did not change for years after the drugs' introduction (Odegaard, 1964; Sedgwick, 1982). It was politics and not drugs that changed the face of mental health care in the late twentieth century. Western governments started to favour locating care in the community in order to reduce costs, and to combat the neglect, brutality and demoralisation that were revealed in some mid-century psychiatric institutions (Grob, 1983). The introduction of the new tranquillisers, however, did provide a convenient justification for this policy, and thereby helped to drive the community care movement forward (Gronfein, 1985).

Ascertaining the long-term outcome of people who experience mental health problems is fraught with difficulty because of changing notions about the nature of these problems and varying definitions of recovery. Thus, people diagnosed with schizophrenia in one era and in one country may have little in common with those in other places or other periods. Although a considerable amount of research has been conducted, 'a clear picture of the long-term outcome in schizophrenia has not emerged' (Warner, 2004, p. 57). Follow-up studies over the course of the twentieth century found little evidence that outcome improved after the introduction of antipsychotics, however. The outlook for someone diagnosed with the disorder in the 1990s was about the same as someone diagnosed in the 1930s (Hegarty, 1994). As we saw in Chapter 6, follow-up studies of patients enrolled in randomised trials of acute treatment also do not confirm that treating a psychotic episode with antipsychotic drugs confers any long-term advantage. Robert Whitaker has proposed that far from improving the ultimate outlook for people diagnosed with psychosis or schizophrenia, long-term antipsychotic treatment may make it worse (Whitaker, 2010). This could explain, he suggests, why two large international studies conducted by the World Health Organization found that people diagnosed with schizophrenia for the first time in the developing world, where drug treatment was often unavailable, had fewer symptoms and functioned better socially a few years later than those in the Western world (Sartorius et al., 1977; Jablensky et al., 1992).

Within Western countries, it has also been found that people who do not take antipsychotics do better than those who do (Lehtinen et al., 2000; Bola and Mosher, 2003; Harrow et al., 2012). Martin Harrow, professor of psychology at Illinois University, has conducted one of the longest follow-up studies of people diagnosed with schizophrenia. Starting in 1975, Harrow recruited 157 young people admitted to one of two psychiatric hospitals in Chicago with an episode of psychosis, and a comparison group comprising 117 patients with 'neurotic' disorders. Sixty-four patients fulfilled criteria for a diagnosis of schizophrenia. All patients were followed up and assessed periodically over the next 20 years. Starting from the 4.5-year follow-up, patients diagnosed with schizophrenia who were not taking antipsychotic drugs had fewer psychotic symptoms and were more likely to meet criteria for 'recovery' (defined as the absence of positive and negative symptoms, and 'adequate' social functioning), than those who were. At the 20-year evaluation, 62% of the patients diagnosed with schizophrenia were taking antipsychotics and only just over 10% of them were considered recovered compared with just over 50% of those who were not taking antipsychotics (Harrow et al., 2012).

Data on the extent to which people showed an all-round recovery, including being able to work and support themselves, as well as remaining symptom-free, suggested that long-term antipsychotic treatment may itself depress outcome. People who were off antipsychotics who were diagnosed with schizophrenia, which is supposed to have the worst outcome of all psychotic syndromes, had a better global outcome than people with other psychotic disorders who were taking antipsychotics. This effect could be seen from around 4 years after enrolment through to the 15-year follow-up, when the data were presented (Figure 7.1) (Harrow and Jobe, 2007).

The authors of this study initially postulated that the differences between drug-treated patients and those who did not receive antipsychotics could be explained by the fact that people who have protracted and severe problems are more likely to receive drug treatment. Only people with the mildest difficulties would be able to avoid contact with services and the drug therapy this usually entails. So it might be the nature of the underlying condition that explains why people on drug treatment appear to fare worse. Harrow and his colleagues looked at some of the factors that might predict recovery and found that people with schizophrenia who were not taking antipsychotics at the 15- and 20-year follow-ups were, indeed, a group with a more favourable outlook, as judged by factors such as their level of achievement prior

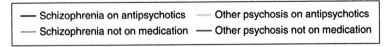

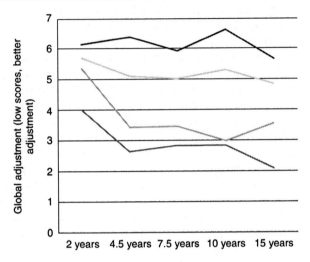

Figure 7.1   Global adjustment of psychotic patients over 15 years of follow-up—low scores indicate better adjustment (data from Harrow and Jobe, 2007)

to the onset of the condition. Comparing only patients with a similar prognostic profile, however, still showed that those who were not taking antipsychotics had a better outcome then those who were (Harrow and Jobe, 2007). This does not rule out the prospect that there are other unmeasured factors about the nature of the disorder that might predict both a poor recovery and the likelihood of taking antipsychotics. It does indicate, however, that the idea that antipsychotic treatment makes people worse has to be considered a possibility, and one which urgently needs to be investigated further.

How antipsychotics negatively affect the outlook of psychotic conditions, if indeed they do, remains uncertain but, as we have seen, it has been proposed that they might make the brain more vulnerable to psychosis by inducing changes in dopamine receptors and other neurotransmitter systems, as in the idea of 'supersensitivity psychosis' (Chouinard and Jones, 1980). This mechanism would predict that some people on long-term treatment would have higher levels of psychotic symptoms than they might have had without that treatment. In terms of general functioning we have seen evidence that antipsychotics can cause a decline in mental abilities, at least in those who develop tardive dyskinesia. As

American psychiatrist Thomas McGlashan put it in an edition of the *Schizophrenia Bulletin*, 'medication may be life-saving in a crisis, but it may render the patient more psychosis-prone should it be stopped and more deficit ridden should it be maintained' (McGlashan, 2006, p. 300).

The other fact that historical studies confirm is that not everyone needs antipsychotics in order to recover from a psychotic episode. Early follow-up studies indicate that there has always been a proportion of people who recover from a psychotic episode eventually, without any modern-day interventions. American psychiatrist Richard Warner surveyed these studies in his book *Recovery from Schizophrenia*. Studies in England, for example, where the diagnosis of schizophrenia remained fairly narrow in contrast to the USA (and in that sense similar to modern-day criteria), found that in the 1930s around 20% of people admitted with a diagnosis of schizophrenia made a full recovery, and this rose to more than 30% in studies of people admitted in the 1940s and early 1950s (Warner, 2004).

Swiss psychiatrist Manfred Bleuler, son of Eugen Bleuler who coined the term 'schizophrenia', followed up 208 psychotic patients admitted to a psychiatric hospital between 1942 and 1943. Twenty-two per cent made a full recovery, which was sustained for at least 5 years, and a further 58% recovered from their initial episode, but had further episodes interspersed with times of remission—and this was more than 10 years before the introduction of antipsychotics (Bleuler, 1974; Modestin et al., 2003). Moreover, Bleuler commented that none of the patients who maintained a sustained recovery after the introduction of antipsychotics received long-term drug treatment after the resolution of their acute symptoms (Bleuler, 1974). Philip May's study also showed that well over half of the patients treated with psychotherapy or milieu therapy were discharged within a year, and the study had excluded people with milder conditions or protective factors that suggested they might be able to recover without drug treatment (May, 1968).

Projects that have been set up with the aim of minimising the use of antipsychotic drugs also confirm that some people can recover from a psychotic episode without them. The Soteria project in the USA was established by psychiatrist Loren Mosher and funded by the National Institute of Mental Health. It consisted of a therapeutic community, staffed by non-professionals, but overseen by Mosher and the research team, and it was designed to minimise the use of antipsychotics by providing a supportive and accepting environment. In order to evaluate the project a trial was set up in which people with an early episode of psychosis (their first or second episode) were randomly or alternatively allocated either to the Soteria project or to receive standard treatment at the local hospital. A limitation of the experiment, however, was that people who were judged to be unmanageable in the Soteria setting were excluded from allocation to the Soteria group and a few more patients dropped out during the early stages of the experiment. The data suggest, however, that the Soteria project was at least as good as 'usual care' in terms of outcomes at 2 years for patients in the study (Bola and Mosher, 2003). Forty-three per cent of the patients treated in the Soteria facility received no antipsychotic treatment at all, and two thirds (66%) had used anti-psychotics either not at all or only occasionally, compared with only 5% of the group admitted to the local hospital. When the numbers who were excluded from the trial are accounted for, the proportion of Soteria sub-jects who avoided the use of antipsychotics altogether was 32%.

A more recent study in Finland produced similar results. In this study services for people with a first episode of psychosis in certain areas of northern Finland were set up with the express aim of avoiding the use of antipsychotics where possible, and supporting patients instead with a mixture of psychotherapy and family therapy. Results from the assess-ment of 84 patients treated in these 'experimental' areas were com-pared with those from 51 patients treated in other areas where services employed antipsychotics according to usual protocols. Forty-three per cent of patients in the experimental areas received no antipsychotic drugs throughout the study compared with only 6% in the other areas. However, almost a third of potential recruits in the experimental areas dropped out of the study early. If all these patients are assumed to have received antipsychotic treatment, then the proportion who avoided the use of these drugs altogether falls to 34%. The patients who stayed in the study in the experimental areas were less likely to have a prolonged hospital admission than patients from the other areas and their global outcome ratings were superior (Lehtinen et al., 2000). However, the replication of this trial in Sweden failed to achieve such high levels of avoidance of drug treatment, with only 19% of patients remaining drug free (Cullberg et al., 2002).

It is clear therefore that not everyone undergoing a psychotic episode needs antipsychotic medication to recover. Some people recover sponta-neously and can be helped and supported through this process without the need for chemical suppression. The disease-centred model of drug action eclipsed this fact, however, replacing it with the belief that people only recover because they receive the necessary and specific treatment.

Far more research is needed into the effects of taking antipsychotics over long periods before people can judge whether it is beneficial to use them. Many people with psychosis find that the drugs suppress their symptoms, although with the advent of clozapine and its positioning for people who are 'treatment resistant', it started to be admitted that up to 30% of people with schizophrenia are not helped by the standard drugs (Meltzer et al., 1989). But even people who obtain some relief from their symptoms may feel the price of this relief is just too high. Majorie Wallace's survey revealed what she called 'the intolerable choice' faced by sufferers 'between being driven by voices and delusions or drowning in agony and despair' (Wallace, 1994, pp. 34–35). For people who suffer from severe and protracted mental disturbance, who may spend years locked into a frightening private world, cut off from reality and from those who love them, the drug-induced reduction in brain function may be a price worth paying. For others the equation is not so clear.

The balance of pros and cons is particularly difficult to discern in relation to the idea of maintenance treatment. Even if we put aside the difficulties in interpreting the clinical trials and assume that the continuation of antipsychotic medication after an acute episode does reduce the risk of relapse at least somewhat, taking a drug-centred perspective suggests that this benefit may not be sufficient to outweigh the day-to-day impairment the drugs produce, coupled with the serious physical consequences associated with long-term treatment (effects we shall explore further in Chapter 9). As Thomas McGlashan questioned 'Do we free patients from the asylum with D_2 blocking agents only to block incentive, engagement with the world and the *joie de vivre* of everyday life?' (McGlashan, 2006, p. 300).

Despite the lack of well-designed trials, guidelines continue to recommend that people should continue to receive antipsychotic medication for 1–2 years after their symptoms have subsided (National Collaborating Centre for Mental Health, 2010). Although it may be difficult to distinguish who has recovered spontaneously, and who may have residual symptoms that the drugs are effectively suppressing and that might resurface if the treatment was stopped, a drug-centred view would suggest that antipsychotics should be used for the shortest possible period, if they cannot be avoided, and reduced gradually as soon as the individual shows signs of recovery. Only after several episodes of psychotic disturbance or when episodes involve dangerous behaviour would the possible benefits of long-term treatment outweigh their adverse effects. If on-going use of antipsychotics is felt to be unavoidable, we must keep in mind the loss of self this treatment can involve. Peter Wescott poignantly expressed the patient's dilemma when he lamented 'In losing my periods of madness, I have had to pay with my soul and the price of health seems twice as high as Everest' (Wescott, 1979, p. 989).

8
Chemical Cosh: Antipsychotics and Chemical Restraint

The most controversial use of antipsychotic drugs is when they are forcibly given to people to control and subdue agitated, aggressive and threatening behaviour that occurs in medical and psychiatric settings. They have been used in this way since their introduction, when they started to replace the use of older sedatives like barbiturates, and since the 1960s antipsychotics of one sort or another have been the principle agents recommended for the purpose of chemical restraint, or 'rapid tranquillisation' as it has come to be called. Haloperidol is the antipsychotic most closely associated with this situation, and it can be given alone or in combination with others sorts of drugs, most commonly a benzodiazepine. The related drug droperidol, launched in 1980 and withdrawn in 2001 owing to safety concerns, was also popular for behavioural control, and in 1990 an injectable preparation known as Clopixol Acuphase was introduced, whose use soon became one of the staple techniques of emergency sedation in psychiatry.

This use of antipsychotics as chemical restraints has long been a subject of intense criticism by many who have been its victims. Psychologist Rufus May, who was admitted to hospital with a psychotic episode when he was 18 years old, described the 'humiliating' and 'degrading' experience of being pinned down by five or six nurses, having his trousers pulled down and being injected in the buttock with drugs that left him feeling drowsy and groggy for days afterwards (May, 2001). Recipients also perceive the procedure as punitive and unnecessary, and patient-centred organisations all over Europe and the USA have repeatedly protested against the practice of 'forced drugging'.[1]

Until recent years, the use of antipsychotics for behavioural control was so ubiquitous that most people admitted to psychiatric facilities were prescribed injectable haloperidol 'just in case'. Since concerns about haloperidol's dangerous and occasionally lethal effects on the heart were publicised in 2007 (Food and Drug Administration, 2007), a wider range of agents is now recommended, including the anti-histamine drug promethazine. The sole use of benzodiazepines, such as lorazepam, which have long been employed alongside antipsychotics, is also encouraged (Taylor et al., 2009). Haloperidol is still widely used, however, and Clopixol Acuphase continues to be given when other measures fail. It was used in almost a fifth of patients in secure psychiatric facilities in one recent survey (Brown et al., 2010).

Despite the fact that there is now a body of literature and research devoted to techniques of 'rapid tranquillisation', the coercive nature of the practice is rarely acknowledged. Most reviews and guidelines present the activity within a therapeutic framework and studiously avoid discussing the ethics of the situation or examining the pharmacological mechanisms that render antipsychotics suitable agents of chemical restraint. The practice is constructed as a diagnosis-driven activity, whose purpose is to treat an underlying disorder, rather than to modify unwanted behaviour. Consensus guidelines on the management of 'behavioural emergencies' produced by a panel of experts from the USA in 2001, for example, presented emergency sedation for people with mental disorders (as opposed to those with physical diseases like delirium or substance intoxication) as an intervention that should be tailored to the suspected diagnosis. Recommendations for 'medication to treat agitation that appears to be due to a primary psychiatric disturbance depend on the provisional diagnosis' the report stated (Allen et al., 2001, p. 16), before setting out different options for emergency sedation in a range of disorders, including schizophrenia, mania, psychotic depression and post-traumatic stress disorder (PTSD). The panel explicitly rejected the notion that drugs were used for the purposes of control or restraint. 'The panel did not endorse the concept of "chemical restraint"', the report stated, continuing that instead it favoured 'the idea that medications are treatments for target behaviours in behavioural emergencies' (Allen et al., 2001, p. 4).

Other experts have distinguished between the management of aggressive or challenging behaviour when it is exhibited by someone undergoing a psychotic episode, and situations involving people who are not psychotic or have other diagnoses. The UK's National Institute for Health and Clinical Excellence (NICE) review of the 'short-term management of disturbed/violent behaviour' published in 2005 recommended the use of an antipsychotic like haloperidol or olanzapine with or without a benzodiazepine 'when behavioural disturbance occurs in the context of psychosis' and a benzodiazepine alone in other circumstances (National Institute for Health and Clinical Excellence, 2005, p. 100). The American Association for Emergency Psychiatry's wide-ranging review of emergency treatment euphemistically named 'Best Practices in the Evaluation and Treatment of Agitation' published in 2012, made the same distinction, explaining that 'for psychosis driven agitation...antipsychotics are preferred over benzodiazepines because they address the underlying psychosis' (Wilson et al., 2012, p. 30). Although the distinction implies that the use of drugs to modify behaviour is not always a therapeutic activity, the fact that the majority of attention is devoted to the management of people diagnosed with psychosis or schizophrenia means the issue of forced drugging remains firmly within the medical arena, immune from the considerations that would apply if its coercive nature were fully acknowledged. In this way, modern practices can be presented as distinct from the murky history of chaining up lunatics or knocking out mental patients with a chemical cosh (Schleifer, 2011).

It was the ascendance of the disease-centred theory of antipsychotic action that allowed the practice of chemical restraint to be rebranded as a medical treatment, and the belief that the forcible administration of these drugs represented a therapeutic activity in its own right ensured that antipsychotics remained at the heart of emergency procedures for many decades, even though other options, such as promethazine and the benzodiazepines, have long been available. Just as adoption of the disease-centred model of drug action drew the curtain on the modifications of mental experience and behaviour that the drugs produce on a day-to-day basis, so it foreclosed objective discussion about the safest, most effective and least obnoxious method of responding to extreme agitation and aggression.

The Early History of Restraint[2]

Methods of restraint have been employed for at least as long as mankind has been able to describe disturbed or unwanted behaviour. The use of chains, shackles and fetters is documented in chronicles by Aulus Cornelius Celsus (25 BC–50 AD) (Soreff and Bazemore, 2006), and is found in descriptions of the management of people who were considered mad in early modern Britain (Rushton, 1988). Although well-known nineteenth-century psychiatrists tried to introduce humanitarian reforms, with Phillippe Pinel in France famously removing patients' chains, and John Connolley in England opening the doors of the Middlesex asylum, physical restraint remained a central feature of the asylum regime well into the twentieth century. In the memoir of his madness published in 1840, the English aristocrat John Perceval described how he had been tied down to a bed for almost 9 months during his time at the Brislington asylum near Bristol (Perceval, 1961). Straight-jackets, introduced in the late eighteenth century and regarded as kinder than chains, continued to be used in some English and American hospitals until the 1950s, and seclusion was frequently employed to isolate and contain disturbed individuals (Alty and Mason, 1994). Sedative drugs were used with increasing frequency from the second half of the nineteenth century, including opiates, bromides, chloral hydrate and paraldehyde, which were 'welcomed for controlling severely disturbed patients' (Alty and Mason, 1994, p. 28).

Not everyone perceived drugs as preferable to physical methods, however. Like Thomas Szasz more than half a century later, Henry Maudsley, eminent psychiatrist and founder of the Maudsley hospital in London, suggested that drugs were welcomed more because they relieved the guilt of the custodians, than for their benefit to the patient. 'It was deemed better for the patient to let him have the relief and self-respect of pretty free exercise than to keep him tied up like a mad dog', he suggested. But, he continued, 'it may be doubted whether its coarse bonds did as much harm as has been done by the finer means of chemical restraint which have been used to paralyse the brain and to render the patient quiet' (Maudsley, 1895, pp. 554–555, cited in Braslow, 1997).

Contemporary psychiatric literature from the first half of the twentieth century had little to say about practices of control and restraint, however. This reticence is typified by the coverage provided in the first edition of *Henderson and Gillespie's Textbook of Psychiatry*. Although the authors expressed a commendable desire to reduce the use of force in psychiatric practice, there is almost no discussion about how to manage episodes of severely disturbed behaviour. In the chapter on schizophrenia, for example, it was recommended that 'episodes of violence should be treated with explanation, suggestion, analysis or, where necessary, by hydrotherapy[3] or drugs' (Henderson and Gillespie, 1927, p. 224), but no further details were provided about which drugs might be employed for this purpose or how they should be used. The chapter on *Manic-Depressive Psychosis* specifically suggested the use of hyoscine hydrobromide, a sedative drug, for use in emergencies, but no further details were provided.

Pharmaceutical companies, which, by the 1940s, were busy advertising barbiturates and stimulants for the mass market of 'everyday nerves', also apparently had no interest in the use of their products for the management of behavioural problems in people with severe psychiatric disorders prior to the advent of antipsychotics. In the psychiatric literature, the subject of how to manage disturbed behaviour continued to receive little attention throughout the 1950s and 1960s. In 1968 a rare review of the area entitled the *Comprehensive Management of Psychiatric Emergencies* made no mention of the use of drugs or other forms of restraint specifically except to say briefly that patients responded to 'supportive treatment such as talking, rest, sedation and, where indicated, food and fluids' (Frazier, 1968, p. 7).

It is only when looking at retrospective accounts written decades later, or speaking to people who recall the period, that the range of techniques of chemical and physical restraint employed in the first half of the twentieth century is revealed. Authors of an article published in 1972 recalled 'full restraints, maximum security chambers, frequent ECT and heavy sedation' as the 'traditional methods' of control prior to the advent of antipsychotics (Fann and Linton, 1972, p. 478). Retired psychiatrist John Bradley remembered the use of straight-jackets, as well as barbiturates and paraldehyde, from the time when he worked as a psychiatrist in the Royal Air Force in the 1950s. The use of intravenous and oral barbiturates and the sedative drug, paraldehyde, was referred to in later editions of *Henderson and Gillespie's Textbook*, supporting the idea that use of these drugs had been widespread, despite the fact they were not mentioned in earlier editions (Henderson and Gillespie, 1962).

Chemical Control Comes out of the Shadows

From the 1950s onwards, the therapeutic enthusiasm that accompanied the introduction of the physical treatment procedures like ECT and insulin coma therapy encouraged some authors to become more explicit in their descriptions of emergency sedation, while highlighting that the procedure was a precursor to proper therapeutic interventions. The authors of the textbook *Clinical Psychiatry*, who were fervent advocates of physical treatments, stressed in the first edition, published in 1954, that 'since the introduction of insulin and convulsion therapy, the symptomatic use of sedative drugs in schizophrenia has diminished in importance'. However, they believed it was 'still essential to know how to deal with the *emergency of an acute schizophrenic attack* in the patient's home so that he can be transported into an observation ward or a psychiatric hospital' (Mayer-Gross et al., 1954, p. 278, original emphasis). They recommended an intravenous injection of hyoscine for this purpose if the patient refused oral medication, but mentioned various other options, including paraldehyde and barbiturates. They also referred to the use of frequent ECT as a form of sedation for 'acutely excited schizophrenics', which could be applied once the patient had been brought into hospital (Mayer-Gross et al., 1954, p. 278).

The textbook emphasised that chemical sedation had the therapeutic purpose of rendering patients amenable to receive specific, targeted interventions, and, in the first edition, insulin coma therapy was the principle treatment recommended for people who were diagnosed with schizophrenia. By the publication of the second edition in 1960, anti-psychotics were said to be equal in effectiveness to insulin coma therapy as a treatment for schizophrenia (Mayer-Gross et al., 1960). In their description of the management of emergency situations, the authors still recommended hyoscine and other older drugs and, therefore, although the last edition published in 1969 recommended chlorpro-mazine as the first choice of drug in this context (Mayer-Gross et al., 1969), antipsychotics were first introduced as a wholly therapeutic intervention, before their use for behavioural control was considered.

Judging from pharmaceutical advertisements of the time, however, antipsychotics started to be used for purposes of emergency sedation as soon as they came into use. The pharmaceutical industry, having real-ised that the treatment of people with severe mental illness could be a lucrative market, identified behavioural management as an important component of psychiatric practice. The control of aggression or agita-tion started to be listed among the many suggested uses of antipsychot-ics in advertisements from the 1950s. In 1957, an early advertisement for promazine, a close relation of chlorpromazine, made reference to its use in 'controlling acute agitation', among other indications (Promazine advertisement, 1957). In 1957 an advertisement for the new phenothi-azine drug, Pacatal, included the statement that it could be used for 'the control of aggression, impulsiveness and overactivity, particularly in the over-50's' (Pacatal advertisement, 1957).

An early advertisement for the widely used antipsychotic drug Stelazine (trifluoperazine) promoted the drug primarily for behavioural control by featuring an illustration of a 'Squirrel cage'. The caption explained that the cage was used for 'calming mental patients (18th Century)', and the message of the advertisement appears to be that Stelazine had replaced the need for mechanical restraints like the cage (Figure 8.1) (Stelazine advertisement, 1959a). Interestingly, the advertisement was subsequently published in a slightly amended version, with a reference, in small print, to a preliminary report of a trial suggesting that regular oral medication

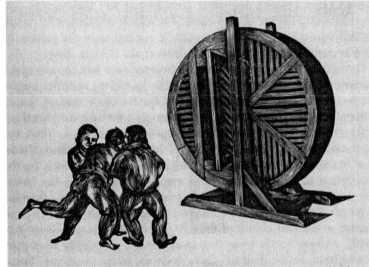

Squirrel cage used for calming mental patients (18th century). Original wood engraving by John De Pole.

STELAZINE

brand of trifluoperazine

the new psychotropic agent
specific for the
hallucinated, delusional, and
aggressive psychotic.

'Stelazine' is the most active phenothiazine available. It has brought about a return to normal in patients who have not responded to any other form of treatment — including not only other phenothiazines, but also insulin and E.C.T.

FORMULA : 2-trifluoromethyl-10-[3'-[3"-methyl piperazinyl-4"]-propyl] phenothiazine dihydrochloride.

Smith Kline & French Laboratories Ltd
Coldharbour Lane, London SE5
SZ.:PA108   'Stelazine' is a trademark

Figure 8.1   Stelazine advertisement
Reproduced with kind permission of GlaxoSmithKline.

with Stelazine was superior to medication given in an emergency or on an occasional basis (Stelazine advertisement, 1959b). This version of the advertisement could be interpreted as suggesting that behavioural control was no longer necessary because of the introduction of effective, therapeutic drug treatment, but, most likely, it was intended to be ambiguous and capture markets for both long-term and emergency treatment.

Subsequently, use of Stelazine for behavioural control was advertised separately from its long-term use, but, nevertheless, all Stelazine advertisements started to associate its use specifically with the treatment of people with a diagnosis of schizophrenia. One advertisement featuring a drawing of a patient being physically restrained by two male mental health staff suggested that 'the first consideration in treating the violently agitated and hostile schizophrenic is to calm, *restore insight, and establish rapport*' (Stelazine advertisement, 1965b, my emphasis) (Figure 8.2). In the 1960s, advertisements also started to portray emergency drug treatment as having the aim of rendering the patient fit to receive more lasting, therapeutic interventions.

Advertisements for haloperidol listed control of aggression among its many uses , and also emphasised its rapidity of action, a vital requirement for any drug that was to be useful in an emergency situation. The advertisements also described the effects of the drug on psychotic symptoms and subsequent outcome, and, by implication therefore, the utility of haloperidol for the management of aggression was suggested to be via its therapeutic effects on the underlying condition. A 1965 advertisement, for example, described how 'Serenace [one of the brand names under which haloperidol was marketed] quickly controls the psychotic manifestations of schizophrenia' (Serenace advertisement, 1965a). Another advertisement from this year prominently presented in large, bold text a quotation from a 1961 study describing how 'A very powerful, restless man, greatly feared by all the staff for his aggressive outbreaks and unreliability...became calm and kindly after receiving the preparation [of haloperidol]. Nowadays he sits with a contented smile and carries out simple hobby tasks' (Serenace advertisement, 1965b).

The use of drugs to control behaviour started to be discussed more frequently in psychiatric journals from the 1970s onwards, but articles adopted various strategies in order to emphasise the therapeutic aspects of emergency drug treatment and play down its coercive function. Many continued to stress that the purpose of emergency sedation was to make the patient more accessible to other, more specific and more lasting forms of treatment. A review of the management of 'acute behavioural disturbance' published in 1975, for example, described the

the first consideration in treating the violently agitated and hostile schizophrenic is to calm, restore insight, and establish rapport

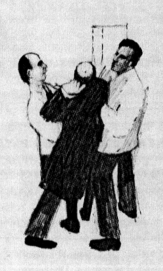

STELAZINE

quickly calms

the major tranquilliser with the invaluable alerting action—proved over the years by a wealth of clinical evidence
Literature containing prescribing information is available on request

SMITH KLINE & FRENCH LABORATORIES LTD Welwyn Garden City, Herts
'Stelazine' (brand of trifluoperazine) is a trade mark

SZ:PA835

Figure 8.2 Stelazine advertisement
Reproduced with kind permission of GlaxoSmithKline.

aim of emergency drug treatment as being the initiation of 'a treatment programme aimed at returning the patient to being a useful and healthy member of society' (Freed, 1975, p. 638).

Mirroring advertisements, recommendations became more diagnosis-specific and antipsychotics were frequently presented as suitable for emergency treatment of people diagnosed with schizophrenia in particular, allowing behavioural control to be aligned with the idea of treatment of the underlying condition. In this situation, emergency drug treatment was often presented as having therapeutic effects in its own right. One of the first papers to use the term 'rapid tranquillisation', for example, described a regime of intensive treatment with oral chlorpromazine, intended to tranquillise the patient within 6 hours. The purpose of the intervention was described as treating or controlling the 'psychotic state' itself, although it was also said to 'allow the patient to sleep as much as he likes'. Ultimately, however, the aim of drug treatment was said to be to enable the patient to undergo intensive 'psychotherapeutic efforts' (Polak and Laycob, 1971, p. 641). The authors of an article from 1974 also described a regime involving the administration of high doses of antipsychotics intended 'to promote the patients' rapid improvement', which they distinguished from the more common practice of general sedation or tranquillisation. They stressed that their method was 'by no means a chemical straightjacket' (Donlon and Tupin, 1974, p. 310).

In 1975, a special issue of the US journal, the *Journal of Nervous and Mental Disease*, was dedicated to the management of violence in psychiatric patients. The issue presented the management of aggression as a diagnosis-driven, therapeutic activity that should be targeted not at the behaviour itself, but at the underlying mental disorder (Lion, 1975). Drug treatment was not to be construed as a 'paralysing chemical straight jacket' but as a specific treatment for the condition that gave rise to the disturbed behaviour in the first place (Monroe, 1975, p. 119). Following an introductory article, the issue was divided up into papers discussing the use of different types of drugs, each relating to different diagnostic categories. The paper on the use of antipsychotics therefore dealt mainly with the treatment of violence in people with schizophrenia and psychotic disorders, although their use in people with dementia was also discussed briefly. Antipsychotics were deemed to be an appropriate treatment for violent behaviour committed by people with schizophrenia because they constituted a specific treatment, and the reduction in aggression that occurred was considered to be 'part of their antipsychotic properties'. The effects of antipsychotics were deemed to be 'due to the effect the drug has on the psychosis and not the aggression itself' (Lion, 1975, p. 76, 79). The paper on benzodiazepines mostly described research on the drugs' effects on hostility occurring in people diagnosed with anxiety, in whom the drugs were thought to exert a disease-specific action (Azcarate, 1975). There was also an article on the use of lithium and anticonvulsants, which proposed that some cases of aggressive behaviour were, like epileptic fits, caused by abnormal electrical discharges in the brain, which could be specifically treated by drugs that lowered the epileptic threshold. In the case of lithium, which is not an anticonvulsant, it was proposed that there was a reduction of the phenomena in some parallel but unspecified manner. The author of this article even denied that these drugs had any sedative or tranquillising properties, even though the well-known benzodiazepine sedative Librium (chlordiazepoxide) was one of the 'anticonvulsant' drugs referred to. The only subjective effect the drugs had, he claimed, was 'the relief sensed by the patient in no longer losing control when he otherwise would' (Monroe, 1975, p. 125).

A paper published in 1972 on the use of the antipsychotic drug perphenazine, subtitled 'The concept of chemical restraint,' was unusual for its time in its explicit description of the mechanism by which antipsychotics control excited and violent behaviour (Fann and Linton, 1972). The authors described how the 'drug-induced rigidity', or the 'Parkinsonoid state', produced by antipsychotics 'may not be deleterious' in emergency situations and that antipsychotics 'offer an excellent alternative to the physical measures that might otherwise be required in acute situations' (p. 479). While still emphasising that the purpose of tranquillisation was for the patient to be rendered able to participate in other therapeutic activities, the authors suggested that the 'ideal agent' for the purpose of chemical restraint 'should permit definite control of the patient's motor activity without reducing his mentation to the point where he cannot participate in ward activities' (p. 479).

They went on to present two case reports by way of illustration. One concerned a 44-year-old man who was said to be extremely 'threatening' to patients and staff. After administration of perphenazine, 'all of his movements became slowed, and though he continued to make verbal threats, he could no longer carry out physical violence...because of markedly reduced movements' (p. 480). The other concerned a 23-year-old man who was extremely hyperactive, and threatening staff and patients with a pool cue and pool balls. After taking perphenazine he showed 'retardation of hyperactive behaviour within 3 to 4 hours' and was described as 'markedly slowed', but able to continue to play pool safely (p. 480).

These descriptions highlight the general lack of coverage, which is evident in the psychiatric literature, of the properties of antipsychotics that make them effective restraining agents. The authors of the paper, however, were careful to draw a distinction between the immediate state of 'behavioural inhibition' that could be produced by the drugs and their 'antipsychotic effect' (p. 479), which was believed to occur more slowly. The idea that the antipsychotic effects of antipsychotic drugs do not start immediately, but occur only after a few weeks of treatment was an article of faith for many years, and calls into question the notion that use of the antipsychotics to induce rapid tranquillisation is a therapeutic intervention in its own right. A recent review of the evidence, however, contradicted this view. Psychotic symptoms are reduced from shortly after antipsychotic drugs are administered, following the same timescale as the sedation and physical restriction the drugs produce (Agid et al., 2003).

Research on 'Rapid Tranquillisation'

Forcing drugs on people to curb disturbing and challenging behaviour is a practice that rightly makes people feel uncomfortable. In the 1975 special issue of the *Journal of Nervous and Mental Disease* one author remarked that if this was the purpose of emergency sedation, it raised 'ethical questions as to when (if ever) it is justified to control behaviour through this type of chemotherapeutic intervention' (Monroe, 1975, p. 125). But the rise of the disease-centred model of drug action, and the idea that antipsychotics work by rectifying an underlying disease, helped to banish the spectre of the chemical straight-jacket and kept the genie of social control firmly inside the psychiatric lantern. Antipsychotics had finally made the practice of forced drugging respectable, and the control of aggression and disruptive behaviour by chemical means could be represented as a therapeutic activity that was part of, or a precursor to, condition-specific, restorative treatment. Neither the introduction of the drug droperidol into the UK in 1980 nor Clopixol Acuphase in 1990, both of which were aimed specifically at the market for short-term sedation, fundamentally altered the mainstream view that the use of drugs to control behaviour was driven and determined, like all psychiatric activity was said to be, by the process of diagnosis and the administration of specific treatment. The fact that in the early 1990s Clopixol Acuphase, a drug rarely given with anyone's consent, could be advertised as 'a harmonious new way to treat acute psychosis' demonstrates the success of the endeavour to reconstruct control and containment as medical treatment (Clopixol Acuphase advertisement, 1990) (Figure 8.3).

STORMS BLOW
FIND THE EYE
WINDS CHANGE
... REFLECT   (Anon)

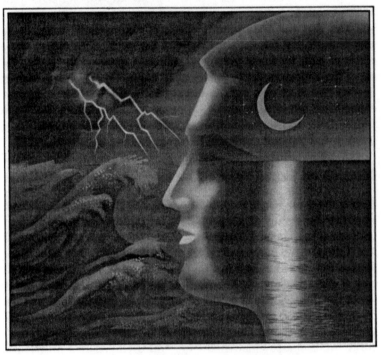

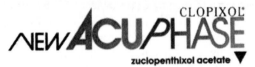

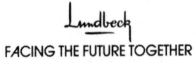

A harmonious new way to treat acute psychosis

FACING THE FUTURE TOGETHER

Further information is available on request from:
Lundbeck Ltd., Lundbeck House, Hastings Street, Luton BEDS LU1 5BE.

Figure 8.3 Clopixol acuphase advertisement
Reproduced with kind permission of Lundbeck.

As with other areas, the conviction that antipsychotics represent a disease-specific treatment for schizophrenia and psychosis meant their use for behavioural control went unexamined for many years. Only recently have large-scale studies been conducted that compare different pharmacological strategies for the management of aggression and disturbed behaviour. The overall results of seven studies comparing an antipsychotic, mostly haloperidol, and a benzodiazepine showed no differences in the ability of the two sorts of drug to produce sedation, reduce aggression and improve behaviour (Volz et al., 2007). Two large trials conducted in Brazil and India compared a benzodiazepine with a combination of haloperidol and promethazine, a cheap and popular mixture in these countries.[4] The Brazilian study found no difference between the haloperidol–promethazine combination and the effects of the benzodiazepine midazolam in achieving rapid tranquillisation, and there was no difference in the proportion of people in both groups who remained in hospital 2 weeks later; in other words, the use of antipsychotics for emergency sedation did not hasten improvement or discharge (TREC Collaborative group, 2003). The Indian study used lorazepam as the comparator and found that results were the same after 4 hours, but that the haloperidol–promethazine combination acted more rapidly, possibly owing to the fact that a relatively large 10-mg dose of haloperidol was used, compared with 5 mg in the Brazilian study. There were no differences in the proportion of people who required additional medication or physical restraint, however, and having a diagnosis of psychosis or schizophrenia did not affect how people responded to the different medications (Alexander et al., 2004). Although few side effects were reported in these particular studies, possibly because of the use of promethazine, in general a higher prevalence of movement abnormalities is associated with the use of antipsychotic drugs for rapid tranquillisation (Gillies et al., 2005). There was one case of potentially life-threatening respiratory depression with midazolam in the Brazilian study, and one epileptic seizure occurred in the haloperidol–promethazine-treated group (TREC Collaborative group, 2003).

There is no doubt that antipsychotic drugs like haloperidol can effectively tranquillise people and eliminate or reduce aggressive behaviour. They are a staple of veterinary medicine, where are also used for purposes of control and restraint, and where their ability to 'decrease motor function and reduce awareness of external stimuli' is well recognised (Bishop, 2005, p. 292). They are not necessarily the safest or most benign drugs to use in this situation, however. Although there have been few instances of cardiac complications in randomised trials of emergency sedation, other data suggest that antipsychotics are associated with sudden cardiac death (Ray et al., 2009), and one study found that the risk of having a cardiac arrest or a serious irregularity of heart rhythm (ventricular arrhythmia) with haloperidol was comparable to that with the antipsychotic thioridazine, whose use was restricted in 2001 owing to concern about its cardiac toxicity (Hennessy et al., 2002). The Maudsley guidelines now recommend that everyone who is commenced on haloperidol should receive an electrocardiogram (ECG), but this is rarely feasible in emergency situations (Taylor et al., 2009). Benzodiazepines appear to be just as effective in reducing disruptive or aggressive behaviour, and there is no evidence that giving antipsychotics ultimately improves outcome in people with a diagnosis of psychosis. Respiratory depression is a concern with the use of benzodiazepines, however, especially midazolam.

Although the ideal agent has yet to be found, overall the evidence does not support the idea that using antipsychotics in the control of aggressive or disruptive behaviour is superior to other pharmacological options for people diagnosed with psychosis or schizophrenia, or for anyone else. Apart from the potential dangers of antipsychotics, they are strongly disliked by recipients, but research has been slow to identify and evaluate alternative strategies. The popularity of antipsychotics for emergency sedation has been sustained by the perception that they are therapeutic agents, which has allowed the dangerous and unpleasant features of the drug-induced state they produce to be overlooked.

As Henry Maudsley suggested, we also need to ask whether chemical restraint is really superior to other strategies for the management of disturbed behaviour, such as mechanical restraints or safely modified seclusion rooms. Since forcing someone to take a drug infringes the integrity of the body and changes the person both physically and mentally, it can be viewed as a more profound violation of an individual's autonomy than putting them in a straight-jacket or a padded cell. Little effort has been paid to establishing patients' views, but one German study conducted in the 1980s found that most patients who had experienced some form of behavioural control clearly preferred the use of seclusion or physical restraint to being forced to take medication. Moreover, patients' opinions were established when they were in remission from the mental disturbance that had led to their confinement, so their views were not clouded by psychotic symptoms or emotional arousal (Schmeid and Ernst, 1983).

We have to ask, therefore, whether chemical sedation became the norm not because it benefitted patients, but because it suited the interests of other people, and of institutions. Chemical restraint is easier for hospital staff, who no longer have to wrestle patients into restraining devices or keep watch on them in isolation rooms, for example. It may be less distressing for relatives and friends not to have to witness the presence of people in manacles or cells, and the public too may prefer not to have to acknowledge that we have the same problems with managing disturbed behaviour as the Victorians had. Hospital staff have the right to be concerned about their vulnerability to violence in emergency departments and psychiatric facilities (Hansen, 1996), and they have a legitimate interest in finding ways to reduce incidents of aggression. We cannot properly evaluate the different options, however, unless we clearly acknowledge that the purpose of the intervention is to control unwanted behaviour, not to treat an illness.

Long-Term Behaviour Control

Although the claim that the forcible administration of drugs in emergency situations is a therapeutic activity that is hard to sustain, there is a more legitimate debate about the nature of antipsychotic treatment when it is given to someone against their wishes on a continuing basis. Psychiatric critics like Thomas Szasz have argued that *all* non-consensual drug 'treatment' should be considered a form of social control and that it consists of the drug-induced modification of behaviour that others find unacceptable. Mainstream opinion, however, regards such activity as medical treatment that is given to improve the patient's 'health', and this is the view that is enshrined in mental health law.

We saw in Chapter 7 how antipsychotic drugs can help to suppress otherwise irresistible psychotic experiences and by doing so can sometimes unlock people from the internal world that had engulfed them. Although some people ultimately welcome these effects, many people find they do not compensate for the state of demotivation and loss of interest the drugs produce. Like Peter Wescott, people sometimes talk of undergoing a personality change while taking the drugs, of becoming someone less interesting and less distinctive than they were before. Moreover, people who are deemed to have severe mental disorders often do not agree that there is anything wrong with their actions, even when their psychotic symptoms have subsided. Where people dislike the effects of the drug more than their symptoms, and where people do not wish to change their behaviour, it is difficult to see how it can be argued that 'treatment' is being imposed in their own interests.

Up until recent times, drugs could only be forced on people against their will while they were in a psychiatric institution or hospital. Once someone had recovered sufficiently to be discharged, they were free agents again and could stop taking their medication if they wished to do so, at least in theory. Research led by Manchester sociologist Anne Rogers showed that even in these circumstances, however, many people felt compelled to continue with their drug treatment when they wished to stop it, even though they were under no legal obligation to do so. The patients who were interviewed revealed that they were cajoled and pestered to take medication by mental health staff, and that they feared they would be taken back to hospital if they refused it. The researchers concluded that some patients had internalised the control that can be exercised through the Mental Health Act, and effectively policed their own medication intake, no longer believing they had any real choice in the matter (Rogers et al., 1998).

Many countries have now introduced legislation that enables people with mental health problems to be legally forced to continue treatment—usually drug treatment—after they are formally discharged from hospital. Community treatment orders were introduced into England and Wales in 2008, and, at first, the government anticipated they would only be applied to only a small fraction of patients. The orders were intended to be applied to the sort of people who had frequent admissions to hospital, sometimes referred to as 'revolving door' patients, and it was estimated that only around 450 orders would be applied in the first year. In reality 2134 orders were made in the first 5 months after the legislation came into force in November 2008. As of the end of March 2011, 10,071 orders had been made, with only 2210 of these being discharged. After taking account of patients who had been recalled to hospital, as well as discharges, 4291 patients remained subject to these powers in the community (NHS Information Centre for Health and Social Care, 2011).

The increasing numbers of people subject to enforced treatment in the community has not resulted in lower rates of compulsory hospital admission, however, despite initial hopes. Numbers of people being forcibly detained in psychiatric inpatient units also rose in the period leading up to 2011, with almost 50,000 compulsory admissions in the period 2010 to 2011 compared with only 46,500 in the 2006 to 2007 statistical year (NHS Information Centre for Health and Social Care, 2011). It appears, therefore, that compulsory community treatment is but one aspect of an increasingly coercive approach to mental health problems. Far from becoming a more voluntaristic enterprise, coercion still 'runs deep and wide' within modern systems of mental health care 'creating an unavoidable yet strangely silent climate of intimidation and acquiescence' (Kirk et al., 2013, p. 304).

The introduction of Community Treatment Orders extends the reach of chemical control far beyond the walls of institutions. The legislation enables mental health services, for the first time in history, to enforce drug treatment on people who have recovered from their mental break-down, who manifest no further symptoms and who are able to function perfectly well in their day-to-day lives. All that is needed to justify the application of an order is the idea that there is a chance that the individual will relapse at some point in the future. Although the threat of being dragged back to hospital hung over patients in the past, they were technically free to make their own choices about medication after they had been properly discharged from hospital, unless they had committed a serious crime and were subject to government supervision.[4] Community treatment orders mean that many people who do not wish to take drugs for the rest of their lives are no longer able to make that decision.

Yet, as we saw in Chapter 6, drug treatment does not eliminate the risk of relapse, it only reduces it, and, in fact, we are not even certain that this is the case owing to the confounding effects of antipsychotic withdrawal in studies of long-term treatment. Even if we assume that antipsychotic treatment does reduce the overall risk of having a relapse, however, this does not mean that everyone benefits from, or requires, long-term treatment. Even after several episodes the course of psychotic conditions is variable, and people may recover, but there is, in any case, no requirement in the law to restrict community treatment orders to people who have had many past episodes. They can be and are, in my experience, sometimes applied to people who have had little previous contact with psychiatric services. Enforcing drug treatment on people who will derive little or no benefit from it produces substantial costs for the individual who has to endure years of dangerous and unpleasant drug-induced stultification, and for society, which has to pay for the consequences of long-term antipsychotic treatment on people's physical health. It is also not clear why patients should not be able to make the choice to lead a drug-free life, accepting the increased risk of occasional episodes of mental illness which that decision might entail. This seems to be a rational and reasonable course of action, and unless there is good reason to think that the individual might commit a serious crime during an episode of mental disturbance, there can be no justification for the enforcement of drug treatment based on considerations of social order. It is only by misconstruing behaviour modification as 'treatment' that denying people this choice can be justified.

The fact that society has endorsed compulsory community psychiatric treatment may have little to do with 'treating' or helping the patient, however. There are economic and social reasons why society does not want people to relapse. It is cheaper to maintain patients in the community with chemical suppression and disability payments than to have to admit them to hospital, and it is less disturbing and more comfortable for the community for people to be subdued by drug treatment than subject to vagaries of mental disorder. Since the final closure of the old asylums in the 1980s and 1990s, there has been a continuing drive to reduce the costly process of treating people in hospital. 'Home treatment' teams were set up in the UK from the late 1990s in order to prevent people being admitted to hospital, and their main function has become persuading and cajoling people to take medication. There is also immense pressure to discharge people who are admitted to inpatient units as soon as possible, and community treatment orders are increasingly used to ensure that people who have not yet recovered from an episode of psychosis can be discharged early and continue to receive drug treatment. Although being allowed to go home may be preferable to the patient, as well as the hospital, they are then subject to on-going restrictions which may never be lifted, as it is notoriously difficult to challenge a community treatment order. If the patient remains well, this is taken as evidence that the order is working, but if the patient is not doing well, this can also be used as an argument that continuing restrictions are necessary.

A Conspiracy of Silence

Accounts of the drug-induced state produced by antipsychotic drugs set out in Chapter 7, and the one rare account of their use as a 'chemical restraint', suggest they are the ultimate chemical straight-jacket. Not only do they decrease arousal, like other sedatives, antipsychotics such as haloperidol restrict and inhibit physical movement itself, and all antipsychotic drugs produce an emotional state of indifference or placidity. Yet there is almost no reference to these qualities in the psychiatric literature, and the use of antipsychotics for rapid tranquillisation is justified instead by the idea that they are an effective and specific treatment for psychosis or schizophrenia. Even where the drastic alteration of behaviour produced by antipsychotics is undeniable, as in their use for emergency sedation, the disease-centred model of drug action has ensured that their psychoactive effects remain invisible.

In their book, *Mad Science*, American academic David Cohen and colleagues described how decreasing attention is paid to the mental and behavioural alterations produced by drugs throughout their course from the laboratory to the clinic. Drug companies test the effects of drugs on animal behaviour early on in their development, but the results of such tests are rarely published. Following this, studies on volunteers, known as phase 1 studies, are required to be performed as part of the licensing process, and some of these involve basic psychological tests, such as reaction times. Again, however, these studies are not frequently published and, when they are, only minimal data on selected physiological measures and test scores are presented. Phase 2 studies consist of randomised trials conducted to assess the efficacy of a drug in reducing symptoms of a particular condition compared to placebo. By focusing on the outcome of the diagnosed disorder, they provide no direct evidence about the alterations produced by the drug or drugs involved. Phase 3 studies consist of long-term safety monitoring that takes place after a drug has been licensed. The book concluded that 'the determination of equivalent or symmetrical psychoactive effects in human subjects as are definitely seen in animals is unsystematic at best, and in most cases of drugs intended for psychiatric use haphazard and possibly non existent' (Kirk et al., 2013, p. 257).

The report by the Medicines and Healthcare products Regulatory Agency, which formed the basis for the approval of risperidone in the UK, illustrates the banishment of psychoactive effects from serious consideration. The only statement about the subjective effects of the drug reads: 'Risperidone induced dose proportional CNS [central nervous system] effects such as tiredness, sedation, lethargy, fatigue, headache, dizziness, disorientation, impaired concentration, and migraine' (MHRA, 1992). No information on the drugs' effects on mood, attention, memory, clarity of thought, mental speed, emotional responsiveness, motivation, creativity or 'any other emotional or intellectual quality' (Kirk et al., 2013, p. 258) was presented, and no further details were provided about the effects described.

It seems extraordinary in the twenty-first century that people should be forced to take drugs which profoundly alter their bodily functions, their emotional life, their behaviour and personality, and that the institutions that instigate and enforce this 'treatment' have no interest in the range of effects the drugs produce and how they make people feel. The misrepresentation of the mental and behavioural modifications produced by psychoactive substances as the targeted reversal of underlying diseases has produced a scientific blind spot that means the full pharmacological effects of psychiatric medications are not properly investigated or appreciated. This ignorance means that the psychiatric community has been historically slow to recognise the serious medical complication that its drugs can produce, as we saw with the emergence of tardive dyskinesia. In the next chapter we shall see how it has been equally tardy in recognising other adverse effects, including those produced by the latest miracle cures, the atypical antipsychotics.

9
Old and New Drug-Induced Problems

As well as understanding the immediate effects produced by antipsychotic drugs and how these might impact on psychological symptoms and challenging behaviour, a drug-centred understanding focuses the spotlight back on the physical alterations that can result from taking these drugs, especially over long periods. Looking at how evidence of the serious complications of antipsychotic use emerged also reveals how modern psychiatry, sometimes, but not always, guided by the pharmaceutical industry, has constructed an agenda that enables it to avoid having to confront the harm its treatments can produce. As we saw with the story of tardive dyskinesia, tactics include blaming the underlying condition and minimising, obscuring or simply ignoring the evidence.

Antipsychotics and Brain Size

A startling example of these strategies can be seen in how research on brain volume has been handled. Despite the fact that evidence implicating antipsychotic use in the smaller brain size observed in people diagnosed with schizophrenia and other severe mental disorders has been available for decades, only in recent years have these findings been given any serious consideration. The significance of these effects is still barely discussed, however, and there has been no discernible impact on the use of these drugs in practice.

The occurrence of tardive dyskinesia confirms that antipsychotics can irreversibly alter the way the brain functions, and, as we saw in Chapter 6, tardive dyskinesia is not simply an isolated abnormality of movement but is associated with more generalised intellectual impairment. Further evidence for the detrimental effects of antipsychotic drugs started to be revealed with the introduction of sophisticated techniques for visualising the brain, beginning with computed tomography (CT) scans, which became available in the 1970s, followed by the technique called magnetic resonance imaging (MRI). Most CT and MRI studies suggest that people diagnosed with long-term schizophrenia have smaller brains and larger brain cavities, or ventricles, than a comparison group, usually consisting of staff from the hospital where the study was conducted. The majority of these studies involved people who had received many years of antipsychotic treatment, but there was a presumption that schizophrenia was the cause of any abnormal findings and a prejudice against any evidence that pointed towards the effects of drugs.

Two studies illustrate this tendency. The first is a well-known study conducted using CT technology in the 1980s by the research group at Northwick park hospital. The study revealed that long-term hospital patients diagnosed with schizophrenia had smaller brains and larger ventricles than patients with 'neurotic' conditions (depression, anxiety, etc.). There was no difference between the brains of people with schizophrenia and long-term patients diagnosed with manic depression (bipolar disorder), however (Owens et al., 1985). As patients with severe manic depression are also likely to be treated with antipsychotics, but those with neurotic disorder are not, this finding itself points to the possible role of drug treatment. In addition to this the strongest predictor of reduced brain volume in this study was the presence of drug-induced movement abnormalities, as measured by two separate scales developed for this purpose. The authors, however, assumed the abnormal movements were a symptom of schizophrenia. Based on a small analysis involving eight patients with schizophrenia, who had never taken antipsychotic drugs and were found not to differ in brain volume from eight fairly similar patients who had, they concluded that there was no relationship between drug treatment and brain volume. The small numbers of patients in this analysis meant only the grossest of differences would have been detected, however.

A more recent study, using MRI, found a similar overlap between patients diagnosed with schizophrenia and those diagnosed with 'bipolar disorder'. In people diagnosed with bipolar disorder, who were the focus of the paper, brain volume reduction was more likely to occur in people on higher doses of antipsychotic drugs ($p = 0.01$), but, again, the authors did not consider the possibility that the drugs directly affect brain size, suggesting instead that antipsychotic drug use was only a 'proxy for a more severe illness' (Arnone et al., 2009, p. 197).

This bias is repeated in longitudinal studies in which changes in brain size are tracked over time. One of the first of these longitudinal studies was conducted by psychiatrist Lynn DeLisi and colleagues based in SUNY University, New York. The study involved 50 patients who had experienced their first episode of a psychosis or schizophrenia-like condition, and a control group consisting of people without any known mental health problems. After 4 years the study revealed that the brain's cerebral hemispheres shrank by an average of 1.4% per year in the group with psychosis compared with 0.7% in the control group. With little consideration of the possible effects of drug treatment, the authors concluded that the study had demonstrated that a 'continual active abnormal process is occurring in the brain after the first episode of psychosis' (p. 136), and the paper was entitled 'Schizophrenia as a chronic active brain process: a study of progressive brain structural change subsequent to the onset of schizophrenia' (DeLisi et al., 1997).

The authors of a similar study, conducted in the Netherlands, examined the role of drug treatment more directly. The study involved 34 people with a first psychotic episode who were starting drug treatment and 36 'carefully matched' controls. The patients with psychosis showed a decline in the total amount of grey matter (nerve cell bodies[1]) in the brain of 2.9% over 1 year compared with the control group who showed a slight *increase* in grey matter volume (1.1%), and the difference was highly statistically significant ($p < 0.001$). There was a strong correlation between the cumulative dose of antipsychotic medication a patient had received over the follow-up year and the amount of reduction of brain grey matter (r = 0.45, df 31, $p = 0.009$) (Cahn et al., 2002). Despite finding this clear and strong association between brain shrinkage and antipsychotic use in the 1-year follow-up of this cohort of patients, reports of 5- and 10-year follow-ups have, surprisingly, not analysed drug treatment. When I queried this with the lead researchers from the group they did not provide an explanation nor did they indicate any intention to publish this information. When I requested the data in order to do it myself, they stopped responding to my enquiries.

Until recently, the effects of drug treatment continued to be dismissed, with researchers still attributing brain deficits to schizophrenia, citing as evidence Owens' eight non-drug-exposed patients, and the older air encephalography studies (Torrey, 2002). These studies, conducted in the middle of the twentieth century, involved injecting air into the brain cavities or ventricles to provide radiographic images of the brain, and some of these studies reported that the brains of long-term mental hospital patients were smaller than might be expected, and their ventricles larger (Lemke, 1936; Huber, 1957). Most studies did not include a control or comparison group , however, and many participants were likely to have endured intensive ECT or insulin coma therapy, procedures which were associated with enlarged ventricles in some studies (Storey, 1966). The one study which involved a comparison between mental hospital patients and a group of people with no known psychiatric disorder found no differences (Storey, 1966) and nor did one which compared patients with different psychiatric diagnoses (Peltonen, 1962).

In 2005 a large study was published which started to fracture the preceding consensus. The study was funded by Eli Lilly as a randomised comparison of olanzapine and haloperidol treatment in a group of patients experiencing their first episode of psychosis, and it was set up partly to examine whether the drugs reversed what was at this time assumed to be an underlying, disease-related process of brain degeneration. As well as 161 patients, a group of 58 healthy controls was recruited, and all participants had MRI scans at the beginning of the study, and then at 12 weeks and 1 year later. The chief investigator was Jeffrey Lieberman, one of the principle figures in academic psychiatry in the USA, and the results of the study were published in the *Archives of General Psychiatry*, the leading American psychiatric journal, in 2005. Considering that this is the largest imaging study ever conducted with people with a first episode of psychosis by a large margin, it received surprisingly little publicity, however.

The study revealed that people treated with haloperidol showed statistically significant shrinkage of the brain's grey matter after just 12 weeks compared with the control group, and at 1 year patients on both haloperidol and olanzapine showed reduced overall grey matter volume, with reductions apparent in most brain areas. However, although the reduction in brain volume in patients on olanzapine compared with controls reached conventional levels of statistical significance ($p = 0.03$), it did not reach the stricter criteria the study imposed to guard against chance findings. Although controlling for random positive outcomes is a worthy thing to do in other circumstances, when looking for potentially important adverse effects of drugs it is preferable to be less, not more, stringent. In this case, using the more restrictive criteria allowed the authors to present the study as if it were only haloperidol that was associated with brain volume reduction. They concluded that olanzapine, but not haloperidol, can prevent an underlying process of brain shrinkage and only briefly did they concede that the findings might indicate, alternatively, that the drugs themselves reduce brain size, although only haloperidol was mentioned in this respect (Lieberman et al., 2005).

Encouraged by the slight superiority demonstrated by olanzapine, Eli Lilly then funded a study using macaque monkeys, hoping that this would confirm that whereas the older drugs like haloperidol might diminish brain size, olanzapine did not. Unfortunately for Lilly the study provided the most incontrovertible evidence yet that both sorts of drugs cause brain shrinkage. The animals were treated with doses of olanzapine or haloperidol that were carefully tailored to be equivalent to the doses used in human patients, and compared with monkeys who were treated with a 'sham' pellet containing no drug. After being treated for between 17 and 27 months the animals were sacrificed and their brains examined. The brains of the monkeys that had been treated with haloperidol were 8.1% lighter than those who had not had drug treatment, and the brains of olanzapine-treated monkeys were 9.6% lighter. The difference between the drug-treated monkeys and non-drug-treated animals was statistically significant ($p = 0.04$), and the differences were present in all parts of the brain, but were most marked in the cerebral hemispheres—the seat of intelligence (Dorph-Petersen et al., 2005).[2]

As a consequence of this study, some researchers started to look at the evidence for a relationship between drug treatment and structural brain changes in human subjects. At last the issue of whether antipsychotics affected brain structure became a question that could be asked, even if people remained hesitant about answering it clearly. Most reviews of the area followed the lead of the Eli Lilly-funded study, suggesting that although the older drugs were associated with brain shrinkage, 'atypical antipsychotics might ameliorate structural changes caused by the disease process underlying schizophrenia' (Scherk and Falkai, 2006, p. 145). Other papers admitted that the drugs had effects on certain circumscribed brain regions, but played down the idea that they might have global effects (Navari and Dazzan, 2009; Smieskova et al., 2009). Much of the literature, however, continued the previous tendency of ignoring evidence of drug-induced effects or suggesting that drug treatment might reverse underlying changes (Hulshoff Pol and Kahn, 2008).

In 2010 I published a paper with a professor of anatomy, Jonathan Leo, which concluded, in typically hesitant academic language, that 'some evidence points towards the possibility that antispsychotics reduce the volume of brain matter and increase the fluid or ventricular space'. We even suggested that 'antipsychotics may contribute to the genesis of some of the abnormalities usually associated with schizophrenia' (Moncrieff and Leo, 2010). It was possible to publish this review because the editor of the journal, psychiatrist Robin Murray, had started to harbour suspicions that antipsychotics diminish brain size, and he published the paper despite opposition from most of the five referees it was sent to.

In 2011, the American group led by Nancy Andreasen, a leading researcher in biological psychiatry and one-time editor of the *American Journal of Psychiatry*, published the latest results of its long-term brain imaging study. These revealed a strong and statistically significant association between the dose of antipsychotic that someone had received over their lifetime and the amount of brain shrinkage detected. In contrast, the severity of symptoms and use of illicit drugs were not strongly associated with brain changes. The authors did not flinch from concluding that antipsychotics have a 'subtle but measurable influence on brain tissue loss over time' (Ho et al., 2011, p. 128). In their next paper, however, the researchers played down these findings, claiming that the process of schizophrenia itself was responsible for brain shrinkage, and barely mentioned the link with antipsychotic treatment demonstrated in the previous paper. The second paper claimed to have parcelled off the effects of drug treatment so that the remaining changes in brain volume could be attributed to the underlying disease (Andreasen et al., 2011). However, the analysis presented in the first paper consisted of a linear analysis of dose levels, which only detects effects that occur in a neatly incremental fashion, and it cannot be assumed to have captured the full effects of drugs. Only a comparison with a non-drug-treated group could reliably discount the impact of drug treatment.

A further animal study was published in the same year that corroborated the earlier macaque monkey study. Rats administered haloperidol or olanzapine in doses equivalent to those given to human patients showed 6–8% greater reductions in brain volume than rats given placebo, particularly in the cerebral cortex. The effects were seen after only 8 weeks, and they were apparent using brain scans and on post-mortem examination (Vernon et al., 2011). It now seems virtually indisputable that antipsychotics shrink the brain.

It is not necessarily the case, however, that a subtle reduction in brain size will inevitably affect mental functioning. The volume of the brain can vary considerably on a day-to-day basis, according to levels of hydration, for example. Several longitudinal and cross-sectional studies have found evidence of an association between impaired performance on mental tests and brain volume changes, however, in people diagnosed with schizophrenia (Sullivan et al., 1996; Gur et al., 1998, 1999; Ho et al., 2003). A recent study of patients with bipolar disorder also found a significant correlation between a reduction in intelligence quotient (IQ) and grey matter density loss in the temporal lobe in patients and controls (Moorhead et al., 2007). In contrast, an early study by Lynn DeLisi found no association between tests of cognitive function and brain volume loss (DeLisi et al., 1991).

Although it continues to be asserted that people with schizophrenia have abnormal brains irrespective of the effects of drug treatment, direct evidence for this claim relies on a small number of studies that have scanned patients with psychosis or schizophrenia prior to them receiving antipsychotic drugs. Despite the fact that these studies have failed to control for effects of intelligence, which is correlated with brain volume (Deary et al., 2010), and likely to differ between patients and controls (Woodberry et al., 2008), most have not reported the sort of global differences in brain size observed between medicated patients and controls. Some have detected differences in various local brain structures, but there is little consistency across studies in the area identified. The largest study with 'drug-naive' patients, for example, which was conducted in China and involved 68 patients and 68 controls, did not report any differences in overall brain matter, grey matter or ventricle volume, but detected some differences in areas of the right temporal lobe of the brain (Lui et al., 2009). This area was not found to be different from controls in three previous studies with antipsychotic-naive subjects, however (Salgado-Pineda et al., 2003; Jayakumar et al., 2005; Chua et al., 2007). The largest study to detect a difference in global brain grey matter and cerebro-spinal fluid volume involved 51 patients in its latest publication (Venkatasubramanian et al., 2008).

The most revealing of these studies are the ones that involved people who had been thought to be suffering from schizophrenia for some time. One of these involved 31 chronically ill, untreated patients in India. Overall, there were no statistically significant differences between patients and controls in the volume of both left and right cerebral hemispheres (which were a little *larger* in patients compared with controls), and left and right ventricular spaces (McCreadie et al., 2002).[3] The study was not reported as negative, however. Instead, the authors focused on some differences between controls and subgroups of patients with and without abnormal movements. Two other studies have been published involving patients who, as a group, had been considered mentally unwell for an average of 4–5 years, and neither reported any difference in global brain volumes (Buchsbaum et al., 1996; Ichimiya et al., 2001). Hence, the only three studies of patients whose duration of illness is comparable with patients who have taken antipsychotic drug treatment for some time report no major differences between patients and controls in the overall volume of the brain matter or brain cavities.

Peter Breggin first raised the possibility that the smaller brains and larger ventricles observed in people diagnosed with schizophrenia might be attributable to antipsychotic drug treatment in the 1980s (Breggin, 1983). Thirty years later, this possibility was finally conceded, but it is still not widely known or accepted. The researchers who uncovered evidence of this effect appear reluctant to discuss its implications, and clinical practice continues much as before. Perhaps this is not surprising as, like tardive dyskinesia, the implications for mainstream psychiatry are devastating. Far from rectifying underlying brain abnormalities, it appears that antipsychotic drugs may actually cause them. The principle treatment for severe mental disorder is not benign, but shrinks the brain and may impair mental functioning as a consequence. Moreover, since brain imaging studies were thought to demonstrate the pathology underlying schizophrenia, the revelation that their findings might be drug induced removes one of the main planks of the argument that schizophrenia is a straightforward brain disease.

Tardive Dyskinesia and 'Atypical' Antipsychotics

Although the significance of tardive dyskinesia has been minimised, as we saw in Chapter 5, it is still regarded as an undesirable condition that should be avoided if possible, and it was hoped and predicted that the new atypical antipsychotics would dispense with the problem. Early studies of people taking atypicals, many of which were conducted by the drug companies, suggested that overall the rate at which people developed tardive dyskinesia was about one quarter of the rate in people on the older drugs (Woods et al., 2010). Clozapine was thought to be particularly safe in this respect, and switching people on the older drugs to clozapine or other atypicals was recommended as a treatment for tardive dyskinesia (Tamminga et al., 1994; Spivak et al., 1997a).

A systematic review published in 2008 summarised the results of studies of tardive dyskinesia in people taking first- and second-generation antipsychotic drugs published since 2004, which had involved more than 28,000 participants in total (Correll and Schenk, 2008). The rate of new cases of tardive dyskinesia among people taking the older antipsychotics was 5.5% per year compared with 4.0% for people taking the newer drugs, but as people on the older drugs were older, and age is known to increase vulnerability to tardive dyskinesia, the difference between the two types of drugs may have been overstated in these data. Another study conducted by researchers at Yale University followed up 352 patients who were confirmed as being free from tardive dyskinesia.

The incidence of new cases over 4 years was around 20%, and there was little difference in rates of onset between people taking the old generation antipsychotics and those on atypicals. Moreover, people who were prescribed an old and a new antipsychotic concurrently were almost twice as likely to develop tardive dyskinesia as people taking the older drugs alone. When the authors compared the results to an older study conducted at the same location using the same methods, they found that the prevalence rate of tardive dyskinesia in the 1980s was 33% compared with 32% in the 2000s (Woods et al., 2010).

Tardive Dementia and Psychosis

Equally worrying, but more difficult to pin down for certain, is the idea that, as well as the movement disorder and accompanying mental decline that constitute tardive dyskinesia, long-term treatment with antipsychotics can lead to general intellectual impairment, behaviour and personality changes, and worsening of psychotic symptoms, even in the absence of tardive dyskinesia.

Evidence on the connection between antipsychotics and intellectual impairment is complex and difficult to interpret, and, again, little research has been dedicated to elucidating the impact of the drugs in comparison to the mountains of studies concerning the putative effects of schizophrenia. Often it is only when new drugs become the centre of attention that the adverse effects of the older ones are acknowledged.

The mental functioning of people who are acutely psychotic improves as their symptoms improve. This may indicate that drug treatment that suppresses psychotic symptoms improves people's ability to sit down and undertake a complex procedure like a test, but it may also reflect what is called a 'practice effect'. This is when subjects perform better the second time they do a test because of having done it before. Claims were made that atypicals were superior to the older antipsychotics in their ability to improve the psychological performance of people diagnosed with schizophrenia, but recent studies that have used more moderate doses of the older drugs suggest there is little difference (Keefe et al., 2006, 2007). However, as we saw in Chapter 8, there is ample evidence that antipsychotics impair mental functioning in animals and volunteers. Moreover, the mental capacity of older people with long-term schizophrenia correlates negatively with the dose of antipsychotic drugs they are taking (Torniainen et al., 2012), and although this may relate to many factors, such as the severity of symptoms, it is consistent with the other evidence that the drugs can impair mental abilities. People with Alzheimer's disease who are treated with an antipsychotic for example—whether of the new or old variety— show greater cognitive decline than those who are not (Schneider et al., 2005). In one study the intellectual deterioration due to antipsychotic treatment was equivalent to the 1 year's worth of dementia-induced decline (Vigen et al., 2011).

Some research also suggests that long-term antipsychotic use may provoke a characteristic change in personality or behaviour, and that it may worsen the symptoms of psychosis. In the 1980s and 1990s a behavioural syndrome was described called 'tardive dysmentia', which was thought to occur with and without the presence of tardive dyskinesia. A paper published in 1983 described the characteristic features as 'unstable mood, loud speech, and inappropriately close approach to the examiner' (Wilson et al., 1983, p. 18), and a later report summarised the features as consisting of excessive emotional reactivity, enhanced responsiveness to environmental stimuli and a reduced awareness of abnormal movements of tardive dyskinesia if these are present (Myslobodsky, 1993). Features such as heightened tension, aggression and a background mood of mild elation were also noted to occur. The researchers suggested that the syndrome was a consequence of organic brain damage induced by long-term antipsychotic treatment, and they pointed to similarities between the characteristics of 'tardive dysmentia' and behaviours associated with brain injury, especially injuries that affect the frontal lobe of the brain. The reduced awareness of abnormal movements is well recognised in tardive dyskinesia and reminiscent of the denial of disability that occurs in other severe brain conditions such as stroke (when it is usually associated with damage to a specific brain region—the parietal non-dominant lobe) and generalised brain diseases, such as neurosyphilis and Korsakoff's disease (Breggin, 1997).

We have already come across evidence that long-term antipsychotic treatment might provoke a psychotic episode either after withdrawal or during the course of long-term treatment. This issue is difficult to investigate because, without starting volunteers on years of antipsychotic treatment, it is impossible to know for certain whether the worsening of psychosis that can occur in later years in some patients who were previously stable, is due to the drug treatment or merely the natural course of their underlying condition. Unlike physical brain changes, it is difficult to investigate in animals because they do not experience psychosis, although behavioural changes in animals subjected to years of antipsychotic exposure might be informative, given that this could not be done in healthy humans. Obviously, it is of the utmost importance to know whether the drug treatment of psychosis ultimately makes the problem worse in some people.

Evidence that long-term antipsychotic treatment might provoke mental decline, personality change and psychotic deterioration should be, but rarely is, a major consideration when starting people on antipsychotic drugs in the first place, and in decisions about whether to continue them or not. For people who recover from their psychotic episodes, these prospects, even if not proven at present, must be a factor in weighing up the pros and cons of continuing to take antipsychotic treatment on a long-term basis. For people who suffer from enduring psychotic symptoms that the drugs help to suppress, there may be no other option.

Metabolic Effects

All antipsychotics cause people and animals to put on weight, although some have a stronger effect than others. In the 1990s it became apparent that some of the newer antipsychotics cause people to put on even more weight than usual, sometimes becoming massively and morbidly obese. The effect was first apparent in relation to clozapine, with clozapine-treated patients putting on weight at an average of 7.7 kg in 6 months in one study (Lamberti et al., 1992) and 3 kg over 3 months in another (John et al., 1995). Indications that patients on clozapine were vulnerable to developing diabetes also started to accumulate, including case reports of people who had developed the severe and life-threatening complication of this condition known as diabetic keto-acidosis (Kamran et al., 1994; Koval et al., 1994). By the late 1990s, it was apparent that other atypical antipsychotics had similar effects, especially olanzapine. In one 6-month study patients on olanzapine gained 4 kg (McQuade et al., 2004). Epidemiological data suggested that atypial antipsychotics in general increased the risk of developing diabetes by a third (Sernyak et al., 2002). There were reports of diabetic keto-acidosis occurring in people started on olanzapine (Goldstein et al., 1999; Lindenmayer and Patel, 1999) and laboratory studies suggesting olanzapine's effects on the body's regulation of glucose were more marked than those of other antipsychotics (Newcomer et al., 2002).

Eli Lilly's attempts to play down the metabolic effects of olanzapine were revealed in an article in the *New York Times* in 2006, based on the content of confidential documents that were obtained in the course of legal proceedings brought by patients who claimed that they had developed diabetes or other medical complications as a consequence of taking olanzapine. The article suggested that even as Eli Lilly continued to claim that scientific evidence had not established that olanzapine causes diabetes, its scientific employees had been concerned about the implications of 'olanzapine-associated weight gain and possible hyperglycaemia' since 1999 (Berenson, 2006). In this year Lilly established an 'executive steering committee' to manage the issues associated with these adverse effects, and, in 2001, an 'action team for quick medical response to customers with Zyprexa safety questions' was proposed (Eli Lilly, 2001a, cited in Spielmans, 2009). The *New York Times* article claimed that sales people were instructed not to introduce the subject of weight gain and diabetes in presentations on Zyprexa, however, unless it was raised by the audience (Berenson, 2006).

Eli Lilly employed another time-honoured tactic that has not been fully exposed, however—blaming the condition. The leaked Zyprexa documents referred to evidence that diabetes is more common in people with mental disorders compared with the general population, and suggested that psychiatric illness might itself be linked to the condition (Eli Lilly, undated). In the early years of the twenty-first century Lilly paid doctors to do 'educational' presentations on the link between schizophrenia and diabetes, some of which I attended. While most academics were writing about the metabolic effects produced by antipsychotic drugs, Eli Lilly employees and consultants produced articles describing schizophrenia as a 'risk factor' for diabetes (Dinan, 2004b; Holt et al., 2005). The company also supported research that reported that there was abnormal glucose metabolism in people with psychosis before starting drug treatment (Ryan et al., 2003), although these findings were later refuted by a larger study published in 2008 (Sengupta et al., 2008).

In October 2003 Eli Lilly sponsored a 'consensus meeting' of academics led by Ted Dinan, professor of psychiatry in Dublin, Ireland, and the meeting resulted in the publication of a supplement of the *British Journal of Psychiatry* entitled 'Schizophrenia and diabetes'. In his introduction to the issue, Dinan barely mentioned the role of antipsychotic drugs except to say that two articles in the supplement challenged the idea of a link between antipsychotics and diabetes (Dinan, 2004a). One of the opening papers reviewed historical evidence, which was claimed to demonstrate that 'diabetes and disturbed carbohydrate metabolism may be an integral part of schizophrenia', although the author admitted that the evidence was anecdotal and inconclusive (Kohen, 2004). Three articles in the supplement, two of which were authored or co-authored by Eli Lilly employees and the other by an academic with financial ties to Lilly, claimed to show that the data suggesting a relationship between antipsychotic treatment and diabetes were flawed, and that data from randomised controlled trials did not indicate a link (Bushe and Holt, 2004; Bushe and Leonard, 2004; Haddad, 2004). As the authors of one of the papers admitted, however, clinical trials are far too short to detect a condition like diabetes, which usually takes years to develop (Bushe and Leonard, 2004).

The concluding statement of the conference reveals its real aims. Entitled a 'Consensus summary', the statement conceded that the 'available evidence supports an association between antipsychotics and impaired glucose metabolism' (Expert Group, 2004, p. S112). However, it continued, the evidence 'does not establish causality' (p. S113). The statement suggested that clozapine might have a stronger relation than other antipsychotic drugs with diabetes and incipient diabetes, but did not mention olanzapine. It was concluded that severe mental illness itself, and the associated unhealthy lifestyle, likely played a more significant role in the high prevalence of diabetes in people with mental illness than antipsychotic drugs (Expert Group, 2004).

Despite these efforts, by 2007 Eli Lilly had paid out $1.2 billion to settle claims made by people who contended that they had developed diabetes or other medical complications through taking olanzapine (Berenson, 2007). The debate about diabetes and schizophrenia took place largely within the academic literature and at professional gatherings, and so this aspect of Eli Lilly's strategy has not been fully appreciated.

Psychiatrists had set a precedent for this tactic with tardive dyskinesia. Just as the gravity of this neurological condition had been minimised, the metabolic effects of the atypical antipsychotics were temporarily obscured by focusing on a possible link with schizophrenia itself, thus minimising the potential backlash that may have occurred as the impact of these drug-induced effects became increasingly apparent. As evidence accumulated that the drugs induce metabolic disturbance in volunteers (Sacher et al., 2008; Albaugh et al, 2011) and people with other diagnoses (Chien et al., 2010; Andrade et al., 2011), it became increasingly difficult to sustain the argument, and in 2008 David Healy and colleagues reported that none of the people treated in hospital for a psychotic disorder between 1894 and 1924 had diabetes on admission, and none were diagnosed with the condition throughout 15 years of follow up. Moreover, no one hospitalised with psychosis between 1994 and 2006 had diabetes at the time of admission, but they developed diabetes at twice the rate of the general population over the next few years (Le Noury et al., 2008). The idea of an intrinsic link between diabetes and schizophrenia faded out of the psychiatric consciousness from around 2005, its plausibility exhausted. Its purposes were already served by this time, however, as Zyprexa had become one of the world's biggest ever selling drugs.

Current data suggest that all antipsychotics, except, perhaps, aripiprazole (Abilify) have a tendency to make people put on weight, an effect that increases with dose, and that it is greatest with olanzapine and clozapine (Rummel-Kluge et al., 2010; Correll, 2011). Most atypicals make people more vulnerable to developing diabetes, but again clozapine, olanzapine and, to a lesser extent risperidone and quetiapine, confer the greatest excess risk (Ramaswamy et al., 2006; Yood et al., 2009). It also appears that interference with the body's mechanisms for sugar and carbohydrate regulation is part of a wider picture of metabolic disruption that antipsychotic drugs induce. They affect fat metabolism as well, for example, leading to increased levels of harmful fats like cholesterol (Rummel-Kluge et al., 2010; Smith et al., 2010; Chaggar et al., 2011). Moreover, studies involving healthy volunteers have demonstrated that the metabolic abnormalities develop rapidly, after short periods of drug treatment and long before weight changes appear (Albaugh et al., 2011).

Children appear to be particularly susceptible to the metabolic complications of the new antipsychotics. They gain more weight and are even more likely to develop diabetes in relation to the norms for their age than adults taking these drugs. Again, clozapine and olanzapine are the worst culprits (De Hert et al., 2011; Pringsheim et al., 2011). A meta-analysis of data from randomised controlled trials found that children started on olanzapine gained an average of 6–7 kg within 8 weeks of starting treatment, and children on risperidone gained 1.7 kg in 12 weeks (Pringsheim et al., 2011). An analysis of a large amount of data from children taking atypical antipsychotics, mostly for behaviour problems and 'mood disorders' rather than schizophrenia or psychosis, found that rates of diabetes were more than three times higher than in children who were not prescribed medication, and more than twice as high as children who were taking antidepressant drugs (Andrade et al., 2011).

Heart Disease and Death

The metabolic effects of antipsychotics are significant not only for the direct discomfort they produce, but because they are recognised risk factors for heart disease, stroke and premature death. People who have what is sometimes called 'metabolic syndrome', for example, which is defined as increased weight and high blood pressure combined with abnormalities in blood glucose and fat concentrations, have twice the risk of developing coronary heart disease over 10 years compared with people without this syndrome (Correll et al., 2006).

As well as disrupting metabolic processes linked with atherosclerotic heart disease (the silting up of the hearts' blood vessels), antipsychotics are also known to interfere with the electrical conductivity of heart muscle, causing prolongation of the 'QT' interval on the electrocardiogram (ECG). This disturbance is known to be associated with irregular heart rhythms, which can lead to sudden death. Studies of people who die suddenly owing to heart disease or malfunction show that people taking antipsychotics have a 2–3-fold higher risk than people who are not taking these drugs, taking into account other relevant factors (Straus et al., 2004; Ray et al, 2001, 2009). The increased risk is the same for people diagnosed with schizophrenia as it is for people who are prescribed the drugs for other diagnoses like dementia (Straus et al., 2004). In one study the rate of 'sudden cardiac death' was found to be similar in users of atypical antipsychotics compared with users of the older antipsychotics, and for all types of drug, except clozapine, there was a strong relationship with dose (Ray et al., 2009) (Figure 9.1). People on the highest doses of atypical antipsychotics, for example, were almost three times more likely to die in this way than non-users, whereas those on the lowest doses were only one and a half times more likely to die (Ray et al., 2009). A dose-related trend of this sort is regarded as one of the strongest indicators of a true causal link in medical research.

Further evidence of the detrimental effects of antipsychotic drugs on the cardiovascular system comes from studies of their use in people with dementia. In the late 1990s and early 2000s several trials were conducted examining the effects of atypical antipsychotics in controlling aggression and disturbed behaviour in people with dementia, many of whom were residents in nursing homes. Most of these studies were never published, but data provided by the manufacturers to the drug regulatory agencies in Canada, the USA and Europe indicated that people in these trials who were randomised to drug treatment rather than placebo had an increased risk of having a stroke or a transient ischaemic attack (a TIA),[4] and were more likely to die during treatment. The early data were derived from trials of risperidone and then olanzapine, but by 2005 there were data from trials of quetiapine and ariprirazole indicating the same trends (Mittal et al., 2011).

Subsequent reviews have confirmed these findings, although most of the data remain unpublished. An analysis of data from 16 studies,

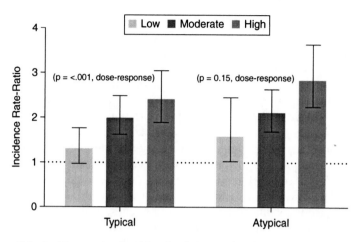

Figure 9.1 Incidence rate of sudden death in people taking antipsychotic drugs compared with people not taking them
From New England Journal of Medicine, *Ray et al. (2009) Atypical antipsychotic drugs and the risk of sudden cardiac death. 260, 225–35. Copyright © 2009 Massachusetts Medical Society, reprinted with permission from Massachusetts Medical Society.*

only five of which had been published in full in peer-reviewed journals, found an increased risk of stroke in people taking atypical antipsychotics, in dementia compared with placebo, and an increased risk of death. Moreover, the drugs produced only a slight improvement in aggressive behaviour, with greater intellectual deterioration in people taking the drugs compared with those on placebo (Schneider et al., 2005, 2006). Only one randomised study included patients who were prescribed the older antipsychotics. This consisted of a withdrawal trial in which people who had already been started on antipsychotics were randomised to two groups, one of which continued on their antipsychotic treatment, and one of which had the drugs gradually withdrawn and replaced by placebo. Patients who continued taking antipsychotics of whatever variety showed increased mortality compared with those who were withdrawn. The study also revealed that the excess mortality in those taking antipsychotics widened with time, so that 12 months after the study began the difference in survival between those taking antipsychotics and those who were switched to placebo was 70% versus 77%, but 24 months after the study began only 46% of those taking antipsychotics were still alive compared with 71% of those who were not taking them. At 3 years the difference was 30% versus 59% (Ballard et al., 2009).

Un-randomised, observational studies also suggest that the older antipsychotics cause stroke and increase mortality in people with dementia, so that it is not an effect that is unique to the new generation of drugs (Mittal et al., 2011). Nevertheless, the atypical antipsychotics have been the main focus of concern, as they were heavily and illegally promoted for the treatment of people with dementia despite the fact that they were never licensed for this indication.

It has been known for a long time that people with severe mental conditions like schizophrenia have a shorter life-span than the general population. The majority of their excess mortality is attributable to heart disease (Osby et al., 2000), and the role of drug treatment in hastening death in this group of people has been the subject of much debate. Undoubtedly, factors such as high rates of smoking and lack of exercise contribute to the problem, but evidence also implicates antipsychotic drugs. Authors of a recent review on the subject concluded that, despite the dearth of research, there was enough evidence to suggest that long-term exposure to antipsychotics is likely to increase the risk of dying prematurely (Weinmann et al., 2009).

Several studies have found that the death rate among people diagnosed with severe mental disorders is proportional to the dose, or to the number, of antipsychotic drugs that patients take (Waddington et al., 1998; Bralet et al., 2000; Joukamaa et al., 2006). A Finnish study revealed that each additional antipsychotic drug taken increased the risk of premature death by two and a quarter times compared with the general population after taking account of some other risk factors, such as smoking (Joukamaa et al., 2006). Another study from Finland, however, reported that people with schizophrenia who had *not* taken antipsychotics had a higher death rate than those who used this medication on a long-term basis. The authors suggested that this surprising result might reflect the ability of drug treatment to reduce the risk of suicide in people diagnosed with schizophrenia (Tiihonen et al., 2009), but the paper has been the focus of much debate. An extensive critique of the study argued that the results were impossible to interpret because a large proportion of deaths were excluded from the analysis because they had occurred in hospital, where data on prescribing were incomplete (De Hert et al., 2010). Moreover, the analysis was complex and opaque, with no figures provided for the actual numbers of deaths in the different groups of patients. The critics also pointed out that although the study reported that a large proportion of patients with schizophrenia had never used antipsychotic drugs, findings from the same research group indicated that data on medication use were highly unreliable.

Between 49% and 96% of patients who were classified as not taking antipsychotics were, in fact, taking them, for at least some of the time (Tiihonen et al., 2006; Haukka et al., 2008).

There is no doubt, therefore, that antipsychotic drugs have dangerous effects. There is substantial evidence that both the old and the new generation of antipsychotics cause irreversible neurological damage in the form of tardive dyskinesia, shrink the size of the brain, cause people to put on weight, disrupt the body's metabolic processes, heighten the risk of heart disease and stroke, and cause premature death, at least in some groups of people. Although the appropriate response to such toxic substances would be to reserve them for the most extreme and irresolvable circumstances, recent trends have been for antipsychotics to be prescribed to increasing numbers of people for increasingly vague and varied problems. This movement has been driven by claims that antipsychotics are good for the brain, but, as we have seen, there is considerable evidence that they are bad for it, and for the body. This is not to say that for someone trapped in the throes of severe mental derangement the drugs might not be the lesser of two evils, but an evil they are nonetheless.

10
The First Tentacles: The 'Early Intervention in Psychosis' Movement

When the new atypical antipsychotics were brought to the market in the 1990s, the first objective from a marketing perspective was to replace the use of the older generation of antipsychotics drugs. Alongside this takeover bid came the desire to expand the market for the drug treatment of schizophrenia to its limits, and in this aspiration was nurtured the 'Early Intervention in Psychosis' movement. The movement was so successful that it ushered in a completely different 'ethical paradigm' in the treatment of people with psychosis (McGlashan, 2005), overturning the previous consensus that symptoms should be given a chance to resolve spontaneously before antipsychotic treatment was started. Instead, it came to be accepted that young people who were experiencing a psychotic episode, or just some psychotic symptoms, or occasionally some vague problems that may or may not be psychotic symptoms, should be started on antipsychotic medication as soon as possible. It was widely believed that early treatment was needed to arrest the progress of a degenerative brain disease, and it became increasingly difficult for patients and their advocates to argue against the use of medication. The balance of considerations was firmly tilted in favour of drug treatment, despite the emerging evidence of its serious and life-threatening consequences.

Treating people early on in the course of their mental condition has been a longstanding obsession of the psychiatric profession and its sponsors. Historically, the idea of 'early intervention' was strongly linked to arguments about the medical nature of mental disturbance—the idea that 'mental illness is a disease like any other'. As insanity was increasingly claimed to arise from a disease of the body or brain, medical intervention was presented as something that could modify the underlying course of the disease, rather than acting as a band-aid that merely suppressed on-going symptoms. Early treatment was a natural corollary of this view, as it is generally thought desirable to arrest a disease process as early as possible. In more recent times, American psychiatrist Jeffrey Lieberman, who became one of the most prominent advocates of early intervention, proposed that the rapid initiation of antipsychotic drugs in people with schizophrenia or psychosis could 'ameliorate the underlying pathophysiology, forestalling the progression of the disease and preventing morbidity from increasing' (Lieberman, 1999a, p. 732). The enthusiasm for early intervention is thus another manifestation of the desire to have specific treatments that target underlying diseases, in other words for a disease-centred model of psychiatric treatment.

The last two decades have witnessed fevered activity in support of the idea of early intervention in incipient psychosis or schizophrenia. Dedicated services have emerged in many parts of the world, publications have proliferated, an international association for early intervention has been formed and a specialist journal was launched in 2007. In 2005, early intervention was declared to be an idea 'whose time has come' that had captured the imagination of clinicians, researchers, families and politicians (McGorry et al., 2005, p. S1). While the recent Early Intervention movement has various drivers, including the commendable desire to offer more support to families, it has been strongly associated with the rise in popularity of the atypical antipsychotics, and the companies that developed these drugs have provided financial support for discussions, conferences, projects and academic organisations concerned with Early Intervention in Psychosis. Critics have emerged, however, who have pointed to the dangers of drawing more and more people into the net of long-term drug treatment (Warner, 2005; Bosanac et al., 2010).

The History of Early Intervention

According to historian Andrew Scull, 'throughout the 19th century, it was an article of faith among those who dealt with lunatics that the deranged were more readily restored in the early stages of the disorder, so that delay in help could prove disastrous' (Scull, 1993, p. 163). One of the decisive arguments in bringing about the country-wide asylum building programme in the UK in the mid-nineteenth century was the idea that properly-run asylums would encourage people to seek help for themselves or their disturbed relatives before they descended into a hopeless and irremediable condition. Later on in the century, when it became apparent that the asylums were silted up with people with chronic, intractable difficulties, and more people died in the asylum than recovered, psychiatrists continued to blame the fact that people did not come to them early enough (Scull, 1993, p. 275).

In the early twentieth century there was increasing interest in public health, and renewed optimism about the possibility of preventing various physical diseases and social problems through early treatment or intervention. The famous Maudsley hospital, set up in London in 1907, was designed specifically to cater for early and acute cases of mental disturbance, and had special exemption from the requirement of the 1890 Lunacy Act for patients to be 'certified' insane prior to admission, in order to avoid delays in treatment. The Macmillan Commission, which reviewed mental health legislation in England in the early 1920s, memorably declared that 'there is no clear demarcation between mental and physical illness' and emphasised the importance of 'prevention and treatment'. The Commission aspired to design a new parliamentary Act that would make it possible to provide treatment for mental illness 'from the very earliest moment of the appearance of its symptoms' (Royal Commission, 1926; cited in Unsworth, 1987, p. 115). These concerns continued to motivate changes in mental health legislation up until the 1959 English Mental Health Act, which, by finally abolishing the role of the magistrate in admission proceedings, was designed to minimise legal bureaucracy and provide more rapid access to treatment (Jones, 1972).

In the nineteenth century early intervention formed one of the principle arguments for the erection of the asylums. In the late twentieth century it was used, among other arguments, to justify the policy of deinstitutionalisation and the replacement of the asylums with community care. The asylums were regarded as outdated and stigmatising, and general hospitals were proclaimed to be the best place to care for people with mental health problems. 'Community care', as visualised by the government of the UK, would provide early intervention and preventive work within the community which would be possible because the looming fear of the asylum would no longer discourage people from obtaining psychiatric help (Boardman, 2005).

The modern early intervention movement has also been associated with an optimistic view of the possibilities of psychiatric treatment. Proponents of the concept wanted to offer people who suffered from psychotic episodes and their families 'a more positive future' (McGorry et al., 2005, p. S1). The services that started to be set up in the 1990s were designed to provide tailored support that would be more acceptable and less stigmatising than intervention from generic mental health teams, with the hope that this would entice more young people into mental health services, and relieve the burden on families struggling to cope with a young person's worrying behaviour. This motivation was combined, however, with the questionable and contentious proposition that psychosis is a 'biologically toxic' process that causes progressive damage to the brain unless averted by selective drug therapy (Wyatt, 1991, p. 347).

In 1991 American psychiatrist Robert Wyatt published a lengthy review of evidence for the impact of drug treatment on the outcome of schizophrenia, concluding that 'early intervention with neuroleptics in first break schizophrenia patients increases the likelihood of an improved long-term course' (Wyatt, 1991, p. 325). None of the numerous studies Wyatt described provided evidence to support this claim, however, and many contradicted it. He cited the Chestnut Lodge study, for example, which showed that in this specialist psychotherapeutic institution people with a short duration of symptoms prior to admission (less than 1 year) had a good long-term outcome despite *not* being treated with antipsychotics, compared with those who had a longer duration of pre-admission symptoms (more than 1 year), who had worse outcomes even though they *did* receive antipsychotics (Fenton and McGlashan, 1987). The only study he cited on early drug treatment was small, excluded people with a poor outcome and was never fully published (Anzia et al., 1988). Nevertheless, Wyatt concluded that the evidence he had mustered suggested there might be 'something about being psychotic that is toxic to the individual beyond the immediate psychotic episode', which, he proposed, could be reversed or prevented by the early initiation of drug treatment (Wyatt, 1991, p. 347).

Despite its deficiencies, Wyatt's paper had a seminal influence on the burgeoning early intervention movement and was repeatedly referred to as a 'landmark' paper (McGorry et al., 2005, p. S2). Wyatt himself became a major player in the International Early Psychosis Association and after his death his colleagues demonstrated their respect by dedicating the third conference of the Association to his memory.

In 1992 a group led by Jeffrey Lieberman followed up 70 patients with a first psychotic episode and found like the Chestnut Lodge study, that those whose symptoms had started a longer while before admission had a worse outcome. They concluded that 'duration of psychosis before treatment could be an important predictor of outcome in first episode schizophrenia. Acute psychotic symptoms could reflect an active morbid process, which if not ameliorated by neuroleptic drug treatment, may result in lasting morbidity' (Loebel et al., 1992, p. 1183). Despite the fact that the prevailing view of the time was that schizophrenia was a 'neurodevelopmental disorder', which was present, although not manifest, from birth, the importance of shortening the 'duration of untreated psychosis' soon became an article of faith, spawning an enormous amount of discussion and research.

By the mid-late 1990s editorials and reviews routinely emphasised the association between duration of untreated psychosis and outcome, and the importance of starting drug treatment early (Wyatt, 1995; Birchwood et al., 1997; Sheitman et al, 1997; Lieberman, 1999b). Lieberman increasingly referred to psychosis itself as a 'degenerative process' that was operative when symptoms were present, but could be curtailed by drug treatment (Lieberman, 1999a, 1999b). He also started to suggest that delaying drug treatment could reduce its effectiveness, so that people who were not treated early would be more likely to become 'treatment resistant' (Lieberman et al., 1998). It was proposed that there might be a 'critical period' of around 5 years when the course of the disorder is most amenable to intervention (Birchwood et al., 1997). In 2005, reviews published in the top two American psychiatric journals concluded that shortening the duration of untreated psychosis by early initiation of drug treatment improved outcome and was an important objective for clinical care (Marshall et al., 2005; Perkins et al., 2005).

There is another simple explanation for Lieberman's original findings, however. It has long been recognised that people who are subsequently diagnosed with schizophrenia, whose symptoms develop slowly over the course of many months, have a worse outlook than those in whom symptoms occur more rapidly. People in whom symptoms appear to be precipitated by a stressful event usually have a particularly good outcome. It used to be believed that people who had a long and gradual decline before their first episode of frank symptoms had an intrinsically more severe and chronically debilitating condition. The 1988 edition of the *Companion to Psychiatric Studies* textbook, for example, stated that there was 'firm agreement on the characteristics of the initial illness' (Kendell and Zealey, 1988, p. 327) that predict outcome, and that one of these was the rapidity of onset of symptoms. Although the association between mode of onset and the subsequent nature of the disorder was widely acknowledged in the early 1990s, it appeared to be forgotten as the concept of 'duration of untreated psychosis' emerged. Moreover, studies that did not detect an association between 'duration of untreated psychosis' and outcome, or found that the association could be explained by other factors, were ignored (Ho et al., 2000). The idea that the fundamental course of a severe mental condition could be modified by treatment appeared to be irresistible, just as it had been in the past.

The 'Neuroprotection' Hypothesis

'Duration of untreated psychosis' was, at best, however, only an indirect manifestation of the hypothesis that psychosis is a toxic brain condition that can be arrested by drug treatment. The hypothesis needed fleshing out and the early intervention enthusiasts were keen to identify neuropathological evidence to support the theory. Findings that were thought to indicate the underlying degenerative nature of psychosis and the recuperative action of drug treatment were consequently drawn together to construct a narrative about how antipsychotic drugs could exert 'neuroprotective' effects. Like other aspects of the antipsychotic story, however, the evidence was more complex, and much of it pointed in the opposite direction, suggesting that antipsychotics were actually neurotoxic.

Most post-mortem studies of brains of people diagnosed with schizophrenia have failed to find any trace of the characteristic changes that occur in people with well-accepted degenerative disorders of the brain, such as Alzheimer's disease (Harrison, 1999). In any case, the studies have mostly included people exposed to years of drug treatment and other potential brain insults like electro-convulsive therapy (ECT). The principle evidence for the idea that schizophrenia is a neurodegenerative process was therefore said to be the subtle diminution of brain matter that had been demonstrated to occur in the magnetic resonance imaging (MRI) studies described in Chapter 9. As we saw, the possibility that the changes might be related to drug treatment was barely considered for many years. By 2007, when researchers had to acknowledge that antipsychotic treatment might account for some of the loss of brain tissue observed in these studies, it was still being claimed that the atypical antipsychotics, at least, 'exert a potential neuroprotective effect' (Jarskog et al., 2007b, p. 57).

By this time a vast amount of research had been conducted into the effects of various psychiatric drugs on aspects of nerve cell survival, and antidepressants, lithium and antipsychotics were all claimed to have neuroprotective properties (Duman et al., 1997; Manji et al., 1999; Hunsberger et al., 2009). Atypical antipsychotics were said to enhance the production of neurotrophic factors (chemicals responsible for promoting nerve cell growth), prevent nerve cell death through various mechanisms and increase the connections between nerve cells (Jarskog et al., 2007a, p. 53). Once again, however, the evidence had been selected and interpreted according to a set of assumptions that the effects of drugs were protective and innocuous. It was possible, as it was with the imaging studies, to tell quite a different story.

It is generally accepted that lithium is the drug with the strongest claim to have neuroprotective properties based on imaging studies where, in contrast to the situation with antipsychotics, lithium treatment is sometimes associated with increased brain volume. Acute lithium treatment enlarges animal brains, but this is thought to reflect the water-retaining properties of lithium (Phatak et al., 2006) and consequent effects on the imaging process (Cousins et al., 2013). A review of 45 studies of people suffering from bipolar disorder, or manic depression, found that the majority of these did not detect an effect of lithium on brain volume, and where such an effect was reported, it only occurred in certain areas and was often marginal (Hafeman et al., 2012). Moreover, if lithium did increase brain volume, it is not clear that this would be any more desirable than the global reduction of brain volume associated with antipsychotics. The older antipsychotics have been shown to enlarge the volume of the basal ganglia in the brain, for example (Chakos et al., 1995), and some, though not all, microscopic studies of post-mortem specimens have found evidence of nerve cell damage and degeneration in this area (Christensen et al., 1970; Jellinger, 1977).

Other evidence cited to support the idea that lithium has a neuroprotective action includes a number of studies suggesting that lithium increases concentrations of a protein involved in preventing nerve cell death, known as beta-cell lymphoma 2 protein, or Bcl-2 (Manji et al., 2000). A study that found that olanzapine and clozapine had similar effects is commonly cited as evidence for the neuroprotective effects of atypical antipsychotics (Bai et al., 2004). But an increase in concentrations of Bcl-2 is characteristic of neurodegenerative disorders like Alzheimer's disease, where it is presumed to indicate a compensatory mechanism employed by the brain to try and counterbalance the underlying disease-related nerve cell loss and damage. So, if lithium and antipsychotics are associated with increased concentrations of Bcl-2, this might just as well indicate that they are *causing* damage to brain cells as protecting them. In any case, a further study found that antipsychotic treatment had no effect on Bcl-2 levels in rats, but it did, to the authors' surprise, increase the activity of a substance called caspase-3—one of the principle agents responsible for nerve cell death (Jarskog et al., 2007a).

Many studies have demonstrated that antipsychotics are toxic to brain cells (Dean, 2006). Numerous laboratory-based investigations show that haloperidol kills and damages nerve cell specimens (Behl et al., 1995; Post et al., 1998; Sagara, 1998). Indeed, some antipsychotics are so effective at killing nerve cells that their use as anti-brain tumour agents has been explored (Gil-Ad et al., 2001). There is less research on the effects of atypical antipsychotics, and some studies suggest lower degrees of toxicity than are seen with haloperidol. One study found that risperidone and sulpiride had no discernible effect on cell death, for example, but clozapine produced even higher rates of cell death than haloperidol (Gil-Ad et al., 2001). Another found that risperidone had weaker effects than haloperidol, but could induce similar levels of nerve cell death at higher doses (Ukai et al., 2004).

With a few exceptions, psychiatric researchers have continued to presume that prescribed drugs are benign and restorative, however, rather than potentially harmful. In the many studies and reviews that cropped up in the first decade of the twenty-first century unambiguous findings of the toxic effects of antipsychotics were swiftly passed over, if they were mentioned at all, and other data were fitted into the preconceived neuroprotective model, even where, like the research on Bcl-2, this was inconsistent with research on other neurological diseases (Berger et al., 2003; Jarskog and Lieberman, 2006; Buckley et al., 2007; Hunsberger et al., 2009). The momentum behind the early intervention movement discouraged critical scrutiny of the neuropathological evidence. Unsubstantiated, unlikely and conflicting claims about the miraculous effects of the atypical antipsychotics and other sorts of drugs continue to abound despite the fact that there is no evidence that could justify the designation of these drugs as 'neuroprotective' agents, and indications that they are, in fact, substantially toxic to brain cells.

Early Intervention in Psychosis Services

Starting in the 1990s, services specialising in the care and treatment of people suffering their first psychotic breakdown started to be developed in different parts of the world. One of these was the pioneering centre in Melbourne, Australia, associated with the charismatic psychiatrist Patrick McGorry. The Melbourne service consisted of a community-based treatment programme known as the Early Psychosis Prevention and Intervention Centre (EPPIC).

In 2001 the UK's Department of Health called for a network of Early Intervention in Psychosis services to be formed across the country (Department of Health, 2001). Within a few years there were more than 100 dedicated teams operating in England alone (Pinfold et al.,

2007). Staff in these teams had a smaller caseload than those in standard community mental health teams and were meant to offer, according to the Department of Health's guidance, expertise in cognitive behavioural therapy, family therapy and treatment of drug and alcohol problems, as well as standard treatments for psychosis (Singh et al., 2003).

Despite the fact that Early Intervention services have now been established throughout the world, only two trials have compared these services with generic mental health care, and neither of these examined the role of drug treatment independently from other aspects of the intervention. The largest study was conducted in Denmark and involved 547 patients with a first psychotic episode who were randomised to specialist Early Intervention or routine care for a duration of 2 years. At the end of this time patients in the specialist intervention group had lower rates of psychotic and negative symptoms, slightly higher levels of functioning and had spent fewer days in hospital. However, both groups received antipsychotic treatment according to Danish government guidelines, with little difference in medication use between the groups (Petersen et al., 2005; Thorup et al., 2005). The patients were followed up again 3 years later, or 5 years after the start of the study, and at this point there were no differences in any of the principle outcomes (Bertelsen et al., 2008).

The Lambeth Early Onset (LEO) study conducted in London enrolled 144 patients with a first or second episode of psychosis. After adjusting for differences in the initial characteristics of participants, the researchers found that people allocated to the Early Intervention service were less likely to be readmitted to hospital than those receiving the ordinary service, but there were no differences in rates of relapse, recovery or the amount of time spent in hospital (Craig et al., 2004). No data on how participants fared after they left the service have been published nor have any details on levels of drug treatment received by each group.

These remain the only studies that offer information about whether providing intensive treatment by specialist teams in the initial phase of a psychotic disorder improves outcome. The Danish study suggested such programmes improve symptoms only while they are running, implying it is the intensive support that is effective, rather than a fundamental modification of the underlying disease that might be attributable to drug treatment. Neither of the two studies examined the role of drug treatment specifically, however, and there remain no trials which assess whether starting antipsychotic medication early on improves outcome of its own accord, despite the fact that this idea was the embryo of the Early Intervention movement.

Early Detection of Psychosis

Participants in the Danish- and London-based trials were already involved with mental health services before taking part in the studies, but other programmes have attempted to draw people into treatment services through public education and mass media campaigns. The rationale for these activities was, again, the unshakeable belief that shortening the duration of untreated psychosis would improve the ultimate outcome of the disorder of schizophrenia. The TIPS (Early Identification and Treatment of Psychosis) programme in Norway was the most extensive of these programmes and consisted of a mass media campaign that included newspaper, cinema and radio advertisements, leaflets posted directly to households, face-to-face training of general practitioners, school teachers and counsellors, and twice-termly presentations in schools. In Canada, an early detection initiative consisted of a public awareness campaign using leaflets, posters, television and cinema advertisements, and training of general practitioners and school counsellors. In Singapore, a similar campaign also involved a 'docudrama' screened on primetime television, and the use of celebrities to endorse the campaign. In Norway and Singapore, it was found that people who presented to services after the early detection programme was instituted had a shorter 'duration of untreated psychosis', than people who presented before, or in areas where it had not yet been launched (Lloyd-Evans et al., 2011).

Only the TIPS programme provided any data on whether early detection affects outcome per se. People who were referred to treatment services in the area where the early detection programme was initiated had milder conditions with lower levels of all types of symptoms and higher rates of illicit drug use, suggesting that the psychotic episodes in this group were more likely to be drug-induced than in the comparison group (Melle et al., 2004; Larsen et al., 2006). Ten years later recovery rates were higher in people who came from the early detection area, but no adjustment was made for the severity of symptoms or differences in illicit drug use at the start of the study. Few details of the characteristics of study participants were presented in any of the study publications and the results of the study are thus rendered quite meaningless. The fact that the authors could, nevertheless, conclude that their findings support the benefits of early intervention illustrates the strength of their underlying assumptions (Hegelstad et al., 2012). The TIPS study merely reveals that people who have less severe symptoms and impairments have a better outcome—a finding that is hardly surprising and in no way demonstrates that earlier institution of treatment has any benefits.

Prevention of Psychosis

In 1995 the Melbourne centre, under the leadership of Patrick McGorry and his colleague Alison Yung, developed a service for identifying young people who might be vulnerable to psychosis at some point in the future. It was known as the Personal Assessment and Crisis Evaluation clinic, or PACE. Motivated by the perceived need to start treatment as early as possible, the aim of the programme was to identify people who might go on to develop psychosis, but who had not yet experienced symptoms that would satisfy diagnostic criteria for a psychotic condition.

In infectious diseases, the initial stage is sometimes referred to as a 'prodrome', which is a state that can only usually be identified retrospectively, as most early signs and symptoms are non-specific. Yung and McGorry drew attention to the early stages of measles, however, where an early sign of the disorder is the appearance of white patches in the mouth known as Koplik spots. Koplik spots, if correctly identified, only occur in measles, and are therefore 100% specific. When looking back at a small group of patients who had experienced a psychotic episode, they noted that although the most common early symptoms were anxiety, depression, irritability, and social withdrawal, closer to the point at which a recognisable psychotic state developed some patients exhibited psychotic-like features such as 'perceptual disturbances', 'delusional mood' and suspiciousness (Yung et al., 1996). They hypothesised, therefore, that there was a pre-psychotic phase that preceded the onset of frank psychosis, which it might be possible to identify and that could be seen as analogous to the Koplik spots of measles. Based on the characteristics of their clients, the PACE team set about constructing a set of criteria which would define this state and help predict the onset of psychosis. A research programme was set up that aimed to identify individuals who were 'at risk' or at 'high risk' of developing psychosis in the near future, in order to initiate antipsychotic treatment and prevent a full-blown psychotic episode from developing.

Early attempts to predict whether an individual would become psychotic were fairly impressive, even if they failed to approach the specificity of Koplik spots. The Melbourne group reported that 41% of

Table 10.1 Melbourne criteria for the 'at risk mental state'

At risk mental state identified if an individual satisfies one of the following three criteria		
Experiences 'attenuated' (low grade) psychotic symptoms, e.g. 'magical thinking', perceptual disturbance, paranoid ideation, odd speech	Experiences brief limited intermittent psychotic symptoms (lasting less than 1 week)	Has a family history of psychosis, schizophrenia, or 'schizotypal personality disorder'[1] combined with a deterioration in the individual's mental state or functioning for at least a month

49 young people identified using their criteria for being in an 'at risk' mental state (Table 10.1) developed a psychotic episode within a year, and they concluded that it was 'possible to accurately identify people at imminent risk of psychosis' (Phillips et al., 2000, p. S164).

The PACE group then proceeded to set up a randomised controlled trial to assess whether instituting treatment in people identified as being at 'high risk' could prevent the onset of psychosis. The trial involved 59 young people who were randomised to two groups: one group received supportive psychotherapy and help with individual problems, which could, and did, include antidepressants and benzodiazepines in many cases, but not antipsychotics; the other group received low-dose antipsychotic treatment using risperidone plus a specially tailored programme of cognitive behaviour therapy. No placebo was used and the study was not conducted blind so that everyone was aware which group individuals had been assigned to. After 6 months of treatment only 10% of people receiving risperidone plus cognitive behaviour therapy had been diagnosed with a full-blown psychotic disorder compared with 36% of the comparison group, a statistically significant difference ($p = 0.03$). However, levels of symptoms, including both positive and negative symptoms of schizophrenia, did not differ between the groups at the end of the treatment period (McGorry et al., 2002). Nevertheless, the trial provoked great excitement and was repeatedly cited as evidence for the benefits of preventive treatment (McGlashan et al., 2006; Marshall and Rathbone, 2011).

Three other trials have subsequently been initiated involving the use of antipsychotic medication, and other studies have tested the efficacy of cognitive behaviour therapy, without antipsychotic medication, as a preventive measure. The PRIME study, conducted at Yale University in the USA, and led by psychiatrist Thomas McGlashan, consisted of a double blind comparison of low-dose olanzapine against placebo in 60 people aged between 12 and 45 years. After a year of treatment 16% of the olanzapine group had developed psychosis compared with 38% of the placebo group, according to the authors' own 'presence of psychosis' scale, a difference that did not quite reach conventional levels of statistical significance. Again, there were no differences and only minimal changes on conventional symptom measures like the Positive and Negative Symptom Scale (PANSS), but people treated with olanzapine gained almost 9 kg during the year of treatment (McGlashan et al., 2006). The researchers blamed the poor result on the fact that recruitment had proved difficult, but McGlashan subsequently distanced himself from this type of research, declaring he did not think that drugs 'could prevent full-blown psychosis, only delay it' and pointing to the fact that the drugs were more likely to induce weight gain than to produce any measurable benefit (Carey, 2006).

Another study, conducted in Germany, involved the use of a combination of amisulpride and cognitive behaviour therapy in a similar design to the Melbourne study. With 124 people randomised in total, it represents the largest trial so far, yet its results have never been properly published. The treatment phase of the study was designed to last 12 months, but only preliminary data collected at 12 weeks have been published so far, suggesting that the group treated with amisulpride and cognitive behaviour therapy had improved levels of positive symptoms and general functioning compared with the comparison group, but that negative symptoms were unaffected (Ruhrmann et al., 2007; Marshall and Rathbone, 2011). To date, no details of rates of onset of psychosis have been published, however, and, given the excitement generated by the results of the Melbourne study, it seems probable that no benefits of drug treatment were detected.

In 2012 results of a further trial conducted by the Melbourne group were published. This trial utilised a placebo and compared the effects of antipsychotic medication plus cognitive behaviour therapy, placebo with behaviour cognitive therapy and placebo alongside non-specific 'supportive' therapy. After a year of treatment only 13% of participants had developed a diagnosable psychotic disorder, and there were no statistically significant differences between the three groups. The authors concluded the study failed 'to provide support for the first-line use of antipsychotic medications in patients at ultra-high risk of psychosis' (McGorry et al., 2013, p. 349). Findings from another US study of people being treated for prodromal symptoms also found that the use of antipsychotic medication had no effect on whether people developed a full-blown psychosis, although this was not a randomised trial (Walker et al., 2009).

Other research groups have failed to replicate the Australian group's early predictive accuracy. In a multi-centre trial, led from Manchester of cognitive behaviour therapy for prevention of psychosis, which used the Melbourne criteria for identifying people at 'high risk', only 8% of the participants went on to develop psychosis, with no difference between those who received cognitive behaviour therapy and those who did not (Morrison et al., 2012). Although a German study found a modest effect of a psychological intervention for people with an 'early initial prodromal state', the rate of onset of psychosis in the control group was still only 17% after a year (Bechdolf et al., 2012). These figures suggest that 80–90% of people in a trial of preventive treatment would be treated unnecessarily. As with so many other miraculous interventions, the remarkable results proclaimed early on have become increasingly marginal in successive studies, and the enterprise of trying to prevent psychosis appears much less feasible than we were led to believe a few years ago.

Criticism of Early Intervention

Despite the lack of evidence to suggest that early intervention fundamentally changes the outlook for people diagnosed with schizophrenia or psychosis, and the questionable effects of preventive interventions, the bandwagon of Early Intervention in Psychosis roles on. The general public continue to be told definitively that 'the sooner a person gets diagnosis and treatment, the better the outcome' (schizophrenia.com, 2012) and that 'early detection of psychosis greatly increases the chance of a successful recovery' (Fraser Health Authority, 2012). Emotive advertising is designed to persuade clinicians that not starting antipsychotic treatment at the earliest possible opportunity consigns people to a life of emptiness and ruin. An advertisement for Risperdal Consta (injectable risperidone) produced in 2007, for example, featured an image of a girl aged around 13 years walking across a playground, dropping a doll and school books in her wake. The caption read 'Prescribe early, because what she loses, she could lose forever', with the obvious implication of a lost childhood without early drug treatment (Risperdal Consta advertisement, 2007).

Despite the results of recent trials of psychosis prevention, several services, especially in the USA, continue to attempt to identify people with possible 'prodromal' symptoms. Maine Medical Centre's PIER (Portland Identification and Early Referral) programme, for example, provides presentations on early warning signs for school students and staff, which it lists as including social withdrawal, decline in performance, difficulty concentrating, loss of motivation and other difficulties that are common in teenagers in a variety of circumstances (Table 10.2).

People considered to be at 'high risk' of going on to develop a full-blown psychotic episode are offered a treatment package that includes medication (PIER, 2012). Columbia University's COPE (Centre of Prevention and Evaluation) programme also aims to attract people with early 'symptoms', listing experiences and behaviour which, like those of the PIER programme, are highly subjective and non-specific (COPE, 2012). The San Francisco-based PREP (Prevention and Recovery in Early Psychosis) programme provides public information on early identification aimed at young people, families, schools, churches and community groups, and explicitly advises people that 'caught very early, it is possible to prevent or delay the onset of a psychotic illness' (PREP, 2012).

The ethics of treating people supposedly at 'high risk' of developing psychosis has now been challenged by several leading researchers and clinicians, however (Bentall and Morrison, 2002; Warner, 2005; Verdoux and Cougnard, 2006; Bosanac et al., 2010). The most accurate predictions of the Melbourne group fall far below the aspiration to identify the Koplik spot of psychosis, but even if the most optimistic predictions are correct, i.e. that about 40% of people identified progress to develop a psychotic episode, so-called preventive treatment means that 60 out of every 100 persons would be exposed to all the risks of antipsychotic treatment without any hope of benefiting from it. It seems likely, however, that the accuracy of prediction is much lower in the real world and that treating people with so-called early signs of psychosis is likely to result in 80 or 90% of people receiving drug treatment unnecessarily.

Even without early detection or prevention programmes, there has been a blurring of the boundaries between full-blown psychosis and its early symptoms, however, which seems likely to increase the rate at which people are diagnosed and treated for having a psychotic episode. As American psychiatrist Richard Warner pointed out, community surveys reveal that there is a large pool of people with psychotic-like symptoms who never require medical or professional attention (Warner, 2005). One such study found that two in every 1000 people fulfilled criteria for a diagnosis of schizophrenia, whereas only a fraction of this number—around 0.24 per 1000—ever come to the attention of traditional mental health services (Tien and Eaton, 1992). Another critic of early intervention services, psychiatrist David Castle, showed that whereas the international World Health Organization studies reported

Table 10.2 PIER (Portland Identification and Early Referral) programme (adapted from PIER, 2012)

'Symptom'	Examples provided
Social withdrawal	Spending more time alone Avoiding friends and family Avoiding groups
Functional decline	Dropping grades Missing classes, school or work Not responding to friends
Behaviour changes	Collecting objects or hoarding Developing a new and unusual interest Developing an odd habit or gesture Taking risks
Concentration difficulty	Having trouble focusing or paying attention Losing abilities in athletics or hobbies Losing track of conversations Forgetting Getting lost Developing difficulty with homework, reading and understanding long sentences
Loss of motivation or energy	Quitting sports, groups or clubs Declining interest in previously enjoyable activities Sleeping more Spending more time inactive Staying home from school
Dramatic sleep and appetite changes	Eating more or less than usual Sleeping more or less than usual Eating only certain foods
Suspiciousness of others	Worrying about what others are thinking Thinking others wish to harm you in some way Watching others with suspicion Feeling fearful or uneasy around people
Unusual or exaggerated beliefs about a person's powers or influences	Thinking you have special or magical powers Believing or fearing you can influence others without their knowledge Believing someone is putting thoughts in your brain
Heightened sensitivity to sights, sounds, smells or touch	Perceiving that lights are brighter and sounds are louder Smelling things that might not be there Avoiding touch Complaining that clothing feels irritating Noticing that senses feel raw

between seven and 14 new cases of psychosis per 100,000 people, the early intervention service in Cambridge, UK, was finding an incidence rate of 50 per 100,000 people. He estimated that the Melbourne service was diagnosing people at a rate of 100 per 100,000 people (Castle, 2012).

As we saw in Chapter 7, some people with full-blown psychosis recover without drug treatment, and it seems likely that early, mild and debateable signs of psychosis are even more likely to resolve spontaneously. Early intervention services may be drawing in people who do not need services, and although receiving general support may not be harmful, long periods of unnecessary antipsychotic treatment certainly are. Ironically, one of Yung and McGorry's early papers documents the existence of transitory psychotic experiences, describing in detail the histories of several young patients who had developed psychotic symptoms, in some cases in response to severely stressful situations, which resolved spontaneously without any specific treatment (Yung et al., 1996).

The height of hubris of the early intervention movement was the proposal for the inclusion of the 'psychosis risk syndrome' as a new and distinct diagnosis in the fifth revision of the American Psychiatric Association's *Diagnostic and Statistical Manual* (*DSM*) of mental disorders. Thankfully, the proposal galvanised psychiatrists who were sceptical of the claims of the early intervention enthusiasts, including such high profile figures as Allen Francis, the head of the previous *DSM* revision taskforce. The proposal was finally jettisoned, but only after considerable deliberation and in the face of a mounting campaign against it (Maxman, 2012).

The Pharmaceutical Industry

The Early Intervention in Psychosis movement has thrived because it fulfils the long-held ambition of the psychiatric profession to have therapeutic interventions that confirm the medical nature of psychiatric activity. It represents the ultimate horizon of the disease-centred model of drug action; the idea that drugs do not just arrest an underlying disease process, but can prevent its emergence in the first place. Early intervention was also eagerly embraced by politicians looking for a quick and simple solution to the costly problem of caring for people with severe mental disorders. This political credulity has led to Patrick McGorry, an energetic and persuasive publicist, becoming what has been described as 'the most powerful psychiatrist in the world' (Francis, 2011). McGorry won over the political establishment of Australia and became influential elsewhere through his messianic approach to early intervention, which enables him to 'defend absolutely indefensible positions with the convincing but inaccurate force of a true believer' (Francis, 2011). Local campaigners, worried about the ethical implications of his expansionist activities, have fought back, however, accusing him of overstating the number of people requiring mental health interventions (Medew, 2010). In return, McGorry has countered his accusers by suggesting they are 'irresponsible' 'merchants of doubt' (McGorry, 2011), whose views deserve 'censure' (McGorry et al., 2010, p. 402).

The success of early intervention is not down to individual efforts, however, any more than it is justified by scientific evidence. The hidden hand of the pharmaceutical industry has been driving the movement since its early days. AstraZeneca, makers of quetiapine, sponsored gatherings of academics that became known as the European First Episode Schizophrenia network, starting in 1995. The Australian group received drug company support through the ORYGEN research centre, and the Melbourne prevention study was funded by Janssen, makers of risperidone. Eli Lilly partially funded the US PRIME trial, and the TIPS early detection programme received funding from Janssen-Cilag, Lundbeck Pharma and Eli Lilly. Conferences organised by the International Early Psychosis Association have been supported by the makers of atypical antipsychotics, and the 2012 conference courted prospective sponsors with a glossy brochure outlining the opportunities for product promotion (International Early Psychosis Association, 2012).

Papers presented at company-sponsored conferences and in company-funded publications have repeatedly stressed the benefits of the atypical antipsychotics, playing down their adverse effects and underlining the 'crude and iatrogenic' effects of the older drugs (McGorry et al., 2005, p. S1; Remington, 2005). In a company-sponsored journal supplement, before the results of the PRIME study became apparent, Thomas McGlashan justified treating people who might never develop psychosis by the argument that the atypical antipsychotics were well-tolerated agents whose harmful effects were 'modest in frequency, and very modest in serious adverse effects' (McGlashan, 2005, p. S114). He did admit, however, that the long-term consequences of treatment were not yet known.

Individual researchers can receive considerable sums of personal income from drug companies for various services, including 'consultancy' and delivering lectures, as well as funding for research. The investigation into the Harvard-based child psychiatrist Joseph Biederman and his colleagues revealed that millions of dollars can be accrued from such activities (see Chapter 11). Patrick McGorry commonly fails to declare any drug company connections in his numerous publications, but when he was forced to by the rigorous 'conflict of interest' policy of the *British Medical Journal* it was revealed that he had 'acted as a paid consultant for, and received speaker fees and travel reimbursement from' Janssen-Cilag, Eli Lilly, Bristol Myers Squibb, AstraZeneca and Pfizer, and that all of these companies, and not just Janssen who funded the risperidone trial, had donated money towards his research activities (McGorry, 2008). The declaration of interests by the authors of the non-randomised longitudinal prodrome study in the USA ran to half a page of small text, with most authors having received research funding, consultancy fees or 'educational fees' from a range of pharmaceutical companies (Walker et al., 2009).

Allen Francis declared that 'the world is a safer place now that "Psychosis Risk" will not be in *DSM 5*. Its rejection saves our kids from the risk of unnecessary exposure to antipsychotic drugs' (Francis, 2012). In a dramatic turnaround, McGorry also recently admitted that antipsychotics might not be justified in people judged to be 'high risk' of developing psychosis, and abandoned plans to launch a preventive trial using quetiapine amid mounting public and professional criticism (Stark, 2011). In many ways, however, the *DSM-5* committee, in considering the proposed diagnosis, was reflecting what had already become normal practice. The concept of psychosis has been profoundly altered by the early intervention movement, expanding to encompass people with all sorts of unusual and troublesome behaviours. Many of these people—who are mostly young—are being started on a course of lifelong treatment with toxic drugs, whose benefit in such marginal situations has not been proven, and whose toxic effects are well documented. Apart from unnecessary exposure to drug treatment, these people will encounter all the difficulties of being labelled a mentally ill person, including the psychological vulnerability and helplessness this often produces. In addition, overstretched services are concentrating resources on people who might have recovered without their help, leaving less support for those with established and severe mental health problems. And the drug companies are laughing all the way to the bank!

11
The Antipsychotic Epidemic: Prescribing in the Twenty-First Century

Having largely replaced the older antipsychotics, and expanded drug treatment for people with schizophrenia or psychosis to its limits through the Early Intervention movement, the makers of atypical antipsychotics set about widening the market for their products beyond the relatively small group of people who suffer from a serious, 'psychotic' disturbance. They achieved this end admirably, deftly combining legal and illegal marketing strategies, and changing and shaping concepts of mental disorder, as well as cleverly managing damaging data about the drugs' adverse effects in ways revealed in Chapter 9. The symbol of the chemical imbalance and the corresponding notion that the drugs restored biochemical harmony, was pivotal to this programme because it allowed these toxic substances to be portrayed, misleadingly, as essentially harmless.

The increasing use of antipsychotic drugs in a whole variety of countries since the late 1990s is a clear testament to the success of these activities (Verdoux et al., 2010). In cases where data are available, it appears that this rising use is driven principally by 'off-label' prescribing for people diagnosed with a variety of common psychological complaints, rather than more severe mental disorders. In the USA, for example, data on medical consultations showed that those involving a prescription of antipsychotics nearly tripled between 1995 and 2006, with the bulk of this increase occurring from 2001 onwards (Alexander et al., 2011). In 2008 only 51% of consultations in which older antipsychotics were prescribed involved people diagnosed with schizophrenia, and less than a quarter (24%) of consultations which resulted in prescriptions of new or atypical antipsychotics. Thirty-four per cent of atypical antipsychotics were prescribed to people diagnosed with some sort of 'bipolar disorder', and most of the rest were prescribed to people with depression, anxiety, dementia and other conditions for which the drugs have not been licenced. Moreover, the rising use of antipsychotics has been paralleled by an increasing tendency for people to be prescribed numerous different psychiatric medications concurrently. Between 1996 and 2003, 87% of consultations involving antipsychotic prescriptions also involved prescriptions of other psychiatric drugs, most commonly antidepressants, 'mood stabilisers' or another sedative (Sankaranarayanan and Puumala, 2007).

The situation in the UK is similar. Between 1991 and 2000 only 10% of newly initiated prescriptions of antipsychotics in general practice were issued to people with a diagnosis of psychosis or schizophrenia. Fifty per cent were prescribed to people with anxiety and depression, and 15% to people with dementia (Kaye et al., 2003). More recent data on prescriptions showed that most of the commonly used antipsychotic drugs, both of the older and newer variety, are prescribed predominantly in low-dose preparations, well below the doses that would be used for people diagnosed with schizophrenia or psychosis (Ilyas and Moncrieff, 2012). Moreover, figures from the USA suggest that antipsychotics are increasingly prescribed by general physicians and family doctors, rather than psychiatrists. In 2002 almost a third of consultations (32.2%) resulting in a prescription of antipsychotics involved physicians who were not mental health specialists, which was more than double the proportion in 1998 (Aparasu et al., 2005).

Data from the USA also show that the rate of antipsychotic prescribing to children and young people increased almost five times between 1995 and 2002. In the year 1995–96 there were 8.6 prescriptions of antipsychotics issued for every 1000 people aged under 18 years in the USA, whereas in 2001–02 this had increased to 39.4 per 1000. The majority of antipsychotic prescriptions issued to this age group were for 'behaviour problems' and mood disorders, and only 14% were given for psychotic conditions (Olfson et al., 2006). Again, almost a third (32.4%) of prescriptions to children were not issued by psychiatrists or mental health specialists (Cooper et al., 2006).

Both legal and illegal strategies have been employed to achieve this expansion in the market for the atypical antipsychotics. Illegal marketing targeted general practitioners and staff of mental health nursing homes in order to increase the use of these drugs in people with dementia, depression and anxiety (Spielmans, 2009). More sinister than the illegal tactics, however, has been the mostly legal manipulation of public and professional understanding of what has come to be called 'bipolar disorder,' the condition previously, and more expressively, known as manic depression. The manufacturers of atypical antipsychotics have set about changing the meaning of this once rare and distinctive condition, expanding its boundaries beyond recognition so that 'bipolar disorder' has become a label that can be attached to a whole myriad of common personal difficulties, which thereby become legitimate targets for antipsychotic treatment.

The New Bipolar Disorder

An article in the British publication *The Psychiatrist* entitled 'I want to be bipolar' describes the relatively recent phenomenon of people actively seeking to be diagnosed with 'bipolar disorder' (Chan and Sireling, 2010). Journalist Patrick Strudwick was one of these people, and he described his story in *The Times* in 2012. After the breakdown of a difficult relationship in 2003, he threw himself into his work, found that he was sleeping less, and had periods when he felt his mind was racing, he was full of energy and over-talkative. He researched his problems on the Internet and decided he had bipolar disorder. Although a friend advised him he most probably did not have the condition, he described how he convinced himself and his doctor that he did. 'I want a label for how I'm feeling and drugs to make it stop'. He recalled 'I read reams about bipolar disorder. Every sensation of the past few months morphs into these descriptions of symptoms. I ignore the ones I don't have'.

When he saw his general practitioner, he described 'only the apex of the hyper moods, the edited highlights. The more complicated reality – that these episodes undulate, subside and sometimes last only an hour or two – I do not describe in case he doesn't take me seriously' (Strudwick, 2012).

Patrick's general practitioner referred him to a psychiatrist who was happy to confirm the diagnosis of bipolar disorder, and Patrick was started on a drug called Depakote (see p. 193). He took this for several years until another psychiatrist questioned the diagnosis, and eventually Patrick started to doubt it himself. Finally tiring of the sedating effects of the drug, he weaned himself off. When he confessed to this episode some years later, two of his friends described how they too had been labelled as having 'bipolar disorder' in the same sort of circumstances. A few days after *The Times* article was published, an old friend of mine contacted me with a similar story. Like the author of the article, my friend had been diagnosed with bipolar disorder and treated for several years with the antipsychotic drug Seroquel (quetiapine) after a life crisis. She had belatedly come to realise that she had been labelled as having a serious, life-long mental condition, which could have untold consequences for her future.

Bipolar disorder was ripe for exploitation. Longstanding associations between manic depression and creativity gave the condition a glamorous image, and it was not linked with the intellectual and social deterioration associated with the concept of schizophrenia. Moreover, experience with the marketing of depression in the 1990s proved that many people were willing to reconceive various social and personal difficulties as arising from a brain-based condition. As Strudwick illustrates, the idea that one's feelings and behaviour constitute an illness or disease can provide a reassuringly concrete explanation for emotional turmoil. Moreover, by locating the problem in defective brain functioning, depression and other illness labels separate the individual's actual, true self from the difficulties they are experiencing, which can therefore be shrugged off and disowned (Stepnisky, 2007). By the late 1990s, however, the label of depression was becoming commonplace, and thereby losing its ability to signal something exceptional. A diagnosis of bipolar disorder was the next step up the ladder, enabling people to retain the feeling that their problems were distinct from ordinary experience, extrinsic to themselves and worthy of regarding as a brain disease.

The 'bipolar' epidemic started in the USA in the 1990s when some academics started to suggest that the disorder was under-recognised (Ghaemi et al., 1999). The condition that had originally been called 'manic depression' is a rare disorder in which the sufferer becomes aroused and over-active over a sustained period lasting weeks at least, and frequently many months. It is easily recognisable because the individual's behaviour is out of character and often out of control, and it usually leads to admission to a psychiatric unit. Most inpatient facilities in the UK see only a handful of such cases a year.

The term 'bipolar disorder' started to be employed in the 1970s, proving attractive to psychiatrists perhaps through its association with electricity and thus with physical science. There were suggestions from this time that there might be a milder form of the condition, which was named 'bipolar II disorder' to distinguish it from the classical form of manic depression, which was referred to as 'bipolar I.' Bipolar II disorder was essentially a variant of depression, in which people were said to suffer principally from episodes of depression with occasional periods of mildly elevated mood. There was little interest in this milder form of the disorder, however, until the mid-1990s, when bipolar disorder became the focus of renewed academic attention, and a whole range of situations and behaviours were swept under its umbrella. The concept of 'bipolar spectrum disorder', which was formulated in 1996, suggested that a tendency for moodiness, or 'lifelong temperamental dysregulation', could be seen as arising from the same biological processes that were thought to give rise to classical manic depression, although, of course, it had to be admitted that these processes were not yet identified (Akiskal, 1996).

The prevalence of bipolar disorder has increased in line with its expanding boundaries. Although classical manic depression was commonly said to affect about 1% of the population, research suggests that fewer than 1 in a 1000 people were hospitalised for a typical episode of mania during the twentieth century (Healy, 2008). An American house-to-house survey conducted in the early 1990s, however, reported that 1.3% of the population suffered from bipolar I disorder (Kessler et al., 1994). By 1998 it was claimed that the prevalence of classical bipolar disorder with full-blown mania was 5% (Angst, 1998). In 2003, an additional 11% of the population was said to suffer from bipolar II disorder, and a total of 24% was thought to show some form of disturbance on the 'bipolar spectrum' (Angst et al., 2003).

Bipolar disorder has been transformed from a readily discernible pattern of behaviour to a highly flexible concept that can be applied to almost any individual in some sort of difficulty. Although all forms of the disorder are proposed to consist of some sort of abnormal variation of mood, there is a world of difference between the sustained periods of heightened arousal, disinhibited behaviour and over-activity characteristic of classical mania, and the periods of increased energy that most people experience from time to time. There is no research evidence that can confirm that these situations are the same phenomena or that they have the same origins. As Patrick Strudwick noticed when he attended the local bipolar support group: 'The others in the group share stories of kaleidoscopic hallucinations, distinctly inappropriate public nudity and policemen fishing them out of reservoirs. My stories do not compare' (Strudwick, 2012).

The Concept of a 'Mood Stabiliser'

Increasing academic interest in bipolar disorder, or the bipolar 'disorders' as they were often referred to, coincided with the first wave of interest from the pharmaceutical industry, which came not from the makers of antipsychotics but from the manufacturer of the drug Depakote (Healy, 2006b). Depakote is the brand name for a newly configured form of the old anti-epileptic drug sodium valproate, and it was released onto the market as a treatment for mania in 1995. Drugs used in epilepsy had been suggested to be useful in manic depression back in the 1980s, based on a misleading analogy between epilepsy and manic depression. As anti-epileptic drugs prevented fits by reducing the brain's nervous excitability, it was proposed that they might quell whatever processes lay behind repeated episodes of manic depression.

Following the release of Depakote the concept of the 'mood stabiliser' started to enter the psychiatric lexicon. Its precise meaning was never clear and psychiatrists could not agree on what the concept referred to (Bowden, 1998; Ghaemi, 2001), but it had popular resonance and people came to believe that drugs referred to as 'mood stabilisers' rectified something awry in the biological basis of emotional regulation. Mood stabilisation became the vague counterpart of the new and equally vague notion of bipolar disorder.

The only research that provided any evidence of the therapeutic potential of Depakote simply consisted of a placebo-controlled trial conducted with people with severe mania. Not surprisingly, in view of Depakote's sedative properties, it performed somewhat better than placebo (Bowden et al., 1994). No research was ever conducted, or at least published, which showed that the drug reduced mood variability, and there remains no evidence that it modifies the biological basis of mood or mood regulation—whatever complex interaction of numerous neurotransmitters that might involve. Moreover, the only published study to have examined the use of Depakote for the long-term prevention of relapse in people with a diagnosis of bipolar I disorder found that neither Depakote nor lithium was superior to placebo (Bowden et al., 2000).

Notwithstanding the evidence, sales of Depakote soared as the concept of mood instability, and the idea that there was a specific treatment for it, infiltrated mental health services (Ilyas and Moncrieff, 2012). Other anti-epileptic drugs were also targeted at the mood disorder market, based on the same rationale, and gabapentin and lamotrigine became widely prescribed in this area, the former through illegal promotion as it was never licenced for this indication (Van Voris and Lawrence, 2010). The manufacturers of the atypical antipsychotics witnessed this development, and in the late 1990s, Eli Lilly set up trials designed to obtain a licence for olanzapine for the treatment of bipolar disorder. Studies were conducted with people with acute mania and showed, again not surprisingly in view of the strong sedation olanzapine induces, that it was superior to placebo and comparable to Depakote and haloperidol in this situation (Tohen et al., 1999, 2002, 2003). In March 2000 olanzapine was granted a licence for use in an episode of mania in people diagnosed with type I bipolar disorder or manic depression.

Marketing Bipolar Disorder

As well as revealing the strategies drug companies use to obscure the nature and severity of adverse events, the opening up of the Zyprexa papers provided an unprecedented insight into Eli Lilly's marketing strategy. It was clear that the company saw Zyprexa (olanzapine) as the natural successor to Prozac, and as the patent on Prozac was about to expire, the company set about devising a strategy to make Zyprexa into the 'most successful pharmaceutical product ever'. The future of the company was seen as riding on the success of this strategy: 'The company is betting the family farm on Zyprexa' the 'Zyprexa Product Team' declared in an internal presentation in 2001. 'The ability of Eli Lilly to remain independent and to emerge as the fastest growing pharma company of the decade depends solely on our ability to achieve *world class commercialisation of Zyprexa*' (Eli Lilly, 2001, cited in Spielmans, 2009, original emphasis). This strategy hinged on the ability of the company to reposition Zyprexa as a treatment for mood disorders that could be marketed to the millions of people who currently thought of themselves as depressed, and could be prescribed not just by psychiatrists but by general practitioners or primary care physicians. The newly flexible concept of bipolar disorder was the link that would enable this to happen. In 1997, for example, the Zyprexa product team predicted that sales projections would increase more than fourfold if olanzapine could be viewed as a 'Depakote like...MOOD STABILISER' rather than a 'Risperdal like...Antipsychotic' (Tollefson, 1997, cited in Spielmans and Parry, 2010, original emphasis).

The repositioning of Zyprexa as a 'mood stabiliser' was achieved through a disease-awareness campaign, similar in nature to previous campaigns that had publicised other vague and expandable mental conditions during the 1990s; conditions like 'social anxiety disorder' and 'premenstrual dysphoric disorder' (Koerner, 2002). In 2002, Eli Lilly ran an advertisement on US television which began, according to David Healy's description,

> ...with a vibrant woman dancing late into the night. A background voice says, 'your doctor never sees you like this'. The advertisement cuts to a shrunken and glum figure, and the voice-over now says 'this is who your doctor sees.' Cutting again to the woman, in active shopping mode, clutching bags with the latest brand names, we hear: 'That is why so many people with bipolar disorder are being treated for depression and aren't getting any better – because depression is

only half the story.' We see the woman depressed, looking at bills that have arrived in the post before switching again to see her energetically painting her apartment, 'That fast talking, energetic, quick tempered, up-all-night you,' says the voice-over, 'probably never shows up in the doctor's office' (Healy, 2008, p. 190)

The advertisement did not mention Zyprexa, or any other drug, but encouraged people to log onto the website of the 'Bipolar Help Centre', sponsored by Eli Lilly, and to take a 'bipolar test'. It concluded by showing the heroine filling in the questionnaire, and recommended viewers take the test to their doctor to obtain a 'correct diagnosis'.

Material aimed at general practitioners again intended to change perceptions about people who might previously have been diagnosed with depression. Eli Lilly formulated the idea of 'complicated mood' to delineate a group of people with common symptoms like irritability, anxiety, disturbed sleep and mood swings, suggesting these were indications of incipient and previously unrecognised bipolar disorder. The concept of 'complicated mood' helped to bridge the gap between the serious mental conditions that were normally associated with the use of antipsychotics, and the sort of mental distress that general practitioners saw on an everyday basis (Spielmans, 2009). To underline this reorientation, sales representatives were instructed to focus on 'symptoms and behaviours' (Eli Lilly, 2000, cited in Spielmans, 2009), rather than diagnoses, to emphasise the broad action of olanzapine, and to encourage general practitioners to identify and prescribe to 'higher functioning' people at 'the low to middle end' of bipolar severity (Porat, 2002, cited in Spielmans and Parry, 2010). Eli Lilly provided a number of patient profiles for use by its sales representatives, ten of which were revealed in the Zyprexa papers. The majority of these described people with common and subjective problems such as those included under the rubric of 'complicated mood,' as well as others like distractibility, 'a tendency to be over-talkative' and 'erratic behaviour' (Eli Lilly, undated, 2001, both cited in Spielmans, 2009).

Wider experience with direct to consumer advertising in the USA and New Zealand proved that patients themselves could provide a useful marketing tool. In 2002, for example, it was estimated that one out of every five medical consultations was instigated by a patient who had seen an advertisement for a product or condition (Mintzes et al., 2002). Associations between drug companies and patient support groups have also provided a vehicle for changing opinions about the nature and frequency of bipolar disorder and the role of drug treatment. In the UK the

Manic Depression Fellowship promoted the use of 'mood diaries' constructed by Eli Lilly, which encourage people to focus on their mood in minute detail by rating it hour-to-hour. Measurement techniques of this sort, which are available on numerous websites, uncover normal emotional variations that occur in everyone. Once translated into numerical and visual form, however, the fluctuations can appear unusual and worrying, and can easily be construed as incipient bipolar disorder (Healy and Le Noury, 2007).

Eli Lilly and the Manic Depression Fellowship also teamed up to produce leaflets and booklets whose message was 'bipolar disorder is a lifelong illness needing lifelong treatment...people feel better because the medication is working'. Anyone who might consider stopping their medication was warned that 'almost everyone who stops taking medication will get ill again' and that 'the more episodes you have the more difficult they are to treat' (cited in Healy and Le Noury, 2007, p. 211).

Information produced by drug companies, patient groups and professional organisations also emphasises the idea that the disorder is caused by 'chemical imbalances in the brain' (AstraZeneca, 2012) that can be rectified with drugs. In 2011, for example, the Geodon website (an atypical antipsychotic made by Pfizer) stated that 'current medicines are designed to help correct these imbalances', accompanied by a picture of a young woman sitting cross-legged, with her hands carefully positioned on her knees, in a perfectly symmetrical and 'balanced' position (Pfizer, 2011). The Manic Depression Fellowship, now renamed the Bipolar Organisation, describes on its website how antipsychotics work by altering the 'balance of a brain chemical called dopamine which is known to be abnormal in mania and psychosis' (Bipolar UK, 2012).

In the early years of the twenty-first century, the media was flooded with stories about bipolar disorder. In 2006 the BBC (British Broadcasting Company) screened a documentary in which the well-known comedian Stephen Fry explored bipolar disorder and 'owned up' to having been diagnosed with the condition himself. The programme won a prestigious Emmy award and did more to glamorise and popularise the condition than any advertising campaign could wish to accomplish. Fry interviewed a number of celebrities diagnosed with the condition, including Hollywood actors, British comedians and television personalities, and many other successful and enthralling characters. 'Manic types do well in Hollywood, in all of show business' he mused. Describing his own problems, Fry admitted to feeling ambivalent, hating the feelings of depression, but also describing the 'huge buzz' and 'sense of adventure' he experienced during his 'manic' periods. 'I love my condition too' he stated at one point, continuing, 'it has tormented me all my life with the deepest of depressions, while giving me the energy and creativity that perhaps has made my career'. One of his interviewees, a former businessman and imprisoned fraudster, wrote on the bipolar support website he had set up: 'still suffering in bliss and agony' (BBC, 2006).

Despite these alluring aspects of the so-called disorder, Fry stressed that the condition is a 'serious' 'disease of the brain' and claimed that four million people in the UK have the disorder—a staggering 8% of the adult population. He explored a number of forms of treatment, including drugs, electro-convulsive therapy (ECT) and cognitive behavioural therapy, and although he was unsure about the necessity or benefits of receiving treatment himself, he seemed delighted with the diagnosis. 'I wouldn't live a normal life' he declared, 'not for all the tea in China'. The programme repeatedly emphasised the importance of early detection, claiming that the condition was often unrecognised, and Fry saw his mission as de-stigmatising the disorder so that more people would be willing to identify themselves or those around them as 'being bipolar' (BBC, 2006). In this manner, ordinary people were encouraged to aspire to this emblem of celebrity culture: the exciting, stylish and tragic condition of the gifted and troubled soul.

Further Expansion

Following studies involving people with an acute episode of mania, Eli Lilly set up a trial to examine the effects of long-term treatment with olanzapine. It found that olanzapine was superior to placebo in preventing a relapse of mania or depression in people who had recovered from an episode of acute mania, but it has been criticised because all the participants were taking olanzapine prior to entering the study, and the results suggest that a discontinuation effect occurred. Half of the placebo group relapsed within 22 days of randomisation, for example, and almost all of them had relapsed within 3 months of the trial commencing, suggesting relapse was constituted or precipitated by the effects of medication withdrawal (Tohen et al., 2006). Even among the olanzapine-treated group, 47% of participants relapsed within a year. Research that has examined the natural history of bipolar I, or manic depression, in the era before supposedly specific drugs like lithium were introduced has found that around 50% of people recently recovered from an episode suffered a relapse over the following 2–3 years (Winokur, 1975; Harris et al., 2005). In other words, people treated with olanzapine in the Eli Lilly study relapsed in under half the time of the natural history of the condition.

Although a partial explanation may lie in the loose definitions of relapse employed in modern clinical trials, the evidence provides little reassurance that long-term olanzapine therapy is better than no treatment at all.

Nevertheless, on the basis of this one trial olanzapine received a licence for the prophylactic treatment of bipolar I disorder and the National Institute for Health and Clinical Exellence's (NICE) guideline on the treatment of bipolar disorder published in 2006 recommended olanzapine alongside lithium and sodium valproate as the first choice of medication for the long-term management of people with the condition (National Institute for Health and Clinical Excellence, 2006). The guideline also recommended quetiapine for the management of people with recurrent depressive symptoms, and depression has since become a major market for this drug. Although the process of instituting prolonged drug treatment for people under the increasingly expandable bipolar umbrella was already well underway by this time, official approval of atypical antipsychotics as the principle agents of treatment provided further momentum to commercial efforts to ensure the migration of these drugs out of the arena of severe mental disorder into the much larger market of people with everyday ups and downs.

The case of quetiapine, or Seroquel, also illustrates the on-going transformation of the market for antipsychotics. Although initially launched as a treatment for schizophrenia and psychosis on the basis of trials revealing mostly modest differences between the drug and placebo (Leucht et al., 2008), it has since been promoted for use in mania and, more recently, as a treatment for depressive symptoms, both in people diagnosed with bipolar disorder and with simple depression. In 2009 AstraZeneca applied to the United States Food and Drug Administration (FDA) for a licence to treat depression and anxiety, which, if obtained, would have opened up a market estimated to consist of more than 20 million Americans (USA Today, 2009). Following advice from a panel of experts, the FDA rejected the application because of concerns about the adverse effects of the drug, particularly its metabolic effects and cardiac toxicity. It endorsed the use of Seroquel as an adjunctive treatment for depression in people who have not responded to other drugs, however, and, as the majority of people treated with antidepressants continue to experience chronic or recurrent symptoms—85% of participants in the large STAR*D (Sequenced Treatment Alternatives to Relieve Depression) study, for example (Rush et al., 2012), this still represents an immense opportunity for extending the drug's reach.

Although some randomised controlled trials have found quetiapine to have superior effects to a placebo for people diagnosed with depression, scrutinising depression trials reveals that the majority of the response to drug treatment is attributable to the placebo effect (Kirsch et al., 2002). Moreover, any drug with psychoactive properties, including many other antipsychotics, appears to demonstrate an effect on depression in one clinical trial or another, suggesting the portion of the response attributable to drug treatment is the non-specific result of being in an altered, drug-induced state (Moncrieff, 2001). As with antidepressants, however, the effects of quetiapine are trivial. Trials involving people diagnosed with depression or with a depressive bipolar episode have typically found differences between the drug and placebo of only 2–3 points on the Montgomery–Åsberg Depresson Rating Scale (MADRS), which has a maximum score of 60 (Bauer et al., 2009; Weisler et al., 2009; McElroy et al., 2010; Bortnick et al., 2011). The large size of the studies, which mostly involved several hundred people, has ensured that these small differences are statistically significant, even though they do not represent a clinically significant effect. Meanwhile, AstraZeneca is busy reaping the rewards of the depression market, while propagating the adverse effects that the FDA panel expressed concern about.

Paediatric Bipolar Disorder

Although it is the adult market that accounts for the bulk of sales of atypical antipsychotics, it is the use of these drugs in children alongside the emergence of the diagnosis of paediatric bipolar disorder that best illustrates the way in which a severe mental disorder can be morphed into a label for common or garden difficulties, as well as the role that money plays in this process. As with adults who seek a bipolar diagnosis to avoid confronting various personal or social difficulties, the concept of paediatric bipolar disorder can appeal to parents because, like attention deficit disorder (ADHD), autism, Asperger's and numerous other diagnoses, it provides a seemingly concrete label for difficult and challenging behaviour. Moreover, by locating the problem in the brain of the child, it seemingly detaches it from the situation within the family. The story of Rebecca Riley, who died aged 4 after being diagnosed with bipolar disorder and 'ADHD', and whose parents were convicted of her murder, illustrates the potentially tragic consequences of this medicalisation of young children's behaviour.

Rebecca Riley was found dead on her parents' bedroom floor in the town of Hull, Massachusetts, in the USA in 2006. At the time of her death she had been prescribed quetiapine along with Depakote, and another sedative drug, clonidine. On the night she died her parents admitted to giving her extra doses of clonidine, along with an over-the-counter cold remedy. The District Attorney's medical examination determined that she died from the combined effects of her prescription medicine and the drugs contained in the cold remedy, and that her heart and lungs were damaged by previous prolonged use of the pre-scribed medication. Rebecca's preschool reported that prior to her death she was so drugged she had to be helped up the stairs and propped up in her chair (Able, 2007).

Prosecutors alleged that Rebecca's parents used prescription drugs to keep their three children quiet and in order to obtain disability benefits, and they were noted to be applying for benefits for Rebecca at the time of her death. A year before Rebecca's death, her mother had been found by the local social services department to have neglected her children and her father had been accused of sexually abusing his 13-year-old step-daughter (Able, 2007).

In 2010, both parents were convicted of Rebecca's murder by 'inten-tional overdose', and received long prison sentences. Rebecca's psy-chiatrist, Kayoko Kifuji, was defended by her employer, Tufts Medical Centre, for practising appropriately and 'within responsible professional standards' (Carey, 2007). The judge at the trial of Rebecca's father dis-agreed: 'If what Dr Kifuji did in this case is the acceptable standard of care for children in Massachusetts' he concluded, 'then there is some-thing very wrong in this State' (Wen, 2010).

Before the tragic death of Rebecca Riley, the American media had been reporting the increase in the diagnosis of bipolar disorder among children as a positive development, whereby an unrecognised, but real, condition was being uncovered. In an article entitled 'Young and bipolar' *Time Magazine* reported on how manic depression or bipolar disorder was not as rare as previously thought and that 'Doctors ...are coming to the unsettling conclusion that large numbers of teens and children are suffering from it as well'. The article stressed the need for prompt diagnosis and treatment, and expressed concern that without it 'plenty of kids are suffering needlessly' (Kluger and Song, 2002).

David Healy and colleagues have convincingly deconstructed the diagnosis of bipolar disorder in children. Prior to the turn of the last century, as they point out, true bipolar disorder, or manic depression, was thought to be vanishingly rare in children. From 2000 onwards, however, a variety of popular books and publications on the 'bipolar child' started to appear, which described children with a variety of com-mon behaviour problems, including temper tantrums, irritability and poor sleep, finally being 'recognised' as displaying signs of childhood bipolar disorder. Academic psychiatry fuelled this craze, with added financial incentive from the pharmaceutical industry, but, in 2007, when Healy's paper was published, the scale of this liaison had not been revealed (Healy et al., 2007).

In the 1990s, a group led by child psychiatrist Joseph Biederman, who was based at Massachussets General Hospital and the prestigious Harvard Medical School, started to suggest that children could manifest 'mania' or bipolar disorder, but that it was frequently missed because it was often co-existent with other childhood problems like ADHD and 'antisocial' behaviour (Faraone et al., 1998). In a paper published in 1996 the group suggested that 21% of children attending their clinics with ADHD also exhibited 'mania', which was diagnosed on the basis of symptoms such as over-activity, irritability and sleep difficulties (Biederman et al., 1996). A year later the group were referring to bipolar disorder in children as if it were a regular, undisputed condition, and emphasised the need for 'an aggressive medication regime' for children with the diagnosis (Bostic et al., 1997).

As Healy observed, the more bipolar disorder in children was written and spoken about, the more it appeared to be a legitimate condition (Healy, 2008). In 2003 another group of academics formulated official 'treatment guidelines', which were published in the leading American journal of child psychiatry. Like Biederman's group, the authors of the guidelines stressed the importance of 'early diagnosis and aggressive treatment' (Kowatch et al., 2005, p. 214). They acknowledged that children with bipolar disorder did not meet official diagnostic criteria because they did not have clearly defined episodes and their 'symptoms' were not prolonged and severe. In fact, the discussion makes it plain that the condition being considered was quite different from bipolar disorder or manic depression as it presents in adults. Children with bipolar disorder do not have discrete periods of mania, the guidelines stated, but rather have 'frequent daily mood swings that have been occurring for months to years' (p. 214). Moreover, the 'mood swings' are most commonly characterised, not by elation and excitement, as in a classical manic episode, but by 'intense mood lability and irritability' (p. 14). Instead of drawing the obvious conclusion that the behaviours being diagnosed as 'bipolar' in children have no relation to the protracted episodes of over-arousal and euphoria characteristic of typical adult mania, the guideline authors suggested that different or adapted criteria were necessary. They recommended treatment with antipsychotics, lithium and other 'mood stabilisers', and regimes involving combinations of two or more drugs were suggested to be needed in the frequent cases where a single drug produced only a 'partial' response. Moreover, additional medication was said to be required for the frequently occurring concurrent disorders like attention deficit disorder and anxiety.

The guidelines were the product of a two-day meeting held under the auspices of the Child and Adolescent Bipolar Foundation, which was sponsored by Abbott Laboratories, AstraZeneca, Eli Lilly, Forest Pharmaceuticals, Janssen, Novartis and Pfizer. In the same year that the guidelines were published, several companies sponsored a symposium at the American Psychiatric Association's annual meeting in San Francisco on 'juvenile bipolar disorder', which featured four talks by Biederman's group (Healy, 2008). By this time, the group had started to run trials of various antipsychotics for the treatment of bipolar disorder in children, sponsored by the manufacturers of the drugs involved. By 2012, risperidone, olanzapine, ariprirazole and zisprasidone had been investigated, mostly in small-scale studies that were not conducted double blind. The drugs were said to have beneficial effects on symptoms of 'mania', which is most likely attributable to their sedative properties, and the researchers concluded that larger double blind studies were justified. One of these studies was aimed at pre-school children aged between 4 and 6 years (Biederman et al., 2005), and children were recruited to these trials through advertisements that told parents that challenging behaviour and aggression in young children might stem from bipolar disorder (Healy, 2008). The trials revealed high rates of adverse effects, including substantial weight gain, especially with olanzapine. In one study children gained 5 kg after only 8 weeks of olanzapine treatment (Frazier et al., 2001), but instead of stopping the research in its tracks, the researchers added more drugs to the mix in an attempt to combat the metabolic effects of the antipsychotic (Wozniak et al., 2009).

These trials were run from the Johnson & Johnson Centre for Paediatric Psychopathology Research, which was set up with money from Janssen Pharmaceuticals, the makers of risperidone, at the request of Joseph Biederman. Documents relating to the centre's objectives were released during litigation brought by parents who alleged their children had been harmed by antipsychotic drugs. The centre's annual report of 2002 stated that the centre's research should satisfy three criteria: it should improve psychiatric care for children, have high standards and 'move forward the commercial goals of J&J'. The report went on to state that the activities of the centre would lead to 'safer, more appropriate and *more widespread* use of medications in children' (my emphasis) and that without the data the centre could produce 'many clinicians question the wisdom of aggressively treating children with medications, especially those like neuroleptics, which expose children to potentially serious adverse events'. An e-mail from a Johnson & Johnson executive stated that the rationale of the centre was to 'generate and disseminate data supporting the use of risperidone' in children and adolescents (Harris and Carey, 2008).

In 2008, just before these reports were made public, an investigation by the Republican senator Charles Grassley revealed that Biederman and some of his colleagues had failed to declare millions of dollars of personal income they had received in consultancy fees from drug companies. When pressed by Senator Grassley, Biederman belatedly admitted to receiving $1.6 million from drug companies between 2000 and 2007, and his Harvard colleagues, psychiatrists Timothey Wilens and Thomas Spencer, admitted to receiving $1.6 and $1 million respectively. Even these figures may be an underestimate, however, as information provided to Senator Grassley by the drug companies indicated even higher payments (Harris and Carey, 2008). The fact that the researchers had failed to declare the extent of their income violated the conditions of the substantial federal funds they had received to conduct research and their programme was temporarily suspended.

Before the scandal erupted, the head of psychiatry at Harvard assured reporters that Biederman would not be influenced by his association with drug companies: 'For Joe, it is his ideas and mission that drive him, not the fees' (Allen, 2007). This was before the extent of these 'fees' became public, but even afterwards it seems that Harvard did not see the incident as meriting serious punishment. The only sanctions levied against the three offenders were that they had to refrain from conducting company-sponsored research for 1 year, and subsequently submit proposals to conduct such research for approval for a further 2 years. They were also told that they might face a delay in consideration for promotion, but as all three were already at professorial level, it is not clear that this would affect their prestige or income in any way (Yu, 2011).

Biederman continues to publish numerous papers on the drug treatment of childhood conditions, including so-called paediatric bipolar disorder. In 2011 his group published a major review of drug treatments for the condition, in which they declared that 'pediatric bipolar disorder is a chronic, severe, and often disabling psychiatric condition', with no reference to any criticism of the concept (Liu et al., 2011, p. 749). In 2012 the group published a study of the antipsychotic quetiapine for 'bipolar spectrum disorder' in preschool children aged

4–6 (Joshi et al., 2012). The restrictions imposed by Harvard seem hardly to have dented Biederman's research activities, which currently receive support from the drug companies Janssen, Shire and Next Wave pharmaceuticals (Joshi et al., 2012).

Neither Harvard nor Massachusetts General Hospital, nor any other psychiatric or medical institution has commented on the fact that prominent academics were found to be enriching themselves to the tune of millions of dollars through researching and promoting the use of dangerous and unlicensed drugs in children and young people. Although some individual psychiatrists have expressed misgivings (Able, 2007), academic papers continue to discuss the diagnosis, treatment and outcome of bipolar disorder in children as if no controversy existed, with more than 100 papers on the subject published in Medline-listed journals between 2010 and 2012. Notwithstanding the death of Rebecca Riley and the disgrace of Joseph Biederman, the practice of diagnosing children with bipolar disorder and treating them with antipsychotics remains alive and kicking.

Off-Label Prescribing

Papers released during recent court actions have revealed that several drug companies deliberately engaged in illegal strategies to market atypical antipsychotics in situations in which their use was not licenced, particularly in nursing homes for use in elderly people with dementia. According to the Zyprexa papers, people with dementia were one of the principle targets for the promotion of olanzapine (Spielmans, 2009). At first it appears that Eli Lilly and some other companies intended to obtain a licence for the use of atypical antipsychotics in dementia to manage psychotic symptoms along with agitation and behaviour problems. Unfortunately, although trials of risperidone and ariprirazole showed small reductions in the occurrence of challenging behaviours, olanzapine did not perform any better than placebo, and it soon became apparent that the use of any of these drugs hastened death in this group of vulnerable elderly people whose nervous systems were already compromised (Schneider et al., 2005, 2006). Moreover, as we saw in Chapter 9, the studies revealed that antipsychotics worsen rather than improve cognitive function in people with Alzheimer's disease or dementia (Schneider et al., 2005). A study involving people with learning disability and behavioural problems also found that neither haloperidol nor risperidone improved aggression more than a placebo over a 4-week period (Tyrer et al., 2008). So although antipsychotics are undoubtedly effective for the immediate containment of challenging and aggressive behaviour (see Chapter 8), the evidence suggests that they are not particularly useful when used continuously over longer periods.

In 2008 the British government commissioned a report into the use of antipsychotic drugs in people with dementia. The report concluded that while 180,000 people with dementia received these drugs, less than a fifth of them derived any benefit, and that around 1800 excess deaths were caused by their use in England alone each year (Banergee, 2009).

Eli Lilly appeared to abandon its attempts to obtain a licence for the use of Zyprexa in dementia by 2003, but, like other atypical manufacturers, the company was not deterred from continuing to promote the drug illegally, as the Zyprexa papers suggest it had been doing since the 1990s (Spielmans, 2009). In 2009 Eli Lilly was fined $1.4 billion for these activities, the largest corporate fine in US legal history at the time. The United States Justice Department stated that the drug had been marketed for behavioural problems in people with dementia, as well as for 'generalised sleep disorder' and depression in the general population (United States Department of Justice, 2009). Later that year an even bigger fine of $2.3 billion was levied against Pfizer for illegal marketing of several drugs, including its antipsychotic Geodon (zisprasidone), which was the fourth time Pfizer had been fined for such practices in 5 years (Harris, 2009). In 2010 AstraZeneca was fined $520 million for promoting Seroquel for unapproved uses, including aggression, dementia, anger management, anxiety, attention deficit disorder, post-traumatic stress disorder and sleeplessness (United States Department of Justice, 2010). Johnson & Johnson agreed to pay the US government $2.2 billion in 2012 as a penalty for allegations of illegal marketing of Risperdal and other drugs, including the claim that it had provided financial inducements to the nursing home pharmacy company, Omnicare Inc., to recommend Risperdal (Fisk et al., 2012). Later in the year it was ordered to pay a further $1.2 billion by the state of Texas for illegal promotion of Risperdal (Thomas, 2012).

When a company seeks a licence for a product it has to demonstrate that, for a particular problem in a particular group of people, giving the drug concerned is better than doing nothing. Although the placebo-controlled trials that are thought to provide this evidence have many drawbacks, as we saw in Chapter 6, the licensing process at least involves an attempt to evaluate the pros and cons of drug treatment. When drugs are used for situations in which approval has not been obtained, there may be no evidence that the drug is of any use at all, let alone safe.

Once tardive dyskinesia was well and truly forgotten, antipsychotics could be launched at the general population, including the ever expanding number of people who struggle at one time or another to meet the demands of modern life—the population that had been delineated by the popularity of Prozac and the other new antidepressants. Although regulatory agencies tried to stop overtly illegal marketing practices, and governments and professionals condemned the use of these drugs as chemical pacifiers in nursing home patients, they were no match for the tsunami of money the companies threw behind promoting their newest blockbusters. In bipolar disorder, companies found a diagnosis that allowed them to present their drugs as a specific treatment for a serious disorder, while simultaneously thrusting them at a wide cross section of the populace. Bipolar disorder proved to be as flexible as labels like depression and anxiety had been in the past, allowing the use of antipsychotics in the general population to creep up without provoking the backlash that eventually arose against unlicenced use in conditions like dementia. Given the brain damage, diabetes and heart disease associated with the use of antipsychotic drugs, not to mention the sexual impairment, weight gain, mental clouding and emotional suppression, this unfounded and increasingly unrestrained prescribing represents a serious threat to the public health of Western nations.

12
All is not as it Seems

The conventional history of antipsychotics presents them as the miracle drugs that finally banished the dark days of straight-jackets and lobotomies, and allowed psychiatry to rise out of its ambivalent position straddling medicine, social work and criminal justice to become a fully-fledged member of the medical sciences. Antipsychotics were proclaimed to be the first intervention that worked in a truly medical manner, not just suppressing symptoms but targeting an underlying disease, and this belief seemingly confirmed the psychiatric profession's longstanding contention that mental disorders arise from distinct, biological anomalies just like other medical conditions. The fact that now-discredited interventions, such as insulin coma therapy, had also been regarded as acting in a disease-specific manner was soon forgotten, and antipsychotics, along with other drugs developed since the 1950s, came to be seen as a completely new and unique sort of treatment, quite different from anything that went before.

The early antipsychotics ushered in the age we now inhabit, in which drugs have come to be seen as 'magic bullets' that can eradicate all sorts of unwanted experiences and behaviours. The 'antidepressants', which followed close on their heels, were claimed to remedy the ancient state of melancholy or despair, 'anxiolytics' apparently abolished the tendency for worry and fear, and stimulants could rectify children's unruly behaviour. More recently it has been claimed that drugs can make us happier (Kramer, 1993), cleverer (Greely et al., 2008) and will finally prevent us from aging (Cooper, 2011).

From the beginning, however, the story of the antipsychotics is not as it seems. From the 'creation myth', where it transpires that the heroic surgeon Laborit was a quack with 'screwy ideas about the treatment of shock' (Swazey, 1974, p. 272), to the clinical trial evidence that shows that the drugs do not reduce psychotic disturbance much more than a placebo, most of the cherished beliefs about these drugs do not stand up to scrutiny. Most traditional accounts give no hint that Laborit's idea that shock should be treated by counteracting the body's physiological reactions had long been rejected by the majority of his profession, and that his anaesthetic cocktails designed to produce a state of total bodily shut-down were unusual and highly dangerous. With a track record of such hazardous procedures as insulin coma therapy, 'deep sleep therapy' and lobotomy, safety was, in any case, no impediment to psychiatry's acceptance of a new intervention at that time. The conventional account presents the pioneers of modern drug treatments as fighting a heroic battle against the entrenched forces of psychoanalysis (Swazey, 1974; Healy, 1996), but in reality it appears little resistance was offered, and psychiatry, which was already adept at interfering with the body, was ripe for the introduction of a new physical technique, especially one that could be administered as easily as a drug.

By the 1970s if not before, the idea that antipsychotics target the basis of an underlying brain disease or abnormality was widely accepted, although there was no evidence that could confirm such a notion. Even now, there remains almost no research which could, or does establish that antipsychotics have a disease-centred mechanism of action in schizophrenia, psychosis or any other disorder. The desire to have disease-specific treatments was so overwhelming, however, that the mere suggestion that antipsychotics could act in this way was embraced enthusiastically and more or less without debate. The aspirations of the psychiatric profession united with political ambitions to reduce the bill for the care of the mentally disabled, to make the myth of a disease-specific therapy into a seeming and unquestioned reality. Once adopted, the psychiatric community chose to forget that there was any other way to understand the action of its drugs. By the 1990s the disease-centred model was so entrenched that no one even thought it necessary to describe or explore the psychoactive and physical state induced by the new, 'atypical' antipsychotics introduced at the time.

The psychiatric establishment has had to make strenuous efforts to suppress alternative ways of thinking about the action of its drug treatments, however, and although the usual response to any countervailing view is to ignore it, when critics gain publicity the reaction can be harsh. The American Psychiatric Association (APA) and the pro-drug National Alliance for the Mentally Ill (NAMI) combined forces against Peter Breggin, for example, after he appeared on the Oprah Winfrey show in 1987. Acting on transcripts handed over by the APA, NAMI lodged an official complaint about Breggin's medical licence with the Maryland State licencing authority, alleging his appearance on the programme had encouraged patients to stop taking their psychiatric medication. The complaint referred to some final, informal remarks Breggin had made to Oprah on the subject of how to obtain help, when he suggested that people in distress should seek a psychotherapist instead of a psychiatrist, and should not take drugs if they were offered them. At no point did he recommend that anyone should stop taking a medicine they were already prescribed. Breggin was completely vindicated by the licencing board, which agreed with him that his accusers had attempted to curtail his right to free speech (Anonymous, 1987; International Center for the Study of Psychiatry and Psychology, 2009).

British-based psychiatrist David Healy was the victim of a similar attack during his long-standing campaign to draw attention to the drug-induced effects of the selective serotonin reuptake inhibitor antidepressants (SSRIs) and their ability to drive some people to think of, or attempt, suicide (Healy, 2006a). More common than malicious attempts to discredit individuals and deprive them of their livelihoods, however, is the elimination of dissent through silence. Breggin has been making his argument about the nature of psychiatric drugs since the 1980s, based on a detailed analysis of the scientific evidence, but there has been no debate about his views in the mainstream literature and no attempt to refute them. The refusal to acknowledge that there are other ways of conceptualising how psychiatric medications produce their effects means that many mental health professionals, and much of the wider public, have the impression that the disease-centred model of psychiatric drug action is the only credible, or even possible, way of thinking about what these drugs do.

Although not all psychiatrists subscribe to a disease-centred view of their drug treatments, nevertheless, the drug-centred model presents a fundamental threat to the beliefs that underpin the biologically oriented psychiatry that has been on the ascendance since the 1970s. Although the drug-centred model does not in itself involve any supposition about the nature of mental disorders, challenging the disease-centred model of drug action can be perceived as undermining the very basis of modern psychiatry because the idea that present-day drugs target underlying biological abnormalities is believed to represent the strongest evidence that mental disorders are diseases 'like any other'. As part of an intellectual debate the drug-centred view is tolerated because it can be ignored, but when it is taken to the people the argument has to be silenced in case the weakness of the medical model of mental disturbance is exposed.

The Effects of Antipsychotics

The adoption of the disease-centred model of antipsychotic action in the 1950s and 1960s led research to focus increasingly on the effects of the drugs on the proposed disorder or disease. The result was an abundance of clinical trials, which created the impression that we know a great deal about these drugs. The message that emerged was that antipsychotics make people better in the short-term, and prevent relapse in the longer term. People in general fare better when treated with antipsychotics than they would do without them. It turns out that these studies can throw little light on the question of whether it is better to take antipsychotics than not to, however, nor on whether taking antipsychotics improves the long-term outlook for people diagnosed with schizophrenia or psychosis. Looking at these studies in detail reveals that the vast majority were conducted with people who were already established on antipsychotic drugs. In fact, most studies involved people who had been taking medication for many years—including the initial studies of the atypical antipsychotics.

These studies only tell us what happens when someone stops taking antipsychotics, not what effects the drugs have when they are first started. Astoundingly, no proper clinical trials have *ever* been conducted involving only people who had not previously been exposed to antipsychotic medication. There is reasonable evidence from early trials that antipsychotics reduce the symptoms of an acute psychotic disturbance for a short period, but other than this fairly predictable observation, the thousands of studies that have been conducted since the 1950s and 1960s tell us almost nothing about the ultimate value of antipsychotic treatment.

Moreover, randomised clinical trials provide little information about what the drugs are actually doing when they reduce symptoms, and the rich descriptions provided by people who have taken the drugs themselves and the careful clinical observations made by early researchers, have been lost from the scientific literature because the presumption that the drugs work in a disease-specific manner renders them uninteresting and unimportant. In modern textbooks and journal articles we can only glimpse the nature of these drugs through sterile lists of 'side effects'. Yet, first-person accounts indicate how antipsychotics can dampen down psychotic thoughts and experiences along with most other aspects of mental and physical functioning. It is a state that is usually found to be unpleasant, but may be judged as preferable to being assailed by intense psychotic phenomena.

What is politically useful and at the same time most dangerous about the disease-centred view of drug action is the way it obscures the pharmacological nature of antipsychotics and other psychiatric drugs. By focusing attention on the disease the drugs are thought to treat, rather than the drugs themselves, the model diverts attention away from the dangerous and debilitating effects the drugs induce. Because antipsychotics are construed not as toxins, like recreational drugs, but as medicines, it is assumed that their effects are necessarily benign, and there is a corresponding tendency to dismiss or ignore their adverse effects, especially if these are linked to their desired, therapeutic actions. The saga of tardive dyskinesia—the minimisation of its prevalence, attempts to blame the condition and the almost complete eclipse of research suggesting it involves general mental impairment as well as involuntary movements—was repeated in many of its elements in subsequent decades. Drug companies mirrored the psychiatric profession's approach to tardive dyskinesia by seeding the idea that the metabolic toxicity caused by some of the atypical antipsychotics might be attributable instead to the condition of schizophrenia. This strategy helped to delay the backlash against these drugs long enough to establish their position as market leaders, even though the pronounced obesity they cause is plain for everyone to see.

In a similar way, the fact that people diagnosed with schizophrenia are often found to have smaller brains than other people was, for many years, presented as incontrovertible evidence that schizophrenia is rightly thought of as a brain disease. A small number of researchers now quietly admit that the evidence suggests that long-term antipsychotic treatment is what shrinks brains, although the idea that 'schizophrenic' brains are somehow different appears to be hard to relinquish completely. But evidence on the effects of antipsychotics has been available for decades now, and for decades Peter Breggin has been pointing it out.

The lack of interest in clarifying the long-term effects of antipsychotics is perhaps most striking given that long-term treatment is the norm for almost all situations in which antipsychotics are used. We do not know the extent to which people and animals become 'tolerant'[1] to the immediate effects of antipsychotics, despite research that demonstrates that the body starts to increase the sensitivity of dopamine receptors within days of starting on a drug like haloperidol (Samaha et al., 2007). We have little information on the nature and range of withdrawal effects, and we know almost nothing about the impact of long-term antipsychotic use on intellectual function, even though it has been well demonstrated that short-term use impairs the mental abilities of human volunteers and animals. Although some evidence suggests that long-term antipsychotic treatment may, in itself, increase an individual's vulnerability to having a psychotic episode or relapse (including what is sometimes referred to as 'supersensitivity psychosis'), we are no nearer confirming whether this effect exists and, if so, how frequently it occurs and by what mechanism. In fact, we remain ignorant of the mechanism behind many of the drugs' most common and profound effects, including the sedation they produce, the metabolic disturbance and tardive dyskinesia.

An almost religious commitment to the disease-centred view of psychiatric drug action has created a blind spot to the serious physical consequences that long-term ingestion of toxic substances is likely to produce, and drug companies are still able to present antipsychotic drugs as innocuous and restorative agents that work by balancing the brain's 'natural chemicals' (Eli Lilly, 2011). The history of antipsychotics illustrates how far the Hippocratic oath, 'first do no harm', is from being followed, and how strong is the opposite inclination to view interventions visited on 'patients' by 'doctors' as an inevitable and undiluted blessing.

Antipsychotics and Diagnosis

The rise of the disease-centred model of drug action has gone hand-in-hand with the application of medical-type systems of diagnosis to the troubles of the mind. Starting in the 1970s, as a response to challenges to mainstream psychiatry from the antipsychiatry movement and economic competition from non-medically-qualified therapists, the conception of mental illness was thoroughly 'remedicalised' (Wilson, 1993). The new orientation was expressed in the third edition of the American Psychiatric Association's *Diagnostic and Statistical Manual (DSM)* published in 1980, which expunged the psychoanalytic influence of previous editions and adopted a seemingly objective and explicit approach to assigning labels to disordered behaviour (American Psychiatric Association, 1980a). The new approach was intended to parallel medical taxonomy and numerous distinct disorders were devised, each defined by lists of characteristic behaviours and experiences. Subsequent editions of the manual have grown, with more and more disorders being added and some being taken out, just as homosexuality was famously removed in the 1970s. The latest version, *DSM-5*, came close to including a diagnosis for a situation in which someone *might* develop a disorder in the future. Even without the proposed 'psychosis risk syndrome', however, the new edition expands the net of medicalisation further over ordinary experience, with critics claiming that it will pathologise 'mild eccentricity, loneliness, shyness, sadness and much else' (P. Kinderman cited in Watts, 2012)).

The credibility of the modern *DSM* and similar systems (the *International Classification of Diseases version 10*, for example) lies in the implication that the various labels they propose indicate the presence of an underlying disease, which particular treatments can target and rectify. In fact, faith in the specificity of drug treatment formed one of the foundations of the new approach to psychiatric classification. The architect of *DSM-3*, psychiatrist Robert Spitzer, defended the validity and utility of psychiatric diagnosis against its critics in the 1970s by citing the 'superiority of major tranquilisers [antipsychotics] in schizophrenia, of electro-convulsive therapy in depression, and more recently of lithium carbonate for the treatment of mania' (Spitzer, 1975, p. 450).[2] Indeed, as Spitzer recognised, if the process of diagnosis cannot direct the choice of treatment, then it has no practical or convincing purpose. The idea that the new drugs worked by attacking the underlying disease process provided the new diagnostic systems with the legitimacy they needed. In turn, these new systems helped to construct the use of mindaltering drugs as medical treatments rather than chemical suppressants. Psychiatric theory became a self-perpetuating cycle, with the illness model of mental disturbance justified by the disease-centred model of drug action, which was itself bolstered by the idea that mental disorders are properly thought of as discrete, biologically-based 'diseases'.

The concept of schizophrenia illustrates this interaction and the way that a drug-centred approach threatens the biological conception of psychiatry and its activities. The idea that the drugs used to treat people with schizophrenia and psychosis act by targeting an underlying, brain-based abnormality is considered as evidence that these conditions are manifestations of a discrete disease. Following from this belief in the disease-centred nature of drug action, the biochemical effects of the drugs, such as their ability to reduce dopamine activity, were presumed to point to the basis of the proposed disease. Because the assumption of disease-specific drug action was not perceived to be an assumption, it came to be believed that abnormal dopamine function lay at the root of schizophrenic or psychotic symptoms, and this dopamine 'hypothesis' then appeared to constitute evidence that antipsychotic drugs work by targeting the underlying disease. Challenging the disease-centred model of drug action therefore removes one of the foundations for the current case that schizophrenia and psychosis should be regarded as bona fide brain diseases in the same sense as conditions like epilepsy or encephalitis. Of course, other evidence might still be found to support the idea that these disorders originate from identifiable brain lesions, and disease-centred treatments might eventually be discovered. The fact that current treatments do not work by targeting a disease process does not mean that there is no disease to be uncovered. But it does reveal that we have not found it yet.

Antipsychotics and Psychiatric Care

Examining the history of antipsychotics from a drug-centred perspective helps to resolve the debate between those who claim that the introduction of antipsychotic drugs was responsible for emptying the asylums, and those who maintain that community care was driven by political imperatives. It would be surprising, from what we have learnt, if the use of antipsychotics did not reduce levels of disturbed behaviour such that people could more easily be accommodated outside the confines of a large institution, and in that sense the drugs can be credited with having hastened the decline in the mental hospital population, even if they did not initiate it. It is doubtful that more people are living independently now than in the era before the introduction of modern drugs, however, and people diagnosed with schizophrenia still occupy more hospital beds, for longer periods, than people with any other medical or psychiatric condition (Pillay and Moncrieff, 2011). David Healy and colleagues found that people with severe psychiatric disorders, such as those diagnosed with schizophrenia, currently spend several more years in an institution of some sort (including supported accommodation like residential homes) than they did 100 years ago (Healy et al., 2005). A process referred to as the 're-institutionalisation' of mental health care has been documented across Europe since the 1990s, with reductions in ordinary psychiatric hospital beds compensated for by an increase in places in residential and nursing homes, alongside a rise in the provision of privately-run, secure facilities (Priebe et al., 2005). The head of the National Institute of Mental Health, American psychiatrist Thomas Insel, even admitted that 'despite five decades of antipsychotic medication and deinstitutionalisation, there is little evidence that the prospects for recovery have changed substantially in the past century' (Insel, 2009, p. 130).

Through the ages the manner in which society supports its dependent members has varied, and the period of herding large numbers of people together in institutions has passed, along with the advantages and disadvantages of this type of care. Further financial incentives to reduce public spending will undoubtedly result in more people living in independent accommodation with the support of welfare payments and visiting carers. There is no evidence, however, that the introduction of antipsychotic drugs has substantially changed the financial and social burden associated with caring for people with the problems we refer to as severe mental disorders. Recent scandals suggest that the move to smaller, privately-run, community-based institutions may also not prevent the demoralisation among staff and abuse of inmates that was once associated with the asylum system (Brindle, 2011). Nevertheless, the drugs can be credited with providing the justification and momentum for a policy that changed the face of psychiatric care. The idea of a simple intervention that could relieve the mentally disturbed of troubling and dangerous thoughts, and might restore them to normal, was a convenient way of selling the potentially unpopular policy of returning the mentally ill to their communities (Gronfein, 1985).

In a similar way, an uncritical faith in the benefits of drug treatment facilitated the introduction of laws that allow people to be forced to continue psychiatric medication after they have been discharged from hospital. Dressed up as a process of enabling people to receive a necessary medical intervention, compulsory community treatment enforces drug-induced suppression beyond the bounds of a 'bricks and mortar' institution, creating a virtual net of control and containment. Although a randomised controlled trial of the use of Community Treatment Orders found that they did not reduce hospital admissions (Burns et al., 2013), they appear to be increasingly employed to enable people to be discharged from hospital earlier than they would have been otherwise. In this way compulsory community treatment reduces the financial costs of providing for the mentally distressed, while helping to maintain the peace of mind of the community at large. The price is borne by those who lose their liberty and autonomy maybe for ever, but perhaps also by all of us, as the principle of self-determination is gradually whittled away.

The Patients' Predicament

Understanding antipsychotic drugs through a drug-centred lens also helps to explain how they can be both the scourge of modern psychiatry—the 'drug prison' described by some of those who have been forced to take them (Breggin, 1993a, p. 57)—and a useful intervention that can reduce unwelcome thoughts and emotions, particularly in people suffering from what is currently labelled as psychosis or schizophrenia. As we saw in Chapter 7, the mental suppression and emotional restriction the drugs produce can help drive intrusive and preoccupying psychotic experiences into the background, and dissipate their intensity and significance, at the same time allowing 'sane' modes of thinking and behaving to re-emerge from psychotic turmoil. Severe mental disturbance can blight a person's whole existence and in this situation antipsychotic treatment, despite its many drawbacks, may be able to provide a quality of life that might not otherwise have been possible. The drugs do not always work, however. People can continue to be preoccupied with internal phenomena, and some prefer to remain in a psychotic world that is vibrant and intense than be transported back into a muted and stifled version of reality. For many people, as illustrated by the stories in Appendix 2, the drugs may reduce the intensity of psychotic experiences and lessen the distress they produce, but symptoms and difficulties persist, often compounded by the noxious effects of the drugs.

What we are to make of the near universal practice of prescribing these drugs for years upon end is the most pressing question we face. Are the experts who made up the Schizophrenia Commission right that antipsychotic drugs are the 'cornerstone of treatment for schizophrenia and psychosis', and the 'foundation upon which personal recovery is based', or should we heed Robert Whitaker's warning that long-term drug treatment has created an iatrogenic epidemic of adverse effects and increased dependency (Whitaker, 2010; Schizophrenia Commission, 2012, p. 29)? Is the treatment worse than the cure, as even some high-profile psychiatrists now seem to be suggesting (McGlashan, 2006; Tyrer, 2012)? There are indications that some people diagnosed with an episode of psychosis, and even with full blown schizophrenia, might function better in the long run by not taking antipsychotics, at least not continuously over long periods. We certainly know from historical data that not everyone who experiences a psychotic breakdown requires long-term medication. We also know that people who develop tardive dyskinesia undergo a decline in their mental abilities. What is less certain is whether long-term antipsychotic use leads to other types of deterioration, including behavioural changes, worsening psychosis and more generalised intellectual impairment, all of which might cancel out any beneficial effects the drugs might have in terms of reducing symptoms or risk of recurrence. We urgently need to clarify how antipsychotics impact on the ultimate course of psychotic conditions such as 'schizophrenia', and whether their long-term use contributes to the poor outcome of people given this diagnosis in the Western world.

While accepting the necessity of using antipsychotics in some circumstances, the data presented in this book suggest they are dangerous substances that should be avoided where possible. Current mental health services provide little opportunity for severe mental disorders to be managed without recourse to prolonged drug treatment, yet experiments like the Soteria project and the Finnish study demonstrate that this is possible within a supportive environment or network. A minority of people can endure a psychotic episode without any antipsychotic treatment and many others require only small amounts of medication on a temporary basis. Helping people in this way is likely to be more labour intensive, costly and protracted than the short, sharp solution that antipsychotics offer, however, and as bed numbers shrink and funds are squeezed, mental health services are more reliant than ever on drugs. There needs to be a radical change of attitude and practice before alternative approaches could be countenanced and implemented effectively within mainstream services, and the political commitment would need to be in place to provide the resources and the assurance to underpin the necessary changes. Many patients and carers want to see alternative approaches to the treatment of severe mental disturbance, however, in which antipsychotic medication is avoided or minimised.[2]

Where antipsychotics are used to treat an acute and severe psychotic episode, a policy of discontinuing antipsychotic medication after someone has recovered from their symptoms—and not many months or years afterwards—may offer the best chance of avoiding all the dangers associated with long-term treatment. In this way, people who would never have had another breakdown are not consigned to a lifetime of unnecessary exposure to harmful substances. Although people may need support to withdraw from antipsychotics safely, the costs of allowing people to continue on these toxic drugs may greatly outweigh the expenses incurred in enabling people to stop them. Not everyone will succeed, but every person that does reduces the considerable burden of drug-related disease and death, and for the individual there is also relief from sexual impairment, mental slowing, emotional suppression and agitation to name just a few of the unpleasant and debilitating effects that antipsychotics produce.

Without recognising that discontinuation may itself provoke unwanted effects, however, the process of medication withdrawal may simply entrench the view that long-term treatment is indispensable. People need to be given the chance to see if post withdrawal difficulties resolve with time or with other temporary measures, rather than being told, as many now are, that their attempt to stop medication has failed and that they were foolish to want to try it in the first place. People inevitably make different choices and some may opt to accept on-going drug treatment, especially if their symptoms are severe or disruptive. Yet others may decide to accept the risk of future relapses rather than embarking on a lifetime of chemical subjection. The important point is that people should be free to make their own choices about antipsychotic medication unless there are good legal reasons why they should not.

It should be acknowledged that in many circumstances antipsychotic drugs are not used because the individual finds them helpful, in fact, but because other people, or society in general, cannot tolerate the person's behaviour. Framing this situation as the treatment of a medical condition confuses and obscures the reality of what is involved—the forcible modification of behaviour using drugs. The disease-centred theory of antipsychotic action has played a major part in the obfuscation of the social control function that has always been embedded at the heart of psychiatric practice. The idea that antipsychotics target an underlying disease means that even when people are pinned down to the ground to be forcibly injected, they can be said to be receiving a therapeutic intervention administered for their own benefit. When the practice of forced drugging is portrayed honestly, it is clear that it requires open, transparent and democratic debate and scrutiny, none of which can occur properly while it is dressed up as a medical treatment. It is also apparent that physical measures might be preferable from the point of view of the individual on the receiving end of pacification techniques. It may be less frightening to be restrained or placed in a seclusion room than to have your mind and body invaded by a foreign chemical substance. Physical methods also brook no denial about the nature of the situation. It is not necessarily wrong to make people change their behaviour if it is seriously antisocial, threatening or dangerous. It is imperative, however, that as a society we should feel a sense of guilt and responsibility about trying to do so, and be prepared to think honestly about the methods we use to do it.

The Creeping Expansion

Although antipsychotics have a place, in my opinion, in the treatment of people with serious mental disorders like psychosis or schizophrenia, the same balance of considerations does not apply in people with other, less devastating conditions. We should be particularly concerned about the recent epidemic of antipsychotic prescribing that has been encouraged by the pharmaceutical industry. Not only have the boundaries of psychosis been stretched so far that any teenager with unusual behaviour might qualify as having early signs of psychosis or schizophrenia, antipsychotics have spread their tentacles out into the realm of what David Healy once called 'everyday nerves' (Healy, 2004). Antipsychotics are now frequently prescribed for depression and anxiety, and packaged under the less frightening name of 'mood stabilisers' they are promoted for the vague, new version of bipolar disorder—a diagnosis that can now be applied to almost anyone.

In many of these situations the drugs have not been properly tested and, where trials have been conducted, it is impossible to tell whether they have any real benefit over and above the sedative effects they are known to produce. What is certain is that the metabolic impairment, cardiac toxicity and neurological damage they induce can occur in anyone, regardless of the individual's diagnosis or the nature of their problems. It is highly unlikely therefore that the benefits of antipsychotics outweigh the risks in people who do not suffer from the most severe forms of mental disturbance. The increasingly indiscriminate prescribing of these noxious substances represents a substantial public health problem waiting to happen. The vision of a population incapacitated by prolonged chemical toxicity may yet be realised if we don't wake up to the real nature of antipsychotic drugs.

Notes

1 Cure or Curse: What Are Antipsychotics?

1. Receptors are chemicals on the outside of brain cells to which neurotransmitters attach and through which they effect their actions.
2. Laing's precise phrasing was 'a perfectly rational adjustment to an insane world'.

3 Magic Bullets: The Development of Ideas on Drug Action

1. I am indebted to other accounts that have noted how a disease-centred view of antipsychotic action emerged during the 1950s and 1960s, especially those of David Healy, Robert Whitaker and Sheldon Gelman (Gelman, 1999; Healy, 2002; Whitaker, 2002).
2. The 'extrapyramidal' system denotes the brain centres responsible for the *involuntary* control and regulation of movement, and is so named to contrast with the 'pyramidal' system, which is a pyramid-shaped tract of nerves that is directly involved in *voluntary* movement.

4 Building a House of Cards: The Dopamine Theory of Schizophrenia and Drug Action

1. The technique involves the injection of a radioactively-labelled chemical called a 'ligand' that binds to the receptor site; the positrons emitted by the ligand are detected by the radioactivity scanner.

5 The Phoenix Rises: From Tardive Dyskinesia to the Introduction of the 'Atypicals'

1. I am indebted to other accounts of the emergence of tardive dyskinesia (Tarsy, 1983; Breggin, 1993; Gelman, 1999).
2. The term 'tardive dyskinesia' literally means late-onset (tardive) abnormal movement (dyskinesia).
3. The basal ganglia is a group of nerve cell nuclei located below the cerebral hemispheres, which form part of the extrapyramidal system. They include the striatum (the name for the caudate nucleus and the putamen), and are sometimes referred to as the striatum or striatal system.

8 Chemical Cosh: Antipsychotics and Chemical Restraint

1. The Mindfreedom and Psychrights organisations have organised demonstrations against forced drugging in the USA; the Kissit campaign and Beyond

Bedlam have been active in the UK, Mad Pride in Eire and We Shall Overcome in Norway.
2. I am grateful to Dr Laura Allison who undertook some of the research for this chapter during the course of her studies for an MSc in Psychiatric Research at University College London.
3. Hydrotherapy involved prolonged immersion in cold or hot baths and was practised in asylums from the late nineteenth century.
4. Under Section 41 of the Mental Health Act of England and Wales people who have committed serious offences are made subject to government supervision after discharge from hospital.

9   Old and New Drug-Induced Problems

1. The brain consists of grey matter, which comprises the nerve cell bodies, and white matter, which consists of the projecting and connecting fibres.
2. The cerebral hemispheres (also known as the cerebral cortex) are the largest part of the brain and responsible for higher intellectual abilities.
3. These overall differences between patients and controls were not provided in the paper, but could be calculated from other data provided.
4. A transient ischaemic attack (TIA) occurs when there is a temporary loss of blood supply to part of the brain causing a temporary neurological deficit.

10   The First Tentacles: The 'Early Intervention in Psychosis' Movement

1. Schizotypal personality disorder is defined as 'a pervasive pattern of social and interpersonal deficits marked by acute discomfort with, and reduced capacity for, close relationships, as well as by cognitive and perceptual distortions or eccentricities of behaviour beginning in early adulthood and present in a variety of contexts' (American Psychiatric Association, 1980a).

12   All is not as it Seems

1. 'Tolerance' is a pharmacological term referring to the phenomena in which the body produces alterations that help to combat the effects of a drug when it is taken on an on-going basis.
2. The quotation cited is from one of two articles that Spitzer wrote in response to the famous Rosenhan experiment, in which psychology students posed as potential patients by presenting at accident and emergency departments saying they heard a voice saying 'thud'. All were admitted as psychiatric inpatients and discharged with a diagnosis of schizophrenia or schizophrenia 'in remission'. The experiment sparked accusations that psychiatrists could not distinguish the mad from the sane, and added to other criticisms of the reliability and validity of psychiatric diagnosis (Rosenhan, 1973).
3. The Soteria Network, for example, is a group of professionals, patients and carers interested in developing alternative services for those with severe mental disorders in the UK. The network supports small independent initiatives, as well as working with mainstream services (http://www.soterianetwork.org.uk/).

Appendix 1: Common Antipsychotic Drugs

	Approximate year of introduction into UK	Chemical class	Principle or original manufacturer	
First generation, oral antipsychotics				
Chlorpromazine (Largactil, Thorazine)	1954	Phenothiazine (aliphatic side chain)	Rhône-Poulenc (now Sanofi Aventis) and Smith Kline & French (now GlaxoSmithKline)	
Droperidol (Droleptan)	1980	Butyrophenone	Janssen	Withdrawn in UK in 2001
Flupentixol (Depixol)	1970s	Thioxanthene	Lundbeck	
Fluphenazine	1970s	Phenothiazine with piperazine side chain	Sanofi Aventis	
Haloperidol (Haldol, Serenace)	1958	Butyrophenone	Janssen	
Perphenazine (Fentazin)	1957	Phenothiazine with piperazine side chain	Allen & Hanburys (absorbed by Glaxo in 1958)	
Sulpiride (Dolmatil)	1983	Benzamide	Sanofi Aventis	
Thioridazine (Melleril)	1960	Phenothiazine with piperidine side chain	Sandoz (now Novartis)	Withdrawn in UK in 2005
Trifluoperazine (Stelazine)	1958	Phenothiazine with piperazine side chain	Smith Kline & French	

(continued)

Appendix 1 Continued

	Approximate year of introduction into UK	Chemical class	Principle or original manufacturer
Zuclopenthixol (Clopixol)	1962	Thioxanthene	Lundbeck
First-generation, long-acting injectable antipsychotics			
Flupentixol decanoate (Depixol)	1972	Thioxanthene	Lundbeck
Fluphenazine decanoate (Modecate)	1968	Phenothiazine with piperazine side chain	Sanofi Aventis
Haloperidol (Haldol)	1982	Butyrophenone	Janssen
Pipotiazine palmitate (Piportil)	1983	Phenothiazine	Sanofi Aventis
Zuclopenthixol decanoate (Clopixol)	1978	Thioxanthene	Lundbeck
Second-generation oral antipsychotics			
Amisulpride (Solian)	1997	Benzamide	Sanofi Aventis
Aripiprazole (Abilify)	2004	Quinalone	Bristol-Myers Squibb
Clozapine (Clozaril)	1990	Tricyclic dibenzodiazepine	Novartis
Olanzapine (Zyprexa)	1996	Thienobenzodiazepine	Eli Lilly & Co.
Quetiapine (Seroquel)	1997	Dibenzothiazepine	AstraZeneca
Risperidone (Risperdal)	1993	Benzisoxazole	Janssen

| Zisprazidone (Geodon) | Not licenced in UK; licenced in US in 2001 | | Pfizer |

Second-generation long-acting, injectable antipsychotics

Olanzapine embonate (ZypAdhera)	2008	Thienobenzodiazepine	Eli Lilly
Paliperidone palmitate (Xeplion)	2011	Benzisoxazole	Janssen
Risperidone (Risperdal Consta)	2002	Benzisoxazole	Janssen

Appendix 2: Accounts of Schizophrenia and Psychosis

The following three accounts are abridged versions of stories found in the National Institute for Health and Clinical Excellence's (NICE) guideline on the treatment of schizophrenia (National Institute for Health and Clinical Excellence, 2002).

Story 1
Mr A described how he started to develop symptoms while he was at University. He was hearing voices and 'reading strange meanings into what was going on'. He was referred to a psychiatrist, but managed to persuade the psychiatrist that there was nothing wrong, and he recovered without any intervention and went on to finish his degree. Later, in his mid-20s, while he was working as a research scientist, he started to hear voices and also to see things, and he was hospitalised after he took an overdose triggered by his distress at what was happening. He was started on an antipsychotic drug in hospital, which he describes as the start of a 'vicious cycle'. He would be put on drugs, find it difficult to function at work, stop taking them and end up being readmitted to hospital. Eventually, he had to give up work, and after 20 years, and despite being on antipsychotic treatment, he describes how the 'voices are still awful when they are really loud. They discuss me, put me down, shout obscenities, comment on what is happening to me and tell me to do things that put me in danger. It is very difficult to remain communicating in the real world, and doing this leaves me exhausted. In addition, I often end up seeing the world in a very different and frightening way and at the time I'm having these delusions I really believe them. I can still get very distressed by it all but these days living with schizophrenia is easier than it was when I was first ill'.

Story 2
Mr B developed symptoms at the age of 33 years. He felt 'wonderfully excited as though I was the only person in the country to be let in on a great secret' and recounted how he spent the summer travelling around in search of more 'delusional excitement', and thought he had 'become involved in the peace process in Northern Ireland'. At the end of the summer he was admitted to hospital after an outburst in which he caused a considerable amount of damage to property. In hospital he was prescribed an antipsychotic, which made him 'suicidally depressed' and he stopped taking it as soon as he was discharged. He spent the next 10 years in a cycle of 'gradually getting ill', which he usually enjoyed, 'getting arrested, being sectioned, and feeling suicidal because of the side effects of the drugs'. At the time he said his 'benchmark for happiness' was 'not being medicated' and when he was psychotic he felt 'positive and purposeful'. Eventually, he accepted drug treatment, encouraged by a supportive relationship with a community psychiatric nurse who was

willing to listen to his point of view and he had not had an admission for 4 years at the time of writing.

Story 3

Mrs C was diagnosed with schizophrenia a few years after she was married. Her husband described how, during her psychotic episodes, she would wonder the streets in a disturbed state, frequently being picked up by the police and ending up in hospital, sometimes for many months. He felt that drug treatment pacified her, but at the cost of destroying her personality and curtailing her enjoyment of life: 'My wife is naturally a very lively and stimulating person to be with and seeing her pacified by the side effects of medication was heartbreaking'. Eventually, his wife was prescribed a low dose of medication, which appeared to control her symptoms without too many adverse effects, and allowed her and her husband to lead 'as normal a life as possible' despite her condition.

The fourth story is taken from Bert Kaplan's book *The Inner World of Mental Illness*, a collection of first-person accounts of episodes of mental disturbance published in 1964 (Anonymous, 1964).

Story 4

A middle-class, professional woman who had worked as a social worker before having children described having three attacks of psychotic experiences in her late 30s. At the age of 36 years she started having an intense affair, and, in order to deal with the strength of her emotions, she started to write poetry and prose. Her writing became increasingly compulsive, and she lost interest in and neglected her children and the 'practical details of living'. She became convinced that she had discovered the secrets of the universe and that she could prove the existence of God. She also thought there had been a world catastrophe, and she thought her children had died; she had a general sense of fear and dread, as well as some unusual religious and sexual ideas. She was taken to hospital in 1948 in a 'rigid catatonic condition' where she was given a barbiturate and discharged after 5 months. Her second episode occurred 1 year later, and she was admitted in much the same state for 3 months and recovered spontaneously. The third episode started in 1951, and she was in hospital on this occasion for over a year. During this episode she developed the idea that she should kill her youngest son and some other people, although she did not act on these thoughts. She was treated with ECT twice during this admission, and up until the time that the book was compiled in the early 1960s, she had had no further episodes. Looking back at the time the account was written she felt that the experience had reduced her anxiety, helped her gain confidence, freed up her intellectual capacities and enabled her to change 'from a non-religious to a religious orientation'.

References

Able, D. (2007) 'Hull parents arrested in girl's poisoning death', *Boston Globe*, 6 Feb.

Ackner, B., Harris, A. and Oldham, A. J. (1957) 'Insulin treatment of schizophrenia: controlled study', *Lancet*, 2, 607–11.

Adler, C. M., Elman, I., Weisenfeld, N., Kestler, L., Pickar, D. and Breier, A. (2000) 'Effects of acute metabolic stress on striatal dopamine release in healthy volunteers', *Neuropsychopharmacology*, 22, 545–50.

Agid, O., Kapur, S., Arenovich, T. and Zipursky, R. B. (2003) 'Delayed-onset hypothesis of antipsychotic action: a hypothesis tested and rejected', *Arch Gen Psychiatry*, 60, 1228–35.

Akiskal, H. S. (1996) 'The prevalent clinical spectrum of bipolar disorders: beyond DSM-IV', *J Clin Psychopharmacol*, 16, 4S–14S.

Albaugh, V. L., Singareddy, R., Mauger, D. and Lynch, C. J. (2011) 'A double blind, placebo-controlled, randomized crossover study of the acute metabolic effects of olanzapine in healthy volunteers', *PLoS One*, 6, e22662.

Alexander, J., Tharyan, P., Adams, C., John, T., Mol, C. and Philip, J. (2004) 'Rapid tranquillisation of violent or agitated patients in a psychiatric emergency setting. Pragmatic randomised trial of intramuscular lorazepam v. haloperidol plus promethazine', *Br J Psychiatry*, 185, 63–9.

Alexander, G. C., Gallagher, S. A., Mascola, A., Moloney, R. M. and Stafford, R. S. (2011) 'Increasing off-label use of antipsychotic medications in the United States, 1995–2008', *Pharmacoepidemiol Drug Saf*, 20, 177–84.

Allen, S. (2007) 'Backlash on bipolar diagnoses in children', *Boston Globe*, 17 Jun.

Allen, M. H., Currier, G. W., Hughes, D. H., Reyes-Harde, M. and Docherty, J. P. (2001) 'The expert consensus guideline series: Treatment of behavioural emergencies', *Postgrad Med*, 1–88.

Alty, A. and Mason, T. (1994) *Seclusion in Mental Health* (London: Chapman & Hall).

American Psychiatric Association (1980a) *Diagnostic and Statistical Manual of Mental Disorders*, 3rd edn. (Washington, DC: American Psychiatric Association).

American Psychiatric Association (1980b) *Task Force Report: Tardive Dyskinesia* (Washington, DC: American Psychiatric Association).

American Psychiatric Association (1996) *Schizophrenia* (Washington, DC: American Psychiatric Association).

American Psychiatric Association (2005) *Lets Talk Facts About Depression* (Washington, DC: American Psychiatric Association).

Andrade, S. E., Lo, J. C., Roblin, D., Fouayzi, H., Connor, D. F., Penfold, R. B., et al. (2011) 'Antipsychotic medication use among children and risk of diabetes mellitus', *Pediatrics*, 128, 1135–41.

Andreasen, N. C., Nopoulos, P., Magnotta, V., Pierson, R., Ziebell, S. and Ho, B. C. (2011) 'Progressive brain change in schizophrenia: a prospective longitudinal study of first-episode schizophrenia', *Biol Psychiatry*, 70, 672–9.

Angermeyer, M. C., Loffler, W., Muller, P., Schulze, B. and Priebe, S. (2001) 'Patients' and relatives' assessment of clozapine treatment', *Psychol Med*, 31, 509–17.

Angst, J. (1998) 'The emerging epidemiology of hypomania and bipolar II disorder', *J Affect Disord*, 50, 143–51.

Angst, J., Gamma, A., Benazzi, F., Ajdacic, V., Eich, D. and Rossler, W. (2003) 'Toward a re-definition of subthreshold bipolarity: epidemiology and proposed criteria for bipolar-II, minor bipolar disorders and hypomania', *J Affect Disord*, 73, 133–46.

Anonymous (1964) 'An autobiography of a schizophrenic experience', in Kaplan, B. (ed.) *The Inner World of Mental Illness*, pp. 89–115 (New York: Harper & Row).

Anonymous (1965) 'Irreversible side effects of phenothiazines', *JAMA*, 191, 333–4.

Anonymous (1987) 'Psychiatrist is cleared in ethics case', *New York Times*, 13 Oct.

Anonymous (1990) *Warley Hospital Brentwood. the First Hundred Years 1853–1953 Incorporating Into the Second Century 1953–1963* (Brentwood: Warley Hospital).

Anonymous (2009a) 'Comment on olanzapine', available at: www.askapatient.com (accessed 14 April 2013).

Anonymous (2009b) 'Comment on Riserpdal', available at: www.askapatient.com (accessed 14 April 2013).

Anton-Stephens, D. (1954) 'Preliminary observations on the psychiatric uses of chlorpromazine (largactil)', *J Ment Sci*, 100, 543–57.

Anzia, N., Okazaki, Y., Miyauchi, M., Harada, S.-I., Kanou, Y., Sasaki, T., et al. (1988) 'Early neuroleptic medication within one year after onset can reduce risk of later relapses in schizophrenia patients', *Annu Rep Pharmacopsychiatry Res Found*, 19, 258–65.

Aparasu, R. R., Bhatara, V. and Gupta, S. (2005) 'U.S. national trends in the use of antipsychotics during office visits, 1998–2002', *Ann Clin Psychiatry*, 17, 147–52.

Apud, J. A., Egan, M. F. and Wyatt, R. J. (2003) 'Neuroleptic withdrawal in treatment-resistant patients with schizophrenia: tardive dyskinesia is not associated with supersensitive psychosis', *Schizophr Res*, 63, 151–60.

Arnone, D., Cavanagh, J., Gerber, D., Lawrie, S. M., Ebmeier, K. P. and McIntosh, A. M. (2009) 'Magnetic resonance imaging studies in bipolar disorder and schizophrenia: meta-analysis', *Br J Psychiatry*, 195, 194–201.

AstraZeneca (2011) 'Seroquel XR for schizophrenia', available at: www.seroquelxr.com/schizophrenia/index.aspx?ux=t (accessed 14 April 2013).

AstraZeneca (2012) 'Bipolar disorder', available at: http://www.seroquelxr.com/bipolar-disorder/index.aspx?ux=t (accessed 14 April 2013).

Austin, S. C., Stolley, P. D. and Lasky, T. (1992) 'The history of malariotherapy for neurosyphilis. Modern parallels', *JAMA*, 268, 516–19.

Azcarate, C. L. (1975) 'Minor tranquilizers in the treatment of aggression', *J Nerv Ment Dis*, 160, 100–7.

Bai, O., Zhang, H. and Li, X. M. (2004) 'Antipsychotic drugs clozapine and olanzapine upregulate bcl-2 mRNA and protein in rat frontal cortex and hippocampus', *Brain Res*, 1010, 81–6.

Baldessarini, R. J. and Viguera, A. C. (1995) 'Neuroleptic withdrawal in schizophrenic patients', *Arch Gen Psychiatry*, 52, 189–92.

Baldessarini, R. J., Tondo, L. and Viguera, A. C. (1999) 'Discontinuing lithium maintenance treatment in bipolar disorders: risks and implications', *Bipolar Disord*, 1, 17–24.

Ballard, C., Hanney, M. L., Theodoulou, M., Douglas, S., McShane, R., Kossakowski, K., et al. (2009) 'The dementia antipsychotic withdrawal trial

(DART-AD): long-term follow-up of a randomised placebo-controlled trial', *Lancet Neurol*, 8, 151–7.

Banergee, S. (2009) *The Use of Antipsychotic Medication for People With Dementia: Time for Action* (London: Department of Health).

Barany, S., Ingvast, A. and Gunne, L. M. (1979) 'Development of acute dystonia and tardive dyskinesia in cebus monkeys', *Res Commun Chem Pathol Pharmacol*, 25, 269–79.

Bartholini, G., Haefely, W., Jalfre, M., Keller, H. H. and Pletscher, A. (1972) 'Effects of clozapine on cerebral catecholaminergic neurone systems', *Br J Pharmacol*, 46, 736–40.

Batki, S. L. and Harris, D. S. (2004) 'Quantitative drug levels in stimulant psychosis: relationship to symptom severity, catecholamines and hyperkinesia', *Am J Addict*, 13, 461–70.

Bauer, M., Pretorius, H. W., Constant, E. L., Earley, W. R., Szamosi, J. and Brecher, M. (2009) 'Extended-release quetiapine as adjunct to an antidepressant in patients with major depressive disorder: results of a randomized, placebo-controlled, double-blind stud', *J Clin Psychiatry*, 70, 540–9.

Baumeister, A. A. and Francis, J. L. (2002) 'Historical development of the dopamine hypothesis of schizophrenia', *J Hist Neurosci*, 11, 265–77.

BBC (2006) 'Stephen Fry: the secret life of the manic depressive', Broadcast 19 and 26 September (London: British Broadcasting Corporation).

Beasley, C. M., Jr, Sanger, T., Satterlee, W., Tollefson, G., Tran, P. and Hamilton, S. (1996a) 'Olanzapine versus placebo: results of a double-blind, fixed-dose olanzapine trial', *Psychopharmacology (Berl)*, 124, 159–67.

Beasley, C. M., Jr, Tollefson, G., Tran, P., Satterlee, W., Sanger, T. and Hamilton, S. (1996b) 'Olanzapine versus placebo and haloperidol: acute phase results of the North American double-blind olanzapine trial', *Neuropsychopharmacology*, 14, 111–23.

Bechdolf, A., Wagner, M., Ruhrmann, S., Harrigan, S., Putzfeld, V., Pukrop, R., et al. (2012) 'Preventing progression to first-episode psychosis in early initial prodromal states', *Br J Psychiatry*, 200, 22–9.

Behl, C., Rupprecht, R., Skutella, T. and Holsboer, F. (1995) 'Haloperidol-induced cell death—mechanism and protection with vitamin E in vitro', *Neuroreport*, 7, 360–4.

Bentall, R. and Morrison, A. P. (2002) 'More harm than good: The case against using antipsychotic drugs to prevent severe mental illness', *J Mental Health*, 11, 351–6.

Berenson, A. (2006) 'Eli Lilly said to play down risks of top pill', *New York Times*, available at: http://www.nytimes.com/2006/12/17/business/17drug.html?pagewanted=all (accessed 14 April 2013).

Berenson, A. (2007) 'Lilly settles with 18,000 over Zyprexa', *New York Times*, available at: http://query.nytimes.com/gst/fullpage.html?res=9F00E5DB1430F936A35752C0A9619C8B63 (accessed 14 April 2013).

Beresford, V., Jenkins, D., Marshall, S. B., Montgomery, V., Swan, H. and Wilson, J. N. (1956) 'Experimental hemorrhage: the deleterious effect of hypothermia on survival and a comparative evaluation of plasma volume changes', *Ann Surg*, 144, 696–714.

Berger, G. E., Wood, S. and McGorry, P. D. (2003) 'Incipient neurovulnerability and neuroprotection in early psychosis', *Psychopharmacol Bull*, 37, 79–101.

Berridge, C. W. (2006) 'Neural substrates of psychostimulant-induced arousal', *Neuropsychopharmacology*, 31, 2332–40.

Bertelsen, M., Jeppesen, P., Petersen, L., Thorup, A., Ohlenschlaeger, J., Le Quach, P., et al. (2008) 'Five-year follow-up of a randomized multicenter trial of intensive early intervention vs standard treatment for patients with a first episode of psychotic illness: the OPUS trial', *Arch Gen Psychiatry*, 65, 762–71.

Biederman, J., Faraone, S., Mick, E., Wozniak, J., Chen, L., Ouellette, C., et al. (1996) 'Attention-deficit hyperactivity disorder and juvenile mania: an overlooked comorbidity?', *J Am Acad Child Adolesc Psychiatry*, 35, 997–1008.

Biederman, J., Mick, E., Hammerness, P., Harpold, T., Aleardi, M., Dougherty, M., et al. (2005) 'Open-label, 8-week trial of olanzapine and risperidone for the treatment of bipolar disorder in preschool-age children', *Biol Psychiatry*, 58, 589–94.

Bipolar UK (2012) 'Medications for bipolar: a short description and resource guide', available at: http://www.bipolaruk.org.uk/assets/uploads/documents/information_leaflets/bipolar_uk_introduction_to_medical_treatment.pdf (accessed 14 April 2013).

Birchwood, M., McGorry, P. and Jackson, H. (1997) 'Early intervention in schizophrenia', *Br J Psychiatry*, 170, 2–5.

Bishop, Y. (2005) *The Vetinary Formulary*, 6th edn. (London: Pharmaceutical Press).

Bleuler, E. (1911) 'Dementia praecox oder gruppe der schizophrenien', in Aschaffenburg, G. (ed.) *Handbuch der Psychiatrie* (Leipzig: Franz Deuticke).

Bleuler, E. (1951) 'Autistic thinking', in Rapoport, D. (ed.) *Organisation and Pathology of Thought. Selected Sources*, pp. 397–437 (New York: Columbia University Press).

Bleuler, M. (1974) 'The long-term course of the schizophrenic psychose', *Psychol Med*, 4, 244–55.

Bloch, H. S. (1970) 'Brief sleep treatment with chlorpromazine', *Compr Psychiatry*, 11, 346–55.

Boardman, J. (2005) *New Services for Old – An Overview of Mental Health Policy* (London: Sainsbury Centre for Mental Health).

Bola, J. R. and Mosher, L. R. (2003) 'Treatment of acute psychosis without neuroleptics: two-year outcomes from the Soteria project', *J Nerv Ment Dis*, 191, 219–29.

Borison, R. L. and Diamond, B. I. (1978) 'A new animal model for schizophrenia: interactions with adrenergic mechanisms', *Biol Psychiatry*, 13, 217–25.

Borison, R. L. and Diamond, B. I. (1983) 'Regional selectivity of neuroleptic drugs: an argument for site specificity', *Brain Res Bull*, 11, 215–18.

Borison, R. L., Diamond, B. I., Sinha, D., Gupta, R. P. and Ajiboye, P. A. (1988) 'Clozapine withdrawal rebound psychosis', *Psychopharmacol Bull*, 24, 260–3.

Bortnick, B., El Khalili, N., Banov, M., Adson, D., Datto, C., Raines, S., et al. (2011) 'Efficacy and tolerability of extended release quetiapine fumarate (quetiapine XR) monotherapy in major depressive disorder: a placebo-controlled, randomized study', *J Affect Disord*, 128, 83–94.

Bosanac, P., Patton, G. C. and Castle, D. J. (2010) 'Early intervention in psychotic disorders: faith before facts?', *Psychol Med*, 40, 353–8.

Bostic, J. Q., Wilens, T., Spencer, T. and Biederman, J. (1997) 'Juvenile mood disorders and office psychopharmacology', *Pediatr Clin North Am*, 44, 1487–503.

Bowden, C. L. (1998) 'New concepts in mood stabilization: evidence for the effectiveness of valproate and lamotrigine', *Neuropsychopharmacology*, 19, 194–9.

Bowden, C. L., Brugger, A. M., Swann, A. C., Calabrese, J. R., Janicak, P. G., Petty, F., et al. (1994) 'Efficacy of divalproex vs lithium and placebo in the treatment of mania. The Depakote Mania Study Group', *JAMA*, 271, 918–24.

Bowden, C. L., Calabrese, J. R., McElroy, S. L., Gyulai, L., Wassef, A., Petty, F., et al. (2000) 'A randomized, placebo-controlled 12-month trial of divalproex and lithium in treatment of outpatients with bipolar I disorder. Divalproex Maintenance Study Group', *Arch Gen Psychiatry*, 57, 481–9.

Braden, W., Fink, E. B., Qualls, C. B., Ho, C. K. and Samuels, W. O. (1982) 'Lithium and chlorpromazine in psychotic inpatients', *Psychiatry Res*, 7, 69–81.

Bralet, M. C., Yon, V., Loas, G. and Noisette, C. (2000) ['Cause of mortality in schizophrenic patients: prospective study of years of a cohort of 150 chronic schizophrenic patients'], *Encephale*, 26, 32–41 [in French].

Braslow, J. (1997) *Mental Ills and Bodily Cures* (Berkely, CA: University of California Press).

Breggin, P. (1983) *Hazards to the Brain* (New York: Springer).

Breggin, P. (2008) *Brain-Disabling Treatments in Psychiatry*, 2nd edn. (New York: Springer).

Breggin, P. R. (1990) 'Brain damage, dementia and persistent cognitive dysfunction associated with neuroleptic drugs. Evidence, etiology, implications', *J Mind Behav*, 11, 425–64.

Breggin, P. R. (1993a) *Toxic Psychiatry* (London: Fontana).

Breggin, P. R. (1993b) 'Parallels between neuroleptic effects and lethargic encephalitis: the production of dyskinesias and cognitive disorders', *Brain Cogn*, 23, 8–27.

Breggin, P. R. (1997) *Brain Disabling Treatments in Psychiatry: Drugs Electroshock and the Role of the FDA* (New York: Springer).

Breggin, P. R. (2006) 'Intoxicatrion anosognosia: the spellbinding effect of psychiatric drugs', *Ethical Human Psychol Psychiatry*, 8, 201–15.

Breier, A. (1989) 'A.E. Bennett award paper. Experimental approaches to human stress research: assessment of neurobiological mechanisms of stress in volunteers and psychiatric patients', *Biol Psychiatry*, 26, 438–62.

Breier, A. (1995) 'Serotonin, schizophrenia and antipsychotic drug action', *Schizophr Res*, 14, 187–202.

Brill, H. (1956) *The First Years' Experience With Large-scale Use of Chlorpormazine and Reserpine in the Mental Hygiene Institutions of New York State: A Preliminary Report* (Rochester: New York State Hospital).

Brill, H. and Patton, R. E. (1957) 'Analysis of 1955–1956 population fall in New York State mental hospitals in first year of large-scale use of tranquilizing drugs', *Am J Psychiatry*, 114, 509–17.

Brindle, D. (2011) 'Abuse at leading care home leads to police inspections of private hospitals', *Guardian*, 1 Jun.

Brodie, B. B., Spector, S. and Shore, P. A. (1959) 'Interaction of drugs with norepinephrine in the brain', *Pharmacol Rev*, 11, 548–64.

Brooks, G. W. (1959) 'Withdrawal from neuroleptic drugs', *Am J Psychiatry*, 115, 931–2.

Brown, S., Chhina, N. and Dye, S. (2010) 'Use of psychotropic medication in seven English psychiatric intensive care units', *Psychiatrist*, 34, 130–5.

Brunello, N., Masotto, C., Steardo, L., Markstein, R. and Racagni, G. (1995) 'New insights into the biology of schizophrenia through the mechanism of action of clozapine', *Neuropsychopharmacology*, 13, 177–213.

Buchsbaum, M. S., Someya, T., Teng, C. Y., Abel, L., Chin, S., Najafi, A., et al. (1996) 'PET and MRI of the thalamus in never-medicated patients with schizophrenia', *Am J Psychiatry*, 153, 191–9.

Buckley, P. F., Mahadik, S., Pillai, A. and Terry, A., Jr (2007) 'Neurotrophins and schizophrenia', *Schizophr Res*, 94, 1–11.

Bunney, B. S., Walters, J. R., Kuhar, M. J., Roth, R. H. and Aghajanian, G. K. (1975) 'D & L amphetamine stereoisomers: comparative potencies in affecting the firing of central dopaminergic and noradrenergic neurons', *Psychopharmacol Commun*, 1, 177–90.

Burns, T., Rugkasa, J., Molodynski, A., Dawson, J., Yeeles, K., Vazquez-Montes, M., et al. (2013) 'Community treatment orders for patients with psychosis (OCTET): a randomised controlled trial', *Lancet*, 25 March, doi: 10.1016/S0140-6736(13)60107-05 (Epub ahead of print).

Burt, D. R., Creese, I. and Snyder, S. H. (1977) 'Antischizophrenic drugs: chronic treatment elevates dopamine receptor binding in brain', *Science*, 196, 326–8.

Bushe, C. and Holt, R. (2004) 'Prevalence of diabetes and impaired glucose tolerance in patients with schizophrenia', *Br J Psychiatry Suppl*, 47, S67–S71.

Bushe, C. and Leonard, B. (2004) 'Association between atypical antipsychotic agents and type 2 diabetes: review of prospective clinical data', *Br J Psychiatry Suppl*, 47, S87–S93.

Byne, W., White, L., Parella, M., Adams, R., Harvey, P. D. and Davis, K. L. (1998) 'Tardive dyskinesia in a chronically institutionalized population of elderly schizophrenic patients: prevalence and association with cognitive impairment', *Int J Geriatr Psychiatry*, 13, 473–9.

Cahn, W., Hulshoff Pol, H. E., Lems, E. B., van Haren, N. E., Schnack, H. G., van der Linden, J. A., et al. (2002) 'Brain volume changes in first-episode schizophrenia: a 1-year follow-up study', *Arch Gen Psychiatry*, 59, 1002–10.

Carey, B. (2006) 'A career that has mirrored psychiatry's twisting path', *New York Times*, 23 May.

Carey, B. (2007) 'Debate over children and psychiatric drugs', *New York Times*, 15 Feb.

Carlsson, A. (2006) 'The neurochemical circuitry of schizophrenia', *Pharmacopsychiatry*, 39(Suppl. 1), S10–S14.

Carlsson, A., Lindqvist, M. and Magnusson, T. (1957) '3,4-Dihydroxyphenylalanine and 5-hydroxytryptophan as reserpine antagonists', *Nature*, 180, 1200.

Carlsson, A., Rasmussen, E. B. and Krist, J. P. (1959) 'The urinary excretion of adrenaline and noradrenaline by schizophrenic patients during reserpine treatment', *J Neurochem*, 4, 318–20.

Carpenter, W. T., Jr (1995) 'Serotonin-dopamine antagonists and treatment of negative symptoms', *J Clin Psychopharmacol*, 15, 30S–35S.

Carpenter, W. T., Jr, Buchanan, R. W., Kirkpatrick, B. and Breier, A. F. (1999) 'Diazepam treatment of early signs of exacerbation in schizophrenia', *Am J Psychiatry*, 156, 299–303.

Casey, J. F., Lasky, J. J., Klett, C. J. and Hollister, L. E. (1960a) 'Treatment of schizophrenic reactions with phenothiazine derivatives. A comparative study of chlorpromazine, triflupromazine, mepazine, prochlorperazine, perphenazine, and phenobarbital', *Am J Psychiatry*, 117, 97–105.

Casey, J. F., Bennett, I. F., Lindley, C. J., Hollister, L. E., Gordon, M. H. and Springer, N. N. (1960b) 'Drug therapy in schizophrenia. A controlled study of the relative effectiveness of chlorpromazine, promazine, phenobarbital, and placebo', *Arch Gen Psychiatry*, 2, 210–20.

Castle, D. J. (2012) 'The truth, and nothing but the truth, about early intervention in psychosis', *Aust N Z J Psychiatry*, 46, 10–13.

Cazzullo, C. L. and Guareschi, A. (1954) ['Effect of a phenothiazine derivative, largactil, on the electric activity of the brain, in dogs'], *Riv Neurol*, 24, 602–32 [in Italian].

Chaggar, P. S., Shaw, S. M. and Williams, S. G. (2011) 'Effect of antipsychotic medications on glucose and lipid levels', *J Clin Pharmacol*, 51, 631–8.

Chakos, M. H., Lieberman, J. A., Alvir, J., Bilder, R. and Ashtari, M. (1995) 'Caudate nuclei volumes in schizophrenic patients treated with typical antipsychotics or clozapine', *Lancet*, 345, 456–7.

Chan, D. and Sireling, L. (2010) '"I want to be bipolar"...a new phenomenon', *Psychiatrist*, 34, 103–5.

Chen, E. Y., Hui, C. L., Lam, M. M., Chiu, C. P., Law, C. W., Chung, D. W., et al. (2010) 'Maintenance treatment with quetiapine versus discontinuation after one year of treatment in patients with remitted first episode psychosis: randomised controlled trial', *BMJ*, 341, c4024.

Chertok, L. (1982) ['30 years later. The story of the discovery of neuroleptics'], *Ann Med Psychol (Paris)*, 140, 971–6 [in French].

Chien, I. C., Chang, K. C., Lin, C. H., Chou, Y. J. and Chou, P. (2010) 'Prevalence of diabetes in patients with bipolar disorder in Taiwan: a population-based national health insurance study', *Gen Hosp Psychiatry*, 32, 577–82.

Chouinard, G. and Jones, B. D. (1980) 'Neuroleptic-induced supersensitivity psychosis: clinical and pharmacologic characteristics', *Am J Psychiatry*, 137, 16–21.

Chouinard, G., Jones, B., Remington, G., Bloom, D., Addington, D., MacEwan, G. W., et al. (1993) 'A Canadian multicenter placebo-controlled study of fixed doses of risperidone and haloperidol in the treatment of chronic schizophrenic patients', *J Clin Psychopharmacol*, 13, 25–40.

Christensen, E., Moller, J. E. and Faurbye, A. (1970) 'Neuropathological investigation of 28 brains from patients with dyskinesia', *Acta Psychiatr Scand*, 46, 14–23.

Chua, S. E., Cheung, C., Cheung, V., Tsang, J. T., Chen, E. Y., Wong, J. C., et al. (2007) 'Cerebral grey, white matter and csf in never-medicated, first-episode schizophrenia', *Schizophr Res*, 89, 12–21.

Clopixol Acuphase advertisement (1990) Advertisement, Br J Psychiatry, July, backcover.

Clow, A., Theodorou, A., Jenner, P. and Marsden, C. D. (1980) 'Changes in rat striatal dopamine turnover and receptor activity during one years neuroleptic administration', *Eur J Pharmacol*, 63, 135–44.

Cole, J. O. (1959) 'The evaluation of the effectiveness of treatment in psychiatry', in Cole, J. O. and Gerard, R. W. (eds) *Psychopharmacology Problems in Evaluation: Proceedings*, pp. 92–107 (Washington, DC: National Academy of Sciences).

Cole, J. (1996) 'The evaluation of psychotropic drugs', in Healy, D. (ed.) *The Psychopharmacologists Volume I*, pp. 239–64 (London: Chapman & Hall).

Comité Lyonnais de Recherches Therapeutiques en Psychiatrie (2000) 'The birth of psychopharmacotherapy: explorations in a new world – 1952–1968', in Healy, D. (ed.) *The Psychopharmacologists III*, pp. 1–53 (London: Arnold).

Cooper, R. (2011) '"We can live to 150 and stay healthy": Professor says first "wonder drugs" could be ready this decade', *Daily Mail*, 19 Oct.

Cooper, W. O., Arbogast, P. G., Ding, H., Hickson, G. B., Fuchs, D. C. and Ray, W. A. (2006) 'Trends in prescribing of antipsychotic medications for US children', *Ambul Pediatr*, 6, 79–83.

COPE (2012) 'The Centre of Prevention and Evaluation', available at: http://www.copeclinic.org/The_COPE_Clinic_at_Columbia_Psychiatry.html (accessed 14 April 2013).

Correll, C. U. (2011) 'Safety and tolerability of antipsychotic treatment in young patients with schizophrenia', *J Clin Psychiatry*, 72, e26.

Correll, C. U. and Schenk, E. M. (2008) 'Tardive dyskinesia and new antipsychotics', *Curr Opin Psychiatry*, 21, 151–6.

Correll, C. U., Frederickson, A. M., Kane, J. M. and Manu, P. (2006) 'Metabolic syndrome and the risk of coronary heart disease in 367 patients treated with second-generation antipsychotic drugs', *J Clin Psychiatry*, 67, 575–83.

Costall, B. and Naylor, R. J. (1975) 'Detection of the nueroleptic properties of clozapine, sulpiride and thioridazine', *Psychopharmacologia*, 43, 69–74.

Cousins, D. A., Aribisala, B., Nicol Ferrier, I. and Blamire, A. M. (2013) 'Lithium, gray matter, and magnetic resonance imaging signal', *Biol Psychiatry*, 73, 652–7.

Craig, T. K., Garety, P., Power, P., Rahaman, N., Colbert, S., Fornells-Ambrojo, M., et al. (2004) 'The Lambeth Early Onset (LEO) Team: randomised controlled trial of the effectiveness of specialised care for early psychosis.', *BMJ*, 329, 1067.

Crane, G. E. (1956) 'Further studies on iproniazid phosphate', *J Nerv Ment Dis*, 124, 322–31.

Crane, G. E. (1967) 'Tardive dyskinesia in schizophrenic patients treated with neuroleptic drugs', *Aggressologie*, 9, 209–18.

Crane, G. E. (1968) 'Dyskinesia and neuroleptics', *Arch Gen Psychiatry*, 19, 700–3.

Crane, G. E. (1973) 'Clinical psychopharmacology in its 20th year. Late, unanticipated effects of neuroleptics may limit their use in psychiatry', *Science*, 181, 124–8.

Crilley, J. (2007) 'The history of clozapine and its emergence in the US market', *Hist Psychiatry*, 18, 39–60.

Crow, T. J. (1987) 'The dopamine hypothesis survives, but there must be a way ahead', *Br J Psychiatry*, 151, 460–5.

Crow, T. J. and Gillbe, C. (1974) 'Brain dopamine and behaviour. A critical analysis of the relationship between dopamine antagonism and therapeutic efficacy of neuroleptic drugs', *J Psychiatr Res*, 11, 163–72.

Crow, T. J., Owens, D. G., Johnstone, E. C., Cross, A. J. and Owen, F. (1983) 'Does tardive dyskinesia exist?', *Mod Probl Pharmacopsychiatry*, 21, 206–19.

Crow, T. J., MacMillan, J. F., Johnson, A. L. and Johnstone, E. C. (1986) 'A randomised controlled trial of prophylactic neuroleptic treatment', *Br J Psychiatry*, 148, 120–7.

Cullberg, J., Levander, S., Holmqvist, R., Mattsson, M. and Wieselgren, I. M. (2002) 'One-year outcome in first episode psychosis patients in the Swedish Parachute project', *Acta Psychiatr Scand*, 106, 276–285.

Cundall, R. L., Brooks, P. W. and Murray, L. G. (1972) 'A controlled evaluation of lithium prophylaxis in affective disorders', *Psychol Med*, 2, 308–11.

Dale, H. H. and Laidlaw, P. P. (1910) 'The physiological action of beta-iminazolylethylamine', *J Physiol*, 41, 318–44.

Dale, H. H. and Richards, A. N. (1918) 'The vasodilator action of histamine and of some other substances', *J Physiol*, 52, 110–65.

Dale, H. H. and Laidlaw, P. P. (1919) 'Histamine shock', *J Physiol*, 52, 355–90.

Dartalan advertisement (1960) *Journal of Mental Science*, 106, July, xviii.

Davis, J. M. (1980) 'Antipsychotic drugs', in Kaplan, H. I., Freedman, A. M. and Sadock, B. J. (eds) *Comprehensive Textbook of Psychiatry*, 3rd edn, pp. 2257–89 (Baltimore, MD: Williams & Wilkins).

Davis, J. M. and Cole, J. (1975) 'Antipsychotic drugs', in Freedman, D. X. and Dyrud, J. E. (eds) *American Handbook of Psychiatry, Volume 5, Treatment*, 2nd edn, pp. 441–75 (New York: Basic Books).

Davis, K. L., Kahn, R. S., Ko, G. and Davidson, M. (1991) 'Dopamine in schizophrenia: a review and reconceptualization', *Am J Psychiatry*, 148, 1474–86.

De Hert, M., Correll, C. U. and Cohen, D. (2010) 'Do antipsychotic medications reduce or increase mortality in schizophrenia? A critical appraisal of the FIN-11 study', *Schizophr Res*, 117, 68–74.

De Hert, M., Detraux, J., van Winkel, R., Yu, W. and Correll, C. U. (2011) 'Metabolic and cardiovascular adverse effects associated with antipsychotic drugs', *Nat Rev Endocrinol*, 8, 114–26.

Dean, C. E. (2006) 'Antipsychotic-associated neuronal changes in the brain: toxic, therapeutic, or irrelevant to the long-term outcome of schizophrenia?', *Prog Neuropsychopharmacol Biol Psychiatry*, 30, 174–89.

Deary, I. J., Penke, L. and Johnson, W. (2010) 'The neuroscience of human intelligence differences', *Nat Rev Neurosci*, 11, 201–11.

DeGrandpre, R. (2006) *The Cult of Pharmcology. How America became the world's most troubled drug culture* (Durham, NC: Duke University Press).

Delay, J. and Deniker, P. (1952) '38 cas de psychoses traites par la cure prolongee et continue de 4560 R.P.', *C R Congres Med Alien Neurol France*, 50, 503–13.

Delay, J. and Deniker, P. (1953) ['Neuroplegics in psychiatric therapy'], *Therapie*, 8, 347–64.

Delay, J. and Deniker, P. (1955) 'Neuroleptic effects of chlorpromazine in therapeutics of neuropsychiatry', *Int Rec Med Gen Pract Clin*, 168, 318–26.

Delay, J. and Deniker, P. (1956) 'Chlorpromazine and neuroleptic treatments in psychiatry', *J Clin Exp Psychopathol*, 17, 19–24.

Delay, J., Deniker, P. and Harl, J. M. (1952) ['Therapeutic use in psychiatry of phenothiazine of central elective action (4560 RP)'], *Ann Med Psychol (Paris)*, 110, 112–17.

Delay, J., Deniker, P., Green, A., and Mordret, M. (1957) ['Excito-motor syndrome provoked by neuroleptic drugs'], *Presse Med*, 65, 1771–4 [in French].

DeLisi, L. E., Hoff, A. L., Schwartz, J. E., Shields, G. W., Halthore, S. N., Gupta, S. M., et al. (1991) 'Brain morphology in first-episode schizophrenic-like psychotic patients: a quantitative magnetic resonance imaging study', *Biol Psychiatry*, 29, 159–75.

DeLisi, L. E., Sakuma, M., Tew, W., Kushner, M., Hoff, A. L. and Grimson, R. (1997) 'Schizophrenia as a chronic active brain process: a study of progressive brain structural change subsequent to the onset of schizophrenia', *Psychiatry Res*, 74, 129–40.

Denham, J. (1965) 'Clinical use of the phenothiazines', in Marks, J. and Pare, C. M. B. (eds) *The Scientific Basis of Drug Therapy in Psychiatry. Proceedings of a Symposium Held at St Bartholomew's Hospital, London*, pp. 56–61 (London: Pergamon Press).

Denham, J. and Carrick, D. J. (1960) 'Therapeutic importance of extrapyramidal phenomena evoked by a new phenothiazine', *Am J Psychiatry*, 116, 927–8.

Deniker, P. (1956) 'Psychophysiologic aspects of the new chemotherapeutic drugs in psychiatry; some practical features of neuroleptics in order to screen new drugs', *J Nerv Ment Dis*, 124, 371–6.

Deniker, P. (1960) 'Experimental neurological syndromes and the new drug therapies in psychiatry', *Compr Psychiatry*, 1, 92–102.

Deniker, P. (1970) 'Introduction of neuroleptic chemotherapy into psychiatry', in Ayd, F. and Blackwell, B. (eds) *Discoveries in Biological Psychiatry*, pp. 155–64 (Philadelphia: J B Lippincott Company).

Deniker, P. (1983) 'Discovery of the clinical use of neuroleptics', in Parnham, M. J. and Bruinvels, J. (eds) *Discoveries in Pharmcology*, pp. 163–80 (Amsterdam: Elsevier).

Deniker, P. (1989) 'From chlorpromazine to tardive dyskinesia (brief history of the neuroleptics)', *Psychiatr J Univ Ott*, 14, 253–9.

Department of Health (2001) *The Mental Health Policy Implementation Guide* (London: Department of Health).

Depatie, L. and Lal, S. (2001) 'Apomorphine and the dopamine hypothesis of schizophrenia: a dilemma?', *J Psychiatry Neurosci*, 26, 203–20.

DeWolfe, A. S., Ryan, J. J. and Wolf, M. E. (1988) 'Cognitive sequelae of tardive dyskinesia', *J Nerv Ment Dis*, 176, 270–4.

Diamond, B. I. and Borison, R. L. (1986) 'Basic and clinical studies of neuroleptic-induced supersensitivity psychosis and dyskinesia', *Psychopharmacol Bull*, 22, 900–5.

Dinan, T. G. (2004a) 'Schizophrenia and diabetes 2003: an expert consensus meeting. Introduction', *Br J Psychiatry Suppl*, 47, S53–S54.

Dinan, T. G. (2004b) 'Stress and the genesis of diabetes mellitus in schizophrenia', *Br J Psychiatry Suppl*, 47, S72–S75.

Divry, P., Bobon, J. and Collard, J. (1958) ['R-1625: a new drug for the symptomatic treatment of psychomotor excitation'], *Acta Neurol Psychiatr Belg*, 58, 878–88 [in French].

Divry, P., Bobon, J., Collard, J., Pinchard, A. and Nols, E. (1959) ['Study & clinical trial of R 1625 or haloperidol, a new neuroleptic & so-called neurodysleptic agent'], *Acta Neurol Psychiatr Belg*, 59, 337–66 [in French].

Domino, E. F. (1985) 'Induction of tardive dyskinesia in *Cebus apella* and *Macaca speciosa* monkeys: a review', *Psychopharmacology Suppl*, 2, 217–23.

Donlon, P. T. and Tupin, J. P. (1974) 'Rapid "digitalization" of decompensated schizophrenic patients with antipsychotic agents', *Am J Psychiatry*, 131, 310–12.

Dorph-Petersen, K. A., Pierri, J. N., Perel, J. M., Sun, Z., Sampson, A. R. and Lewis, D. A. (2005) 'The influence of chronic exposure to antipsychotic medications on brain size before and after tissue fixation: a comparison of haloperidol and olanzapine in macaque monkeys', *Neuropsychopharmacology*, 30, 1649–61.

Dreifus, C. (2008) 'A conversation with Nancy Andreasen: Using imaging to look at changes in the brain', *New York Times*, 15 Sep.

Druckman, R., Seelinger, D. and Thulin, B. (1962) 'Chronic involuntary movements induced by phenothiazines', *J Nerv Ment Dis*, 135, 69–76.

Dubovsky, S. L., Davies, R. and Dubovsky, A. N. (2001) 'Mood disorders', in Hales, R. E. and Yudofsky, S. C. (eds) *Textbook of Clinical Psychiatry* (Washington, DC: American Psychiatric Association).

Duman, R. S., Heninger, G. R. and Nestler, E. J. (1997) 'A molecular and cellular theory of depression', *Arch Gen Psychiatry*, 54, 597–606.

Ebaugh, F. G. (1943) 'A review of the drastic shock therapies in the treatment of the psychoses', *Ann Int Med*, 18, 294–5.

Ehrhardt, H. (1966) 'Present status of insulin coma and electric convulsive treatment in Germany', in Rinkel, M. (ed.) *Biological Treatment of Mental Illness*, p. 838 (New York: Farrar, Straus & Giroux).

Ehringer, H. and Hornykiewicz, O. (1960) ['Distribution of noradrenaline and dopamine (3-hydroxytyramine) in the human brain and their behavior in diseases of the extrapyramidal system'], *Klin Wochenschr*, 38, 1236–9 [in German].

Eli Lilly (2011) 'How Zyprexa works', available at: www.zyprexa.com/schizophrenia/pages/howzyprexaworks.aspx (accessed 25 March 2011).

Eli Lilly (undated) 'Zyprexa papers', available at: www.furiousseasons.com/zyprexa%20documents/ (accessed 31 January 2011).

Elkes, J. and Elkes, C. (1954) 'Effects of chlorpormazine on the behaviour of chronically overactive psychotic patients', *Br Med J*, ii, 560–5.

Ellis, R. (2006) 'The asylum, the Poor Law, and a reassessment of the four-shilling grant: admissions to the county asylums of Yorkshire in the nineteenth century', *Soc Hist Med*, 19, 55–71.

Emanuel, M. B. (1999) 'Histamine and the antiallergic antihistamines: a history of their discoveries', *Clin Exp Allergy*, 29(Suppl. 3), 1–11.

Evans, J. H. (1965) 'Persistent oral dyskinesia in treatment with phenothiazine derivatives', *Lancet*, 1, 458–60.

Expert Group (2004) '"Schizophrenia and Diabetes 2003" Expert Consensus Meeting, Dublin, 3–4 October 2003: consensus summary', *Br J Psychiatry Suppl*, 47, S112–14.

Fagan, D., Scott, D. B., Mitchell, M. and Tiplady, B. (1991) 'Effects of remoxipride on measures of psychological performance in healthy volunteers', *Psychopharmacology (Berl)*, 105, 225–9.

Fann, W. E. and Linton, P. H. (1972) 'Use of perphenazine in psychiatric emergencies: the concept of chemical restraint', *Curr Ther Res Clin Exp*, 14, 478–82.

Faraone, S. V., Biederman, J., Mennin, D. and Russell, R. (1998) 'Bipolar and antisocial disorders among relatives of ADHD children: parsing familial subtypes of illness', *Am J Med Genet*, 81, 108–16.

Farde, L., Wiesel, F. A., Hall, H., Halldin, C., Stone-Elander, S. and Sedvall, G. (1987) 'No D2 receptor increase in PET study of schizophrenia', *Arch Gen Psychiatry*, 44, 671–2.

Farde, L., Nordstrom, A. L., Wiesel, F. A., Pauli, S., Halldin, C. and Sedvall, G. (1992) 'Positron emission tomographic analysis of central D1 and D2 dopamine receptor occupancy in patients treated with classical neuroleptics and clozapine. Relation to extrapyramidal side effects', *Arch Gen Psychiatry*, 49, 538–44.

Faurbye, A. (1968) 'The role of amines in the etiology of schizophrenia', *Compr Psychiatry*, 9, 155–77.

Faurbye, A., Rasch, P. J., Petersen, P. B., Brandborg, G. and Pakkenberg, H. (1964) 'Neurological symptoms in pharmacotherapy of psychoses', *Acta Psychiatr Scand*, 40, 10–27.

Fenton, W. S. and McGlashan, T. H. (1987) 'Sustained remission in drug-free schizophrenic patients', *Am J Psychiatry*, 144, 1306–9.

Fenton, W. S., Wyatt, R. J. and McGlashan, T. H. (1994) 'Risk factors for spontaneous dyskinesia in schizophrenia', *Arch Gen Psychiatry*, 51, 643–50.

Fenton, W. S., Blyler, C. R., Wyatt, R. J. and McGlashan, T. H. (1997) 'Prevalence of spontaneous dyskinesia in schizophrenic and non-schizophrenic psychiatric patients', *Br J Psychiatry*, 171, 265–8.

Ferguson, A. T., Wilson, J. N., Jenkins, D. and Swan, H. (1958) 'The effect of hypothermia on hemorrhagic shock', *Ann Surg*, 147, 281–8.

Fink, M. and Karliner, W. (2007) 'Primary sources: insulin coma therapy. PBS American Experience', available at: www.pbs.org/wgbh/amex/nash/filmmore/ps_ict.html (accessed 26 April 2013).

Fink, M., Shaw, R., Gross, G. E. and Coleman, F. S. (1958) 'Comparative study of chlorpromazine and insulin coma in therapy of psychosis', *J Am Med Assoc*, 166, 1846–50.

Finlay, J. M. and Zigmond, M. J. (1997) 'The effects of stress on central dopaminergic neurons: possible clinical implications', *Neurochem Res*, 22, 1387–94.

Fischer, E. (1970) 'Biogenic amines and schizophrenia', *Psychosomatics*, 11, 495.

Fisk, M. C., Feeley, J. and Voreacos, D. (2012) 'J&J said to agree to $2.2 billion drug marketing accord', *Bloomberg News*, 11 Jun.

Flugel, F. (1959) 'Neuroleptic treatment in schizophrenia', in Kline, N. S. (ed.) *Psychopharmacology Frontiers*, pp. 45–7 (Boston, MA: Little, Brown & Co).

Food and Drug Administration (2007) 'Information for healthcare professionals: haloperidol (marketed as haldol, haldol decanoate and haldol lactate)', available at: http://www.fda.gov/Drugs/DrugSafety/Postmarket DrugSafetyInformationforPatientsandProviders/DrugSafetyInformation forHeathcareProfessionals/ucm085203.htm (accessed 14 April 2013).

Francis, A. (2011) 'Seven questions for Patrick McGorry', available at: http://www.psychologytoday.com/blog/dsm5-in-distress/201108/seven-questions-professor-patrick-mcgorry (accessed 14 April 2013).

Francis, A. (2012) 'Wonderful news: DSM-5 finally begins its belated and necessary retreat', available at: http://www.psychologytoday.com/blog/dsm5-in-distress/201205/wonderful-news-dsm-5-finally-begins-its-belated-and-necessary-retreat (accessed 14 April 2013).

Frank, L. R. (1978) *The History of Shock Treatment* (San Fransisco, CA: self-published).

Frankenhaeuser, M., Lundberg, U., Rauste, v. W., von Wright, J. and Sedvall, G. (1986) 'Urinary monoamine metabolites as indices of mental stress in healthy males and females', *Pharmacol Biochem Behav*, 24, 1521–5.

Franzen, G. and Ingvar, D. H. (1975) 'Abnormal distribution of cerebral activity in chronic schizophrenia', *J Psychiatr Res*, 12, 199–214.

Fraser Health Authority (2012) 'Psychosis sucks', available at: http://www.psychosissucks.ca/treatment.cfm (accessed 13 December 2012).

Frazier, S. H. (1968) 'Comprehensive management of psychiatric emergencies', *Psychosomatics*, 9, 7–11.

Frazier, J. A., Biederman, J., Tohen, M., Feldman, P. D., Jacobs, T. G., Toma, V., et al. (2001) 'A prospective open-label treatment trial of olanzapine monotherapy in children and adolescents with bipolar disorder', *J Child Adolesc Psychopharmacol*, 11, 239–50.

Freed, E. D. (1975) 'The drug management of acute behavioural disturbances', *S Afr Med J*, 49, 638–40.

Freedman, D. X. (1973) 'Neurological syndromes associated with antipsychotic drug use. A special report', *Arch Gen Psychiatry*, 28, 463–7.

Freeman, D. (2007) 'Suspicious minds: the psychology of persecutory delusions', *Clin Psychol Rev*, 27, 425–57.

Freyhan, F. A. (1955) 'The immediate and long-range effects of chlorpromazine on the mental hospital', in Smith Kline & French Laboratories (ed.) *Chlorpromazine and Mental Health*, pp. 71–87 (Philadelphia, PA: Lea & Febiger).

Freyhan, F. A. (1959) 'Clinical and investigative aspects', in Kline, N. S. (ed.) *Psychopharmaclogy Frontiers. Second International Congress of Psychiatry Psychopharmacology Symposium*, pp. 7–14) (London: J&A Churchill).

Freyhan, F. A. (1964) 'Ten years of clinical psychopharmacology: hopes and frustrations', in *Neuropsychopharmacology Volume 3. Proceedings of the Third Meeting of the Collegium Internationale Neuropsychopharmacologium*, pp. 559–61 (Amsterdam: Elsevier).

Gaddum, J. H. and Hameed, K. A. (1954) 'Drugs which antagonize 5-hydroxytryptamine', *Br J Pharmacol Chemother*, 9, 240–8.

Gaebel, W., Janner, M., Frommann, N., Pietzcker, A., Kopcke, W., Linden, M., et al. (2002) 'First vs multiple episode schizophrenia: two-year outcome of intermittent and maintenance medication strategies', *Schizophr Res*, 53, 145–59.

Gaebel, W., Riesbeck, M., Wolwer, W., Klimke, A., Eickhoff, M., Von Wilmsdorff, M., et al. (2011) 'Relapse prevention in first-episode schizophrenia—maintenance vs intermittent drug treatment with prodrome-based early intervention: results of a randomized controlled trial within the German Research Network on Schizophrenia', *J Clin Psychiatry*, 72, 205–18.

Gardos, G. and Cole, J. O. (1980) 'Overview: public health issues in tardive dyskinesia', *Am J Psychiatry*, 137, 776–81.

Geddes, J., Freemantle, N., Harrison, P. and Bebbington, P. (2000) 'Atypical antipsychotics in the treatment of schizophrenia: systematic overview and meta-regression analysis', *BMJ*, 321, 1371–6.

Gelman, S. (1999) *Medicating Schizophrenia: a history* (New Brunswick, NJ: Rutgers University Press).

Gerlach, J. (1985) 'Pathophysiological mechanisms underlying tardive dyskinesia', *Psychopharmacology Suppl*, 2, 98–103.

Ghaemi, S. N. (2001) 'On defining "mood stabilizer"', *Bipolar Disord*, 3, 154–8.

Ghaemi, S. N., Sachs, G. S., Chiou, A. M., Pandurangi, A. K. and Goodwin, K. (1999) 'Is bipolar disorder still underdiagnosed? Are antidepressants overutilized?', *J Affect Disord*, 52, 135–44.

Gil-Ad, I., Shtaif, B., Shiloh, R. and Weizman, A. (2001) 'Evaluation of the neurotoxic activity of typical and atypical neuroleptics: relevance to iatrogenic extrapyramidal symptoms', *Cell Mol Neurobiol*, 21, 705–16.

Gillies, D., Beck, A., McCloud, A., Rathbone, J. and Gillies, D. (2005) 'Benzodiazepines alone or in combination with antipsychotic drugs for acute psychosis', *Cochrane Database Syst Rev*, CD003079.

Gittins, D. (1998) *Madness in its Place: Narratives of Severall Hospital 1913–1997* (London: Routledge).

GlaxoSmithKline (2009) Available at: www.paxilcr.com (accessed 25 February 2009).

Goerendt, I. K., Messa, C., Lawrence, A. D., Grasby, P. M., Piccini, P. and Brooks, D. J. (2003) 'Dopamine release during sequential finger movements in health and Parkinson's disease: a PET study', *Brain*, 126, 312–25.

Goldberg, E. (1985) 'Akinesia, tardive dysmentia, and frontal lobe disorder in schizophrenia', *Schizophr Bull*, 11, 255–63.

Goldstein, L. E., Sporn, J., Brown, S., Kim, H., Finkelstein, J., Gaffey, G. K., et al. (1999) 'New-onset diabetes mellitus and diabetic ketoacidosis associated with olanzapine treatment', *Psychosomatics*, 40, 438–43.

Gracie, A., Freeman, D., Green, S., Garety, P. A., Kuipers, E., Hardy, A., et al. (2007) 'The association between traumatic experience, paranoia and hallucinations: a test of the predictions of psychological models', *Acta Psychiatr Scand*, 116, 280–9.

Granger, B. and Albu, S. (2005) 'The haloperidol story', *Ann Clin Psychiatry*, 17, 137–40.

Greely, H., Sahakian, B., Harris, J., Kessler, R. C., Gazzaniga, M., Campbell, P., et al. (2008) 'Towards responsible use of cognitive-enhancing drugs by the healthy', *Nature*, 456, 702–5.

Green, M. F., Marder, S. R., Glynn, S. M., McGurk, S. R., Wirshing, W. C., Wirshing, D. A., et al. (2002) 'The neurocognitive effects of low-dose haloperidol: a two-year comparison with risperidone', *Biol Psychiatry*, 51, 972–8.

Greenson, P. R. (2012) 'The therapeutic role of drugs in the process of repression, dissociation and synthesis', *Psychanalytic Quarterly*, 16, 140–1.

Grob, G. (1983) *The Inner World of American Psychiatry 1890–1940* (New Brunswick, NJ: Rutgers University Press).

Grob, G. (1994) *The Mad Among Us* (New York: The Free Press).

Gronfein, W. (1985) 'Psychotropic drugs and the origins of deinstitutionalisation', *Social Problems*, 32, 437–54.

Gualtieri, C. T., Sprague, R. L. and Cole, J. O. (1986) 'Tardive dyskinesia litigation and the dilemmas of neuroleptic treatment', *J Psychiatry Law*, 14, 187–216.

Guillin, O., Abi-Dargham, A. and Laruelle, M. (2007) 'Neurobiology of dopamine in schizophrenia', *Int Rev Neurobiol*, 78, 1–39.

Guiraud, P. and David, C. (1950) 'Treatment de l'agitation mortrice par un antihistaminique (3277 RP)', *C R Congres Med Alien Neurol France*, 48, 599–602.

Gunne, L. M. and Barany, S. (1976) 'Haloperidol-induced tardive dyskinesia in monkeys', *Psychopharmacology (Berl)*, 50, 237–40.

Gur, R. E., Cowell, P., Turetsky, B. I., Gallacher, F., Cannon, T., Bilker, W., et al. (1998) 'A follow-up magnetic resonance imaging study of schizophrenia. Relationship of neuroanatomical changes to clinical and neurobehavioral measures', *Arch Gen Psychiatry*, 55, 145–52.

Gur, R. E., Turetsky, B. I., Bilker, W. B. and Gur, R. C. (1999) 'Reduced gray matter volume in schizophrenia', *Arch Gen Psychiatry*, 56, 905–11.

Gurd, F. N. (1955) 'Current trends in the treatment of shock', *Can Med Assoc J*, 73, 977–80.

Guy, W. E. (1976) 'Clinical Global Impressions Scale', in *ECDEU Assessment Manual for Psychopharmacology Revised* (Rockville, MD: National Institute of Mental Health).

Haase, H. J. (1954) ['Occurrence and interpretation of psychomotor parkinsonism in megaphen or largactil prolonged therapy'], *Nervenarzt*, 25, 486–92 [in German].

Haase, H. J. (1956) ['Definition and mode of action of the psychomotor Parkinson syndrome therapeutically induced by serpasil and largactil'], *Monatsschr Psychiatr Neurol*, 131, 201–14 [in German].

Haase, H.-J. and Janssen, P. A. J. (1965) *The Action of Neuroleptic Drugs* (Chicago, IL: Yearbook Medical Publishers).

Haddad, P. M. (2004) 'Antipsychotics and diabetes: review of non-prospective data', *Br J Psychiatry Suppl*, 47, S80–S86.

Hafeman, D. M., Chang, K. D., Garrett, A. S., Sanders, E. M. and Phillips, M. L. (2012) 'Effects of medication on neuroimaging findings in bipolar disorder: an updated review', *Bipolar Disord*, 14, 375–410.

Hammond, R. C. (1964) 'Problems arising from prescribing trends', *Can Med Assoc J*, 91, 135.

Hamon, J., Paraire, J. and Velluz, J. (1952a) ['Anxiety states and potentialized barbiturates'], *Ann Med Psychol (Paris)*, 110, 403–7.

Hamon, J., Praraire, J. and Velluz, J. (1952b) 'Remarques sur l'action du 4560 R.P. sur l'agitation maniaque', *Ann Med Psychol (Paris)*, 110, 331–5.

Hansen, B. (1996) 'Workplace violence in the hospital psychiatric setting. An occupational health perspective', *AAOHN J*, 44, 575–80.

Harris, G. (2009) 'Pfizer pays \$2.3 billion to settle marketing case', *New York Times*, 2 Sep.

Harris, D. and Batki, S. L. (2000) 'Stimulant psychosis: symptom profile and acute clinical course', *Am J Addict*, 9, 28–37.

Harris, G. and Carey, B. (2008) 'Researchers fail to reveal full drug pay', *New York Times*, 8 Jun.

Harris, M., Chandran, S., Chakraborty, N. and Healy, D. (2005) 'The impact of mood stabilizers on bipolar disorder: the 1890s and 1990s compared', *Hist Psychiatry*, 16, 423–34.

Harrison, P. J. (1999) 'The neuropathology of schizophrenia. A critical review of the data and their interpretation', *Brain*, 122, 593–624.

Harrow, M. and Jobe, T. H. (2007) 'Factors involved in outcome and recovery in schizophrenia patients not on antipsychotic medications: a 15-year multi-follow-up study', *J Nerv Ment Dis*, 195, 406–14.

Harrow, M., Jobe, T. H. and Faull, R. N. (2012) 'Do all schizophrenia patients need antipsychotic treatment continuously throughout their lifetime? A 20-year longitudinal study', *Psychol Med*, 42, 2145–55.

Haukka, J., Tiihonen, J., Harkanen, T. and Lonnqvist, J. (2008) 'Association between medication and risk of suicide, attempted suicide and death in nationwide cohort of suicidal patients with schizophrenia', *Pharmacoepidemiol Drug Saf*, 17, 686–96.

Healy, D. (1996) *The Psychopharmacologists. Interviews by David Healy. Volume I* (London: Chapman and Hall).

Healy, D. (2002) *The Creation of Psychopharmacology* (Cambridge, MA: Harvard University Press).

Healy, D. (2004) 'Shaping the intimate: influences on the experience of everyday nerves', *Soc Stud Sci*, 34, 219–45.

Healy, D. (2006a) 'Academic stalking', available at: http://www.healyprozac.com/AcademicStalking/AcademicStalking.htm (accessed 14 April 2013).

Healy, D. (2006b) 'The latest mania: selling bipolar disorder', *PLoS Med*, 3, e185.

Healy, D. (2008) *Mania: A Short History of Bipolar Disorder* (Baltimore, MD: John Hopkins University Press).

Healy, D. and Farquhar, G. (1998) 'Immediate effects of droperidol', *Hum Psychopharmacol*, 13, 113–20.

Healy, D. and Le Noury, J. (2007) 'Pediatric bipolar disorder: An object study in the creation of an illness', *Int J Risk Safety Med*, 19, 209–21.

Healy, D., Harris, M., Michael, P., Cattell, D., Savage, M., Chalasani, P., et al. (2005) 'Service utilization in 1896 and 1996: morbidity and mortality data from North Wales', *Hist Psychiatry*, 16, 27–42.

Hegarty, J.D., Baldessarini, R.J., Tohen, M., Waternaux, C. and Oepen, G. (1994) 'One hundred years of schizophrenia: a meta-analysis of the outcome literature', *Am J Psychiatry*,151, 1409–16.

Hegelstad, W. T., Larsen, T. K., Auestad, B., Evensen, J., Haahr, U., Joa, I., et al. (2012) 'Long-term follow-up of the TIPS early detection in psychosis study: effects on 10-year outcome', *Am J Psychiatry*, 169, 374–80.

Henderson, D. and Gillespie, R. D. (1927) *Henderson and Gillespie's Textbook of Psychiatry*, 1st edn (Oxford: Oxford University Press).

Henderson, D. and Gillespie, R. D. (1962) *Henderson and Gillespie's Textbook of Psychiatry*, 9th edn (Oxford, Oxford University Press).

Heninger, G., Dimascio, A. and Klerman, G. L. (1965) 'Personality factors in variability of response to phenothiazines', *Am J Psychiatry*, 121, 1091–4.

Hennessy, S., Bilker, W. B., Knauss, J. S., Margolis, D. J., Kimmel, S. E., Reynolds, R. F., et al. (2002) 'Cardiac arrest and ventricular arrhythmia in patients taking antipsychotic drugs: cohort study using administrative data', *BMJ*, 325, 1070.

Herman, Z. S. (1970) 'The effects of noradrenaline on rat's behaviour', *Psychopharmacologia*, 16, 369–74.

Himwich, H. E. (1955) 'Prospects in psychopharmacology', *J Nerv Ment Dis*, 122, 413–23.

Hippius, H. (1999) 'A historical perspective of clozapine', *J Clin Psychiatry*, 60(Suppl. 12), 22–3.

Ho, B. C., Andreasen, N. C., Flaum, M., Nopoulos, P. and Miller, D. (2000) 'Untreated initial psychosis: its relation to quality of life and symptom remission in first-episode schizophrenia', *Am J Psychiatry*, 157, 808–15.

Ho, B. C., Andreasen, N. C., Nopoulos, P., Arndt, S., Magnotta, V. and Flaum, M. (2003) 'Progressive structural brain abnormalities and their relationship to clinical outcome: a longitudinal magnetic resonance imaging study early in schizophrenia', *Arch Gen Psychiatry*, 60, 585–94.

Ho, B. C., Andreasen, N. C., Ziebell, S., Pierson, R. and Magnotta, V. (2011) 'Long-term antipsychotic treatment and brain volumes: a longitudinal study of first-episode schizophrenia', *Arch Gen Psychiatry*, 68, 128–37.

Hoch, P. (1959) 'Drug therapy', in Arieti, S. (ed.) *American Handbook of Psychiatry, Volume II*, 1st edn, pp. 1541–51 (New York: Basic Books).

Hollister, L. E. (1957) 'Complications from the use of tranquilizing drugs', *N Engl J Med*, 257, 170–7.

Holt, R. I., Bushe, C. and Citrome, L. (2005) 'Diabetes and schizophrenia 2005: are we any closer to understanding the link?', *J Psychopharmacol*, 19, 56–65.

Howes, O. D., Kambeitz, J., Kim, E., Stahl, D., Slifstein, M., Abi-Dargham, A., et al. (2012) 'The nature of dopamine dysfunction in schizophrenia and what this means for treatment', *Arch Gen Psychiatry*, 69, 776–86.

Howes, O. D. and Kapur, S. (2009) 'The dopamine hypothesis of schizophrenia: version III—the final common pathway', *Schizophr Bull*, 35, 549–62.

Huber, G. (1957) *Penumoencephalographische und Psychopathologische Bilder bei Endogen Psychosen* (Berlin: Springer Verlag).

Hulshoff Pol, H. E. and Kahn, R. S. (2008) 'What happens after the first episode? A review of progressive brain changes in chronically ill patients with schizophrenia', *Schizophr Bull*, 34, 354–66.

Hunsberger, J., Austin, D. R., Henter, I. D. and Chen, G. (2009) 'The neurotrophic and neuroprotective effects of psychotropic agents', *Dialogues Clin Neurosci*, 11, 333–48.

Hunter, A. R. (1967) 'Old unhappy far off things. Some reflections on the significance of the early work on shock', *Ann R Coll Surg Engl*, 40, 289–305.

Hunter, R., Earl, C. J. and Janz, D. (1964a) 'A syndrome of abnormal movements and dementia in leucotomized patients treated with phenothiazines', *J Neurol Neurosurg Psychiatry*, 27, 219–23.

Hunter, R., Earl, C. J. and Thronicroft, S. (1964b) 'An apparently irreversible syndrome of abnormal movements following phenothiazine medication', *Proc R Soc Med*, 57, 758–62.

Hutton, P., Morrison, A. P., Yung, A. R., Taylor, P. J., French, P. and Dunn, G. (2012) 'Effects of drop-out on efficacy estimates in five Cochrane reviews of popular antipsychotics for schizophrenia', *Acta Psychiatr Scand*, 126, 1–11.

Huttunen, M. (1995) 'The evolution of the serotonin-dopamine antagonist concept', *J Clin Psychopharmacol*, 15, 4S-10S.

Ichimiya, T., Okubo, Y., Suhara, T. and Sudo, Y. (2001) 'Reduced volume of the cerebellar vermis in neuroleptic-naive schizophrenia', *Biol Psychiatry*, 49, 20–7.

Idanpaan-Heikkila, J., Alhava, E., Olkinuora, M. and Palva, I. (1975) 'Letter: Clozapine and agranulocytosis', *Lancet*, 2, 611.

Ilyas, S. and Moncrieff, J. (2012) 'Trends in prescriptions and costs of drugs for mental disorders in England, 1998 to 2010', *British Journal of Psychiatry*, 200, 393–8.

IMS Institute for Healthcare Informatics (2011) 'The use of medicines in the United States: Review of 2010', available at: www.imshealth.com/ (accessed 15 April 2013).

Insel, T. R. (2009) 'Translating scientific opportunity into public health impact: a strategic plan for research on mental illness', *Arch Gen Psychiatry*, 66, 128–33.

International Center for the Study of Psychiatry and Psychology (2009) *The Conscience of Psychiatry: The Reform Work of Peter R. Breggin, MD* (Ithaca, NY: Lake Edge Press).

International Early Psychosis Association (2012) 'Sponsorship Prospectus: 8th international conference on early psychosis', 11–13 October, 2012 San Fransisco, CA, USA, available at: http://www.iepaconference.org/wordpress/wp-content/uploads/2011/07/sponsorship-prospectus.pdf [On-line]. Available: http://www.iepaconference.org/wordpress/wp-content/uploads/2011/07/sponsorship-prospectus.pdf (accessed 15 April 2013).

Iversen, L. (1998) 'Neuroscience and drug development', in Healy, D. (3 ed.) *The Psychopharmacologists*, p. 325 (London: Chapman & Hall).

Jablensky, A., Sartorius, N., Ernberg, G., Anker, M., Korten, A., Cooper, J. E., et al. (1992) 'Schizophrenia: manifestations, incidence and course in different cultures. A World Health Organization ten-country study', *Psychol Med Monogr Suppl*, 20, 1–97.

Jacquy, J., Wilmotte, J., Piraux, A. and Noel, G. (1976) 'Cerebral blood flow patterns studied by rheoencephalography in schizophrenia', *Neuropsychobiology*, 2, 94–103.

Janssen, P. (1998) 'From haloperidol to risperidone', in Healy, D. (ed.) *The Psychopharmacologists Volume II*, pp. 39–70 (London: Chapman & Hall).

Janssen, P. A., Niemegeers, C. J., Awouters, F., Schellekens, K. H., Megens, A. A. and Meert, T. F. (1988) 'Pharmacology of risperidone (R 64 766), a new antipsychotic with serotonin-S2 and dopamine-D2 antagonistic properties', *J Pharmacol Exp Ther*, 244, 685–93.

Jarskog, L. F. and Lieberman, J. A. (2006) 'Neuroprotection in schizophrenia', *J Clin Psychiatry*, 67, e09.

Jarskog, L. F., Gilmore, J. H., Glantz, L. A., Gable, K. L., German, T. T., Tong, R. I., et al. (2007a) 'Caspase-3 activation in rat frontal cortex following treatment with typical and atypical antipsychotics', *Neuropsychopharmacology*, 32, 95–102.

Jarskog, L. F., Miyamoto, S. and Lieberman, J. A. (2007b) 'Schizophrenia: new pathological insights and therapies', *Annu Rev Med*, 58, 49–61.

Jayakumar, P. N., Venkatasubramanian, G., Gangadhar, B. N., Janakiramaiah, N. and Keshavan, M. S. (2005) 'Optimized voxel-based morphometry of gray matter volume in first-episode, antipsychotic-naive schizophrenia', *Prog Neuropsychopharmacol Biol Psychiatry*, 29, 587–91.

Jellinger, K. (1977) 'Neuropathologic findings after neuroleptic long-term therapy', in Roizin, L., Shiraki, H. and Greevic, N. (eds) *Neurotoxicology*, pp. 25–42 (New York: Raven Press).

Jenner, F. A., Monteiro, A. C. D., Zagalo-Cardoso, J. A. and Cunha-Oliveira, J. A. (1993) *Schizophrenia: A Disease or Some Ways of Being Human* (Sheffield: Sheffield Academic Press).

Jeste, D. V., Caligiuri, M. P., Paulsen, J. S., Heaton, R. K., Lacro, J. P., Harris, M. J., et al. (1995) 'Risk of tardive dyskinesia in older patients. A prospective longitudinal study of 266 outpatients'. *Arch Gen Psychiatry*, 52, 756–65.

John, J. P., Chengappa, K. N., Baker, R. W., Gupta, B. and Mortimer, M. T. (1995) 'Assessment of changes in both weight and frequency of use of medications for the treatment of gastrointestinal symptoms among clozapine-treated patients', *Ann Clin Psychiatry*, 7, 119–25.

Johnson, W. (undated) 'An interesting compound' (unpublished: Smith Kline & French).

Johnstone, E. C., Crow, T. J., Frith, C. D., Carney, M. W. and Price, J. S. (1978) 'Mechanism of the antipsychotic effect in the treatment of acute schizophrenia', *Lancet*, 1, 848–51.

Johnstone, E. C., Crow, T. J., Frith, C. D. and Owens, D. G. (1988) 'The Northwick Park "functional" psychosis study: diagnosis and treatment response', *Lancet*, 2, 119–25.

Jones, B. D. (1985) 'Tardive dysmentia: further comments', *Schizophr Bull*, 11, 187–9.

Jones, K. (1972) *A History of the Mental Health Services* (London: Routledge & Kegan Paul).

Joshi, G., Petty, C., Wozniak, J., Faraone, S. V., Doyle, R., Georgiopoulos, A., et al. (2012) 'A prospective open-label trial of quetiapine monotherapy in preschool and school age children with bipolar spectrum disorder', *J Affect Disord*, 136, 1143–53.

Joukamaa, M., Heliovaara, M., Knekt, P., Aromaa, A., Raitasalo, R. and Lehtinen, V. (2006) 'Schizophrenia, neuroleptic medication and mortality', *Br J Psychiatry*, 188, 122–7.

Judah, L. N., Josephs, Z. M. and Murphree, O. D. (1961) 'Results of simultaneous abrupt withdrawal of ataraxics in 500 chronic psychotic patients', *Am J Psychiatry*, 118, 156–8.

Jureidini, J. N., McHenry, L. B. and Mansfield, P. R. (2008) 'Clinical trials and drug promotion: Selective reporting of study 329', *Int J Risk Saf Med*, 20, 73–81.

Kamran, A., Doraiswamy, P. M., Jane, J. L., Hammett, E. B. and Dunn, L. (1994) 'Severe hyperglycemia associated with high doses of clozapine', *Am J Psychiatry*, 151, 1395.

Kane, J. M., Honigfeld, G., Singer, J. and Meltzer, H. (1988) 'Clozapine in treatment-resistant schizophrenics', *Psychopharmacol Bull*, 24, 62–7.

Kapur, S. (2003) 'Psychosis as a state of aberrant salience: a framework linking biology, phenomenology, and pharmacology in schizophrenia', *Am J Psychiatry*, 160, 13–23.

Kapur, S. and Seeman, P. (2001) 'Does fast dissociation from the dopamine d(2) receptor explain the action of atypical antipsychotics?: A new hypothesis', *Am J Psychiatry*, 158, 360–9.

Kapur, S., Remington, G., Zipursky, R. B., Wilson, A. A. and Houle, S. (1995) 'The D2 dopamine receptor occupancy of risperidone and its relationship to extrapyramidal symptoms: a PET study', *Life Sci*, 57, L103–7.

KARN, W. N., Jr and Kasper, S. (1959) 'Pharmacologically induced Parkinson-like signs as index of the therapeutic potential', *Dis Nerv Syst*, 20, 119–22.

Karow, A., Naber, D., Lambert, M. and Moritz, S. (2012) 'Remission as perceived by people with schizophrenia, family members and psychiatrists', *Eur Psychiatry*, 27, 426–31.

Kaye, J. A., Bradbury, B. D. and Jick, H. (2003) Changes in antipsychotic drug prescribing by general practitioners in the United Kingdom from 1991 to 2000: a population-based observational study. *Br J Clin Pharmacol*, 56, 569–75.

Keefe, R. S., Seidman, L. J., Christensen, B. K., Hamer, R. M., Sharma, T., Sitskoorn, M. M., et al. (2006) 'Long-term neurocognitive effects of olanzapine or low-dose haloperidol in first-episode psychosis', *Biol Psychiatry*, 59, 97–105.

Keefe, R. S., Bilder, R. M., Davis, S. M., Harvey, P. D., Palmer, B. W., Gold, J. M., et al. (2007) 'Neurocognitive effects of antipsychotic medications in patients with chronic schizophrenia in the CATIE Trial', *Arch Gen Psychiatry*, 64, 633–47.

Kendall, T. (2011) 'The rise and fall of the atypical antipsychotics', *Br J Psychiatry*, 199, 266–8.

Kendell, R. E. and Zealey, A. K. (1988) *Companion to Psychiatric Studies*, 4th edn (Edinburgh: Churchill Livingstone).

Kendler, K. S. and Schaffner, K. F. (2011) 'The dopamine hypothesis of schizophrenia: an historical and philosophical analysis', *Philosophy Psychiatry Psychol*, 18, 41–63.

Kessler, R. C., McGonagle, K. A., Zhao, S., Nelson, C. B., Hughes, M., Eshleman, S., et al. (1994) 'Lifetime and 12-month prevalence of DSM-III-R psychiatric disorders in the United States. Results from the National Comorbidity Survey', *Arch Gen Psychiatry*, 51, 8–19.

Kestler, L. P., Walker, E. and Vega, E. M. (2001) 'Dopamine receptors in the brains of schizophrenia patients: a meta-analysis of the findings', *Behav Pharmacol*, 12, 355–71.

Kety, S. S. (1974) 'Prologue', *J Psychiatric Res*, 11, ix–xi.

Khin, N. A., Chen, Y. F., Yang, Y., Yang, P. and Laughren, T. P. (2012) 'Exploratory analyses of efficacy data from schizophrenia trials in support of new drug applications submitted to the US Food and Drug Administration', *J Clin Psychiatry*, 73, 856–64.

Khot, V. and Wyatt, R. J. (1991) 'Not all that moves is tardive dyskinesia', *Am J Psychiatry*, 148, 661–6.

Kinross-Wright, V. (1954) 'Chlorpromazine; a major advance in psychiatric treatment', *Postgrad Med*, 16, 297–9.

Kinross-Wright, V. (1956) 'Clinical application of chlorpormazine', in Kline, N. S. (ed.) *Psychopharmacology. A Symposium Organised by the Section on Medical Sciences for the American Association of the Advancement of Science and the American Psychiatric Association*, pp. 31–8 (Washington DC: American Association for the Advancement of Science).

Kirk, S., Gomery, T. and Cohen, D. (2013) *Mad Science; Psychiatric Coercion, Diagnosis and Drugs* (Rutgers, NJ: Transaction Publishers).

Kirsch, I., Moore, T. J., Scoboria, A. and Nicholls, S. S. (2002) 'The emperor's new drugs: an analysis of antidepressant medication data submitted to the US Food and Drug Administration', *Prevention and Treatment*, 5.

Kline, N. S. (1954) 'Use of *Rauwolfia serpentina* Benth. in neuropsychiatric conditions', *Ann N Y Acad Sci*, 59, 107–32.

Kline, N. S. (1956) 'Chemotherapy in psychiatry; recent advances', *Semin Int*, 5, 7–10.

Kline, N. S. (1959) 'Psychopharmaceuticals: effects and side effects', *Bull World Health Organ*, 21, 397–410.

Kline, N. S. (1968) 'On the rarity of 'irreversible' oral dyskinesias following phenothiaziones', *Am J Psychiatry*, 124, 48–51.

Kline, N. S. (1969) 'Nomenclature vs. nature', *Int J Psychiatry*, 7, 292–3.

Kline, N. S. and Stanley, A. M. (1955) 'Use of reserpine in a neuropsychiatric hospital', *Ann N Y Acad Sci*, 61, 85–91.

Kluger, J. and Song, S. (2002) 'Manic depression: young and bipolar', *Time Magazine*, 19 Aug.

Koerner, B. I. (2002) 'Disorders made to order', *Mother Jones*, 27.

Kohen, D. (2004) 'Diabetes mellitus and schizophrenia: historical perspective', *Br J Psychiatry Suppl*, 47, S64–6.

Koval, M. S., Rames, L. J. and Christie, S. (1994) 'Diabetic ketoacidosis associated with clozapine treatment', *Am J Psychiatry*, 151, 1520–1.

Kowatch, R. A., Fristad, M., Birmaher, B., Wagner, K. D., Findling, R. L. and Hellander, M. (2005) 'Treatment guidelines for children and adolescents with bipolar disorder', *J Am Acad Child Adolesc Psychiatry*, 44, 213–35.

Krakowski, M. I., Czobor, P., Citrome, L., Bark, N. and Cooper, T. B. (2006) 'Atypical antipsychotic agents in the treatment of violent patients with schizophrenia and schizoaffective disorder', *Arch Gen Psychiatry*, 63, 622–9.

Kramer, P. D. (1993) *Listening to Prozac* (New York: Viking Penguin).

Kruse, W. (1960) 'Persistent muscular restlessness after phenothiazine treatment: report of 3 cases', *Am J Psychiatry*, 117, 152–3.

Kulenkampff, C. & Tarnow, G. (1956) ['An unusual syndrome in the oral region caused by administration of megaphen'], *Nervenarzt*, 27, 178–80 [in German].

Kulkarni, S. K. and Dhir, A. (2011) 'Animal models of tardive dyskinesia', *Int Rev Neurobiol*, 98, 265–87.

Laborit, H. (1949) 'Etudes experimentale du syndrome d'irritation et application clinique a la maladie post-traumatique', *Therapie*, 4, 126–39.

Laborit, H. (1950) *Physiologie et Biologie du Systeme Nerveux Vegetatif au Service de la Chirurgie* (Paris: G. Doin).

Laborit, H. (1952) ['Artificial hibernation in anesthesiology'], *Anesth Anal*, 9, 1–15.

Laborit, H. and Huguenard, P. (1951) ['Artificial hibernation by pharmacodynamical and physical means'], *Presse Med*, 59, 1329.

Laborit, H., Huguenard, P. and Alluaume, R. (1952) ['A new vegetative stabilizer; 4560 R.P.'], *Presse Med*, 60, 206–8.

Lacoursiere, R. (1976) 'Medical effects of abrupt withdrawal of neuroleptic therapy', *JAMA*, 240, 109.

Laing, R. D. (1965) *The Divided Self* (Harmondsworth: Pelican Books).

Laing, R. D. (1967) *The Politics of Experience and The Bird of Paradise* (Harmondsworth: Penguin Books).

Lamberti, J. S., Bellnier, T. and Schwarzkopf, S. B. (1992) 'Weight gain among schizophrenic patients treated with clozapine', *Am J Psychiatry*, 149, 689–90.

Lane, C. J., Ngan, E. T., Yatham, L. N., Ruth, T. J. and Liddle, P. F. (2004) 'Immediate effects of risperidone on cerebral activity in healthy subjects: a comparison with subjects with first-episode schizophrenia', *J Psychiatry Neurosci*, 29, 30–7.

Largactil advertisement (1965) Advertisement, *Br J Psychiatry*, 111 January, x.

Larsen, T. K., Melle, I., Auestad, B., Friis, S., Haahr, U., Johannessen, J. O., et al. (2006) 'Early detection of first-episode psychosis: the effect on 1-year outcome', *Schizophr Bull*, 32, 758–64.

Laruelle, M., D'Souza, C. D., Baldwin, R. M., Abi-Dargham, A., Kanes, S. J., Fingado, C. L., et al. (1997) 'Imaging D2 receptor occupancy by endogenous dopamine in humans', *Neuropsychopharmacology*, 17, 162–74.

Laruelle, M., Abi-Dargham, A., Gil, R., Kegeles, L. and Innis, R. (1999) 'Increased dopamine transmission in schizophrenia: relationship to illness phases', *Biol Psychiatry*, 46, 56–72.

Lazorthes, G., Campan, L. and Anduze, H. (1952) ['Indication of artificial hibernation in cerebral surgery and in cranial traumatology'], *Rev Neurol (Paris)*, 87, 585–7.

Le Noury, J., Khan, A., Harris, M., Wong, W., Williams, D., Roberts, T., et al. (2008) 'The incidence and prevalence of diabetes in patients with serious mental illness in North West Wales: two cohorts, 1875–1924 & 1994–2006 compared', *BMC Psychiatry*, 8, 67.

Lee, T. and Seeman, P. (1980) 'Elevation of brain neuroleptic/dopamine receptors in schizophrenia', *Am J Psychiatry*, 137, 191–7.

Lehmann, H. E. (1955) 'Therapeutic results with chlorpromazine (largactil) in psychiatric conditions', *Can Med Assoc J*, 72, 91–9.

Lehmann, H. (1959) 'Concepts, rationale and research', in Kline, N. S. (ed.) *Psychopharmacology Frontiers. Second International Congress of Psychiatry Psychopharmacology Symposium*, pp. 21–30 (London: J&A Churchill Ltd).

Lehmann, H. E. (1993) 'Before they called it psychopharmacology', *Neuropsychopharmacology*, 8, 291–303.

Lehmann, H. E. and Hanrahan, G. E. (1954) 'Chlorpromazine; new inhibiting agent for psychomotor excitement and manic states', *AMA Arch Neurol Psychiatry*, 71, 227–37.

Lehtinen, V., Aaltonen, J., Koffert, T., Rakkolainen, V. and Syvalahti, E. (2000) Two-year outcome in first-episode psychosis treated according to an integrated model. Is immediate neuroleptisation always needed? *Eur Psychiatry*, 15, 312–20.

Lemke, R. (1936) 'Untersuchungen ueber die soziale prognose der schizophrenie', *Archiv Psychiatrie*, 104, 89–136.

Leucht, S., Kane, J. M., Etschel, E., Kissling, W., Hamann, J. and Engel, R. R. (2006) 'Linking the PANSS, BPRS, and CGI: clinical implications', *Neuropsychopharmacology*, 31, 2318–25.

Leucht, S., Heres, S., Hamann, J., & Kane, J. M. (2008) 'Methodological issues in current antipsychotic drug trials', *Schizophr Bull*, 34, 275–85.

Leucht, S., Arbter, D., Engel, R. R., Kissling, W. and Davis, J. M. (2009) 'How effective are second-generation antipsychotic drugs? A meta-analysis of placebo-controlled trials', *Mol Psychiatry*, 14, 429–47.

Leucht, S., Tardy, M., Komossa, K., Heres, S., Kissling, W., Salanti, G., et al. (2012a) 'Antipsychotic drugs versus placebo for relapse prevention in schizophrenia: a systematic review and meta-analysis', *Lancet*, 379, 2063–71.

Leucht, S., Tardy, M., Komossa, K., Heres, S., Kissling, W. and Davis, J. M. (2012b) 'Maintenance treatment with antipsychotic drugs for schizophrenia', *Cochrane Database Syst Rev*, 5, CD008016.

Lickey, M. E. and Gordon, B. (1986) *Medicamentos Para las Enfermadades Mentales* (Barcelona: Labor).

Lieberman, J. A. (1999a) 'Is schizophrenia a neurodegenerative disorder? A clinical and neurobiological perspective', *Biol Psychiatry*, 46, 729–39.

Lieberman, J. A. (1999b) 'Pathophysiologic mechanisms in the pathogenesis and clinical course of schizophrenia', *J Clin Psychiatry*, 60(Suppl.12), 9–12.

Lieberman, J. A., Kinon, B. J. and Loebel, A. D. (1990) 'Dopaminergic mechanisms in idiopathic and drug-induced psychoses', *Schizophr Bull*, 16, 97–110.

Lieberman, J. A., Sheitman, B., Chakos, M., Robinson, D., Schooler, N. and Keith, S. (1998) 'The development of treatment resistance in patients with schizophrenia: a clinical and pathophysiologic perspective', *J Clin Psychopharmacol*, 18, 20S–24S.

Lieberman, J. A., Tollefson, G. D., Charles, C., Zipursky, R., Sharma, T., Kahn, R. S., et al. (2005) 'Antipsychotic drug effects on brain morphology in first-episode psychosis', *Arch Gen Psychiatry*, 62, 361–70.

Lindenmayer, J. P. and Patel, R. (1999) 'Olanzapine-induced ketoacidosis with diabetes mellitus', *Am J Psychiatry*, 156, 1471.

Lion, J. R. (1975) 'Conceptual issues in the use of drugs for the treatment of aggression in man', *J Nerv Ment Dis*, 160, 76–82.

Liu, H. Y., Potter, M. P., Woodworth, K. Y., Yorks, D. M., Petty, C. R., Wozniak, J. R., et al. (2011) 'Pharmacologic treatments for pediatric bipolar disorder: a review and meta-analysis', *J Am Acad Child Adolesc Psychiatry*, 50, 749–62.

Lloyd-Evans, B., Crosby, M., Stockton, S., Pilling, S., Hobbs, L., Hinton, M., et al. (2011) 'Initiatives to shorten duration of untreated psychosis: systematic review', *Br J Psychiatry*, 198, 256–63.

Loebel, A. D., Lieberman, J. A., Alvir, J. M., Mayerhoff, D. I., Geisler, S. H. and Szymanski, S. R. (1992) 'Duration of psychosis and outcome in first-episode schizophrenia', *Am J Psychiatry*, 149, 1183–8.

Lu, M. L., Pan, J. J., Teng, H. W., Su, K. P. and Shen, W. W. (2002) 'Metoclopramide-induced supersensitivity psychosis', *Ann Pharmacother*, 36, 1387–90.

Lui, S., Deng, W., Huang, X., Jiang, L., Ma, X., Chen, H., et al. (2009) 'Association of cerebral deficits with clinical symptoms in antipsychotic-naive first-episode schizophrenia: an optimized voxel-based morphometry and resting state functional connectivity study', *Am J Psychiatry*, 166, 196–205.

Maas, J. W. and Garver, D. L. (1975) 'Linkage of basic neuropharmacology and clinical psychopharmacology', in Hamburg, D. A. and Brodie, H. K. H. (eds) *American Handbook of Psychiatry, Volume 6; New Psychiatric Frontiers*, 2nd edn, pp. 427–59 (New York: Basic Books).

McClelland, G. R., Cooper, S. M. and Pilgrim, A. J. (1990) 'A comparison of the central nervous system effects of haloperidol, chlorpromazine and sulpiride in normal volunteers', *Br J Clin Pharmacol*, 30, 795–803.

McCreadie, R. G., Thara, R., Padmavati, R., Srinivasan, T. N. and Jaipurkar, S. D. (2002) 'Structural brain differences between never-treated patients with schizophrenia, with and without dyskinesia, and normal control subjects: a magnetic resonance imaging study', *Arch Gen Psychiatry*, 59, 332–36.

McElroy, S. L., Weisler, R. H., Chang, W., Olausson, B., Paulsson, B., Brecher, M., et al. (2010) 'A double-blind, placebo-controlled study of quetiapine and paroxetine as monotherapy in adults with bipolar depression (EMBOLDEN II)', *J Clin Psychiatry*, 71, 163–74.

McGlashan, T. H. (2005) 'Early detection and intervention in psychosis: an ethical paradigm shift', *Br J Psychiatry Suppl*, 48, s113–s115.

McGlashan, T. H. (2006) 'Rationale and parameters for medication-free research in psychosis', *Schizophr Bull*, 32, 300–2.

McGlashan, T. H., Zipursky, R. B., Perkins, D., Addington, J., Miller, T., Woods, S. W., et al. (2006) 'Randomized, double-blind trial of olanzapine versus placebo in patients prodromally symptomatic for psychosis', *Am J Psychiatry*, 163, 790–9.

McGorry, P. D. (2008) 'Is early intervention in the major psychiatric disorders justified? Yes', *BMJ*, 337, a695.

McGorry, P. (2011) 'Merchants of doubt do no favours for people with mental illness', available at: http://www.patmcgorry.com.au/blog/pmcgorry/merchants-doubt-do-no-favours-people-mental-illnesses (accessed 15 April 2013).

McGorry, P. D., Yung, A. R., Phillips, L. J., Yuen, H. P., Francey, S., Cosgrave, E. M., et al. (2002) 'Randomized controlled trial of interventions designed to reduce the risk of progression to first-episode psychosis in a clinical sample with subthreshold symptoms.', *Arch Gen Psychiatry*, 59, 921–8.

McGorry, P., Nordentoft, M. and Simonsen, E. (2005) 'Introduction to "Early psychosis: a bridge to the future"', *Br J Psychiatry Suppl*, 48, s1–s3.

McGorry, P., Johanessen, J. O., Lewis, S., Birchwood, M., Malla, A., Nordentoft, M., et al. (2010) 'Early intervention in psychosis: keeping faith with evidence-based health care', *Psychol Med*, 40, 399–404.

McGorry, P. D., Nelson, B., Phillips, L. J., Yuen, H. P., Francey, S. M., Thampi, A., et al. (2013) 'Randomized controlled trial of interventions for young people at ultra-high risk of psychosis: twelve-month outcome', *J Clin Psychiatry*, 74, 349–56.

McGowan, S., Lawrence, A. D., Sales, T., Quested, D. and Grasby, P. (2004) 'Presynaptic dopaminergic dysfunction in schizophrenia: a positron emission tomographic [18F]fluorodopa study', *Arch Gen Psychiatry*, 61, 134–42.

Mackay, A. V., Iversen, L. L., Rossor, M., Spokes, E., Bird, E., Arregui, A., et al. (1982) 'Increased brain dopamine and dopamine receptors in schizophrenia', *Arch Gen Psychiatry*, 39, 991–997.

McQuade, R. D., Stock, E., Marcus, R., Jody, D., Gharbia, N. A., Vanveggel, S., et al. (2004) 'A comparison of weight change during treatment with olanzapine or aripiprazole: results from a randomized, double-blind study', *J Clin Psychiatry*, 65(Suppl. 18), 47–56.

Malitz, S. and Hoch, P. (1966) 'Drug therapy: neuroleptics and tranquilizers', in Arieti, S. (ed.) *American Handbook of Psychiatry, Volume III*, 2nd edn, pp. 458–76 (New York: Basic Books).

Manji, H. K., Moore, G. J. and Chen, G. (1999) 'Lithium at 50: have the neuroprotective effects of this unique cation been overlooked?', *Biol Psychiatry*, 46, 929–40.

Manji, H. K., Moore, G. J., & Chen, G. (2000) 'Lithium up-regulates the cytoprotective protein Bcl-2 in the CNS in vivo: a role for neurotrophic and neuroprotective effects in manic depressive illness', *J Clin Psychiatry*, 61(Suppl. 9), 82–96.

Manji, R. A., Wood, K. E. and Kumar, A. (2009) 'The history and evolution of circulatory shock', *Crit Care Clin*, 25, 1–29, vii.

Mapp, Y. and Nodine, J. H. (1962) 'Psychopharmacology. II. Tranquilizers and antipsychotic drugs', *Psychosomatics*, 3, 458–463.

Marder, S. R. and Meibach, R. C. (1994) 'Risperidone in the treatment of schizophrenia', *Am J Psychiatry*, 151, 825–35.

Marshall, M. and Rathbone, J. (2011) 'Early intervention for psychosis', *Schizophr Bull*, 37, 1111–14.

Marshall, M., Lewis, S., Lockwood, A., Drake, R., Jones, P. and Croudace, T. (2005) 'Association between duration of untreated psychosis and outcome in cohorts of first-episode patients: a systematic review', *Arch Gen Psychiatry*, 62, 975–83.

Martinot, J. L., Peron-Magnan, P., Huret, J. D., Mazoyer, B., Baron, J. C., Boulenger, J. P., et al. (1990) 'Striatal D2 dopaminergic receptors assessed with positron emission tomography and [76Br]bromospiperone in untreated schizophrenic patients', *Am J Psychiatry*, 147, 44–50.

Matthysse, S. (1973) 'Antipsychotic drug actions: a clue to the neuropathology of schizophrenia?', *Fed Proc*, 32, 200–5.

Matthysse, S. (1974a) 'Dopamine and the pharmacology of schizophrenia: the state of the evidence', *J Psychiatr Res*, 11, 107–13.

Matthysse, S. (1974b) 'Epilogue', *J Psychiatric Res*, 11, xiii–xvi.

Maudsley, H. (1895) *The Pathology of the Mind* (London: Macmillan).

Maxman, A. (2012) 'Psychosis risk syndrome excluded from DSM-5', *Nature News*, 9 May.

May, P. R., Tuma, A. H., Dixon, W. J., Yale, C., Thiele, D. A. and Kraude, W. H. (1981) 'Schizophrenia. A follow-up study of the results of five forms of treatment', *Arch Gen Psychiatry*, 38, 776–84.

May, P. R. A. (1968) *Treatment of Schizophrenia* (New York City: Science House).

May, R. (2001) 'Taking a stand: Fergus Keane interview with Rufus May', *BBC Radio 4*, 6 Feb.

Mayer-Gross, W., Slater, E. and Roth, M. (1954) *Clinical Psychiatry*, 1st edn (London: Cassell & Co.).

Mayer-Gross, W., Slater, E. and Roth, M. (1960) *Clinical Psychiatry*, 2nd edn (London: Cassell & Co.).

Mayer-Gross, W., Slater, E. and Roth, M. (1969) *Clinical Psychiatry*, 3rd edn (London: Bailliere Tindall).

Medew, J. (2010) 'McGorry "misleading the public"', *The Age*, 9 Aug.

Melander, H., Ahlqvist-Rastad, J., Meijer, G. and Beermann, B. (2003) 'Evidence b(i)ased medicine—selective reporting from studies sponsored by pharmaceutical industry: review of studies in new drug applications', *BMJ*, 326, 1171–3.

Melle, I., Larsen, T. K., Haahr, U., Friis, S., Johannessen, J. O., Opjordsmoen, S., et al. (2004) 'Reducing the duration of untreated first-episode psychosis: effects on clinical presentation', *Arch Gen Psychiatry*, 61, 143–50.

Melleril advertisement (1960) Advertisement, *J Mental Sci*, 106 (April), iii–vii.

Melleril advertisement (1970) Advertisement, *Br J Psychiatry*, 117 (Sept), xii–xiii.

Meltzer, H. Y. (1991) 'The mechanism of action of novel antipsychotic drugs', *Schizophr Bull*, 17, 263–87.

Meltzer, H. Y. (1994) 'An overview of the mechanism of action of clozapine', *J Clin Psychiatry*, 55(Suppl. B), 47–52.

Meltzer, H. Y. (1995) 'The role of serotonin in schizophrenia and the place of serotonin-dopamine antagonist antipsychotics', *J Clin Psychopharmacol*, 15, 2S–3S.

Meltzer, H. Y. and Stahl, S. M. (1976) 'The dopamine hypothesis of schizophrenia: a review', *Schizophr Bull*, 2, 19–76.

Meltzer, H. Y., Matsubara, S. and Lee, J. C. (1989) 'Classification of typical and atypical antipsychotic drugs on the basis of dopamine D-1, D-2 and serotonin2 pKi values', *J Pharmacol Exp Ther*, 251, 238–46.

Meyers, F. H. (1956) 'Pharmacology of chlorpormazine, reserpine and related drugs', in Kline, N. S. (ed.) *Psychopharmacology. A Symposium Held by the Section on Medical Sciences of the American Association for the Advancement of Science and the American Psychiatric Association*, pp. 131–40 (Washington DC: American Association for the Advancement of Science).

MHRA (1992) *Clinical assessment report on ripseridone – Final* (London: obtained through Freedom of Information Act request to Medicines and Healthcare products Regulatory Agency (MHRA)).

Miller, D. D., McEvoy, J. P., Davis, S. M., Caroff, S. N., Saltz, B. L., Chakos, M. H., et al. (2005) 'Clinical correlates of tardive dyskinesia in schizophrenia: baseline data from the CATIE schizophrenia trial', *Schizophr Res*, 80, 33–43.

Mindfreedom (2012) 'Occupy American Psychiatric Association New York City', available at: http://www.mindfreedom.org/as/act-archives/us/new-york/occupy-apa-nyc-2012 (accessed 15 April 2013).

Mintzes, B., Barer, M. L., Kravitz, R. L., Kazanjian, A., Bassett, K., Lexchin, J., et al. (2002) 'Influence of direct to consumer pharmaceutical advertising and patients' requests on prescribing decisions: two site cross sectional survey', *BMJ*, 324, 278–9.

Mittal, V., Kurup, L., Williamson, D., Muralee, S. and Tampi, R. R. (2011) 'Risk of cerebrovascular adverse events and death in elderly patients with dementia when treated with antipsychotic medications: a literature review of evidence', *Am J Alzheimers Dis Other Demen*, 26, 10–28.

Mizrahi, R., Bagby, R. M., Zipursky, R. B. and Kapur, S. (2005) 'How antipsychotics work: the patients' perspective', *Prog Neuropsychopharmacol Biol Psychiatry*, 29, 859–64.

Mizrahi, R., Kiang, M., Mamo, D. C., Arenovich, T., Bagby, R. M., Zipursky, R. B., et al. (2006) 'The selective effect of antipsychotics on the different dimensions of the experience of psychosis in schizophrenia spectrum disorders', *Schizophr Res*, 88, 111–18.

Modestin, J., Huber, A., Satirli, E., Malti, T. and Hell, D. (2003) 'Long-term course of schizophrenic illness: Bleuler's study reconsidered', *Am J Psychiatry*, 160, 2202–8.

Moffat, L. E., Hamilton, D. N. and Ledingham, I. M. (1985) 'To stop his wounds, lest he do bleed to death. A history of surgical shock', *J R Coll Surg Edinb*, 30, 73–81.

Mogilnicka, E. and Braestrup, C. (1976) 'Noradrenergic influence on the stereotyped behaviour induced by amphetamine, phenethylamine and apomorphine', *J Pharm Pharmacol*, 28, 253–5.

Moncrieff, J. (1999) 'An investigation into the precedents of modern drug treatment in psychiatry', *Hist Psychiatry*, 10, 475–90.

Moncrieff, J. (2001) 'Are antidepressants overrated? A review of methodological problems in antidepressant trials', *J Nerv Ment Dis*, 189, 288–295.

Moncrieff, J. (2003) 'Clozapine v. conventional antipsychotic drugs for treatment-resistant schizophrenia: a re-examination', *Br J Psychiatry*, 183, 161–6.

Moncrieff, J. (2006) 'Does antipsychotic withdrawal provoke psychosis? Review of the literature on rapid onset psychosis (supersensitivity psychosis) and withdrawal-related relapse', *Acta Psychiatr Scand*, 114, 3–13.

Moncrieff, J. (2008a) *The Myth of the Chemical Cure: A Critique of Psychiatric Drug Treatment* (Basingstoke: Palgrave Macmillan).

Moncrieff, J. (2008b) 'The creation of the concept of the antidepressant: an historical analysis', *Soc Sci Med*, 66, 2346–55.

Moncrieff, J. (2009) 'A critique of the dopamine hypothesis of schizophrenia and psychosis', *Harv Rev Psychiatry*, 17, 214–25.

Moncrieff, J. and Cohen, D. (2005) 'Rethinking models of psychotropic drug action', *Psychother Psychosom*, 74, 145–53.

Moncrieff, J. and Crawford, M. J. (2001) 'British psychiatry in the 20th century—observations from a psychiatric journal', *Soc Sci Med*, 53, 349–56.

Moncrieff, J. and Cohen, D. (2006) 'Do antidepressants cure or create abnormal brain states?', *PLoS Med*, 3, e240.

Moncrieff, J. and Leo, J. (2010) 'A systematic review of the effects of antipsychotic drugs on brain volume', *Psychol Med*, 40, 1–14.

Moncrieff, J., Cohen, D. and Mason, J. P. (2009) 'The subjective experience of taking antipsychotic medication: a content analysis of Internet data', *Acta Psychiatr Scand*, 120, 102–11.

Monroe, R. R. (1975) 'Anticonvulsants in the treatment of aggression', *J Nerv Ment Dis*, 160, 119–26.

Montgomery, A. J., Mehta, M. A. and Grasby, P. M. (2006) 'Is psychological stress in man associated with increased striatal dopamine levels?: A [11C]raclopride PET study', *Synapse*, 60, 124–31.

Moorhead, T. W., McKirdy, J., Sussmann, J. E., Hall, J., Lawrie, S. M., Johnstone, E. C., et al. (2007) 'Progressive gray matter loss in patients with bipolar disorder', *Biol Psychiatry*, 62, 894–900.

Morrison, A. P., French, P., Stewart, S. L., Birchwood, M., Fowler, D., Gumley, A. I., et al. (2012) 'Early detection and intervention evaluation for people at risk of psychosis: multisite randomised controlled trial', *BMJ*, 344, e2233.

Mukherjee, S. (1984) 'Tardive dysmentia: a reappraisal', *Schizophr Bull*, 10, 151–3.

Muller, P. and Seeman, P. (1978) 'Dopaminergic supersensitivity after neuroleptics: time-course and specificity', *Psychopharmacology (Berl)*, 60, 1–11.

Myslobodsky, M. S. (1993) 'Central determinants of attention and mood disorder in tardive dyskinesia ("tardive dysmentia")', *Brain Cogn*, 23, 88–101.

Naidoo, D. (1956) 'The effect of reserpine (serpasil) on the chronic disturbed schizophrenic: a comparative study of Rauwolfia alkaloids and electroconvulsive therapy', *J Nerv Ment Dis*, 123, 1–13.

National Collaborating Centre for Mental Health (2010) 'Schizophrenia. the NICE guideline on core interventions in the treatment and management of schizophrenia in adults in primary and secondary care – updated', Rep. No. 82 (London: British Psychological Society and Royal College of Psychiatrists).

National Institute for Health and Clinical Excellence (2002) *Schizophrenia: Core Interventions in the Treatment and Management of Schizophrenia in Primary and Secondary Care* (London: National Institute for Clinical Excellence).

National Institute for Health and Clinical Excellence (2005) *Violence: The Short-term Management of Distrubed/Violent Behaviour in In-patient Psychiatric Settings and Emergency Departments* (London: Royal College of Nursing).

National Institute for Health and Clinical Excellence (2006) 'Bipolar Disorder. the management of bipolar disorder in adults, children and adolescents, in primary and secondary care', Rep. No. NICE Clinical Guideline 38 (London: National Institute for Clinical Excellence).

National Institute of Mental Health Psychopharmacology Service Center Collaborative Study Group (1964) 'Phenothiazine treatment in acute schizophrenia', *Arch Gen Psychiatry*, 10, 246–58.

Navari, S. and Dazzan, P. (2009) 'Do antipsychotic drugs affect brain structure? A systematic and critical review of MRI findings', *Psychol Med*, 39, 1763–77.

Newcomer, J. W., Haupt, D. W., Fucetola, R., Melson, A. K., Schweiger, J. A., Cooper, B. P., et al. (2002) 'Abnormalities in glucose regulation during antipsychotic treatment of schizophrenia', *Arch Gen Psychiatry*, 59, 337–45.

Ngan, E. T., Lane, C. J., Ruth, T. J. and Liddle, P. F. (2002) 'Immediate and delayed effects of risperidone on cerebral metabolism in neuroleptic naive schizophrenic patients: correlations with symptom change', *J Neurol Neurosurg Psychiatry*, 72, 106–10.

NHS Information Centre for Health and Social Care (1998–2010) 'Prescription Cost Analysis. London: The Health and Social Care Information Centre', available at: http://www.hscic.gov.uk/searchcatalogue?q=title%3A%22prescription+cost+analysis%22&area=&size=10&sort=Relevance (accessed 26 April 2013).

NHS Information Centre for Health and Social Care (2010) *In-patients Formally Detained in Hospitals Under the Mental Health Act 1983 and Patients Subject to Supervised Community Treatment, Annual Figures, England 2009/10* (London: The Health and Social Care Information Centre).

NHS Information Centre for Health and Social Care (2011) *In-patients Formally detained in Hospitals Under the Mental Health Act 1983 and Patients Subject to Supervised Community Treatment, Annual Figures, England 2010/2011* (London: The Health and Social Care Information Centre).

NHS Prescription Services (2009) *Prescribing Review April–June 2009. Antipsychotic drugs.* (London: NHS Business Services Authority).

Nieoullon, A. and Coquerel, A. (2003) 'Dopamine: a key regulator to adapt action, emotion, motivation and cognition', *Curr Opin Neurol*, 16(Suppl. 2), S3–S9.

Noce, R. H., Williams, D. B. and Rapaport, W. (1954) 'Reserpine (serpasil) in the management of the mentally ill and mentally retarded; preliminary report', *JAMA*, 156, 821–4.

Nozaki, S., Kato, M., Takano, H., Ito, H., Takahashi, H., Arakawa, R., et al. (2009) 'Regional dopamine synthesis in patients with schizophrenia using L-[beta-11C]DOPA PET', *Schizophr Res*, 108, 78–84.

Nyberg, S., Nordstrom, A. L., Halldin, C. and Farde, L. (1995) 'Positron emission tomography studies on D2 dopamine receptor occupancy and plasma antipsychotic drug levels in man', *Int Clin Psychopharmacol*, 10(Suppl. 3), 81–5.

Oaks, D. (2011) 'Users views on coercive treatment', in Kallert, T. W., Mezzich, J. E. and Monahan, J. (eds) *Coercive Treatment in Psychiatry: Clinical Legal and Ethical aspects*, 1st edn, pp. 187–211 (Hoboken, NJ: John Wiley).

Odegaard, O. (1964) 'Pattern of discharge from Norwegian psychiatric hospitals before and after the introduction of psychiatric drugs', *Am J Psychiatry*, 70, 772–8.

Olfson, M., Blanco, C., Liu, L., Moreno, C. and Laje, G. (2006) 'National trends in the outpatient treatment of children and adolescents with antipsychotic drugs', *Arch Gen Psychiatry*, 63, 679–85.

Osby, U., Correia, N., Brandt, L., Ekbom, A. and Sparen, P. (2000) 'Mortality and causes of death in schizophrenia in Stockholm county, Sweden', *Schizophr Res*, 45, 21–8.

Otsuka America Pharmaceutical (2012) 'Understanding bipolar I disorder', available at: http://www.abilify.com/bipolar/about/bipolar-disorder.aspx?tc=89340&utm_source=google&utm_medium=organic_search&utm_term=&sa=t&rct=j&q=&esrc=s&frm=1&source=web&cd=1&ved=0CDAQFjAA&url=http%3A%2F%2Fwww.abilify.com%2F&ei=nAS-UMiwJ8TT0QWBroDgCg&usg=AFQjCNEmuZnhqoRv2cM0IGq_-bFnCG8QJw&sig2=liuonlDgERjWI6SxmKQOKA (accessed 16 April 2013).

Overholser, W. (1956) 'Has chlorpromazine inaugurated a new era in mental hospitals?', *J Clin Exp Psychopathol*, 17, 197–201.

Overton, R. C. and De Bakey, M. E. (1956) 'Experimental observations on the influence of hypothermia and autonomic blocking agents on hemorrhagic shock', *Ann Surg*, 143, 439–47.

Owen, F., Cross, A. J., Crow, T. J., Longden, A., Poulter, M. and Riley, G. J. (1978) 'Increased dopamine-receptor sensitivity in schizophrenia', *Lancet*, 2, 223–6.

Owens, D. G. (1985) 'Involuntary disorders of movement in chronic schizophrenia—the role of the illness and its treatment', *Psychopharmacology Suppl*, 2, 79–87.

Owens, D. C. (2008) 'How CATIE brought us back to Kansas: a critical re-evaluation of the concept of atypical antipsychotics and their place in the treatment of schizophrenia', *Adv Psychiatr Treat*, 14, 17–28.

Owens, D. G., Johnstone, E. C. and Frith, C. D. (1982) 'Spontaneous involuntary disorders of movement: their prevalence, severity, and distribution in chronic schizophrenics with and without treatment with neuroleptics', *Arch Gen Psychiatry*, 39, 452–61.

Owens, D. G., Johnstone, E. C., Crow, T. J., Frith, C. D., Jagoe, J. R. and Kreel, L. (1985) 'Lateral ventricular size in schizophrenia: relationship to the disease process and its clinical manifestations', *Psychol Med*, 15, 27–41.

Pacatal advertisement (1957) Advertisement. *J Mental Sci*, 103, April, vii.

Pariante, C. M., Vassilopoulou, K., Velakoulis, D., Phillips, L., Soulsby, B., Wood, S. J., et al. (2004) 'Pituitary volume in psychosis', *Br J Psychiatry*, 185, 5–10.

Paterson, A. S. (1963) *Electrical and Drug Treatments in Psychiatry* (London: Elsevier).

Paulsen, J., Heaton, R. and Jeste, D. (1994) 'Neuropsychological impairment in tardive dyskinesia', *Neuropsychology*, 8, 227–41.

Paulson, G. W. (2005) 'Historical comments on tardive dyskinesia: a neurologist's perspective', *J Clin Psychiatry*, 66, 260–4.

Pellegrino, E. D. (1979) 'The socio-cultural impact of twentieth century therapeutics', in Vogel, M. J. and Rosenberg, C. E. (eds) *The Therapeutic Revolution*, pp. 245–66 (Philadelphia, PA: University of Pennsylvania Press).

Peltonen, L. (1962) 'Pneumoencephalographic studies on the third ventricle of 644 neuropsychiatric patients', *Acta Psychiatr Scand*, 38, 15–34.

Perceval, J. (1961) *Perceval's Narrative. A Patient's Account of his Psychosis 1830–1832* (Stanford, CA: Stanford University Press).

Peretti, C. S., Danion, J. M., Kauffmann-Muller, F., Grange, D., Patat, A. and Rosenzweig, P. (1997) 'Effects of haloperidol and amisulpride on motor and cognitive skill learning in healthy volunteers', *Psychopharmacology (Berl)*, 131, 329–38.

Perkins, D. O., Gu, H., Boteva, K. and Lieberman, J. A. (2005) 'Relationship between duration of untreated psychosis and outcome in first-episode schizophrenia: a critical review and meta-analysis', *Am J Psychiatry*, 162, 1785–804.

Petersen, L., Jeppesen, P., Thorup, A., Abel, M. B., Ohlenschlaeger, J., Christensen, T. O., et al. (2005) 'A randomised multicentre trial of integrated versus standard treatment for patients with a first episode of psychotic illness', *BMJ*, 331, 602.

Pfizer (2006) Pfizer website, available at: www.geodon.com/s_WhatCauses.asp (accessed 6 February 2002).

Pfizer (2011) 'About bipolar disorder', available at: https://www.geodon.com/what-is-bipolar-disorder.aspx (accessed 16 April 2013).

Phatak, P., Shaldivin, A., King, L. S., Shapiro, P. and Regenold, W. T. (2006) 'Lithium and inositol: effects on brain water homeostasis in the rat', *Psychopharmacology (Berl)*, 186, 41–7.

Phillips, L. J., Yung, A. R. and McGorry, P. D. (2000) 'Identification of young people at risk of psychosis: validation of Personal Assessment and Crisis Evaluation Clinic intake criteria', *Aust N Z J Psychiatry*, 34(Suppl.), S164–9.

PIER (2012) 'The PIER programme', available at: http://www.mmc.org/pier_body.cfm?id=2184 (accessed 16 April 2013).

Pillay, P. and Moncrieff, J. (2011) 'Contribution of psychiatric disorders to occupation of NHS beds: analysis of Hospital Episode Statistics', *Psychiatrist*, 35, 56–9.

Pilowsky, L. S., Costa, D. C., Ell, P. J., Verhoeff, N. P., Murray, R. M. and Kerwin, R. W. (1994) 'D2 dopamine receptor binding in the basal ganglia of antipsychotic-free schizophrenic patients. An 123I-IBZM single photon emission computerised tomography study', *Br J Psychiatry*, 164, 16–26.

Pinfold, V., Smith, J. and Shiers, D. (2007) 'Audit of early intervention in psychosis service development in England in 2005', *Psychiatric Bull*, 31, 7–10.

Pletscher, A., Shore, P. A. and Brodie, B. B. (1955) 'Serotonin release as a possible mechanism of reserpine action', *Science*, 122, 374–5.

Polak, P. and Laycob, L. (1971) 'Rapid tranquilization', *Am J Psychiatry*, 128, 640–3.

Post, A., Holsboer, F. and Behl, C. (1998) 'Induction of NF-kappaB activity during haloperidol-induced oxidative toxicity in clonal hippocampal cells: suppression of NF-kappaB and neuroprotection by antioxidants', *J Neurosci*, 18, 8236–46.

PREP (2012) 'Prevention and recovery in early psychosis', available at: http://www.prepwellness.org/videos.html (accessed 16 April 2013).

Priebe, S., Badesconyi, A., Fioritti, A., Hansson, L., Kilian, R., Torres-Gonzales, F., et al. (2005) 'Reinstitutionalisation in mental health care: comparison of data on service provision from six European countries', *BMJ*, 330, 123–6.

Pringsheim, T., Lam, D., Ching, H. and Patten, S. (2011) 'Metabolic and neurological complications of second-generation antipsychotic use in children: a systematic review and meta-analysis of randomized controlled trials', *Drug Saf*, 34, 651–68.

Promazine advertisement (1957) Advertisement, *J Mental Sci*, 103, October, vi.

Ramaekers, J. G., Louwerens, J. W., Muntjewerff, N. D., Milius, H., de Bie, A., Rosenzweig, P., et al. (1999) 'Psychomotor, Cognitive, extrapyramidal, and affective functions of healthy volunteers during treatment with an atypical (amisulpride) and a classic (haloperidol) antipsychotic', *J Clin Psychopharmacol*, 19, 209–21.

Ramaswamy, K., Masand, P. S. and Nasrallah, H. A. (2006) 'Do certain atypical antipsychotics increase the risk of diabetes? A critical review of 17 pharmacoepidemiologic studies', *Ann Clin Psychiatry*, 18, 183–94.

Rammsayer, T. and Gallhofer, B. (1995) 'Remoxipride versus haloperidol in healthy volunteers: psychometric performance and subjective tolerance profiles', *Int Clin Psychopharmacol*, 10, 31–7.

Randrup, A. and Munkvad, I. (1967) 'Brain dopamine and amphetamine-induced stereotyped behaviour', *Acta Pharmacol Toxicol (Copenh)*, 25(Suppl. 4), 62.

Randrup, A. and Munkvad, I. (1972) 'Influence of amphetamines on animal behaviour: stereotypy, functional impairment and possible animal-human correlations', *Psychiatr Neurol Neurochir*, 75, 193–202.

Randrup, A., Munkvad, I. and Udsen, P. (1963) 'Adrenergic mechanisms and amphetamine induced abnormal behaviour', *Acta Pharmacol Toxicol (Copenh)*, 20, 145–57.

Rauste-von Wright, M. and Frankenhaeuser, M. (1989) 'Females' emotionality as reflected in the excretion of the dopamine metabolite HVA during mental stress', *Psychol Rep*, 64, 856–8.

Ray, W. A., Meredith, S., Thapa, P. B., Meador, K. G., Hall, K. and Murray, K. T. (2001) 'Antipsychotics and the risk of sudden cardiac death', *Arch Gen Psychiatry*, 58, 1161–7.

Ray, W. A., Chung, C. P., Murray, K. T., Hall, K. and Stein, C. M. (2009) 'Atypical antipsychotic drugs and the risk of sudden cardiac death', *N Engl J Med*, 360, 225–35.

Read, J., Agar, K., Argyle, N. and Aderhold, V. (2003) 'Sexual and physical abuse during childhood and adulthood as predictors of hallucinations, delusions and thought disorder', *Psychol Psychother*, 76, 1–22.

Redeptin advertisement (1975) Advertisement, *Br J Psychiatry*, 126 June.

Remington, G. (2005) 'Rational pharmacotherapy in early psychosis', *Br J Psychiatry Suppl*, 48, s77–s84.

Remington, G. (2008) 'Alterations of dopamine and serotonin transmission in schizophrenia', *Prog Brain Res*, 172, 117–40.

Reserpine advertisement (1956) Advertisement, *J Ment Sci*, 102, January vi.

Reynolds, G. P., Riederer, P., Jellinger, K. and Gabriel, E. (1981) 'Dopamine receptors and schizophrenia: the neuroleptic drug problem', *Neuropharmacology*, 20, 1319–20.

Risperdal Consta advertisement (2007) Advertisement, *Br J Psychiatry*, 191, October, backcover.
Ritalin advertisement (1964) Advertisement, *BMJ*, 2.
Roberts, M. H. T. (1973) 'Pharmacology of drugs of importance in psychiatry', in Forrest, A. (ed.) *Companion to Psychiatric Studies Volume 1*, 1st edn, pp. 348–85 (Edinburgh: Churchill Livingstone).
Robertson, M. M. and Trimble, M. R. (1982) 'Major tranquillisers used as antidepressants. A review', *J Affect Disord*, 4, 173–93.
Rogers, A. and Pilgrim, D. (2001) *Mental Health Policy in Britain*, 2nd edn (Basingstoke: Palgrave Macmillan).
Rogers, A., Day, J. C., Williams, B., Randall, F., Wood, P., Healy, D., et al. (1998) 'The meaning and management of neuroleptic medication: a study of patients with a diagnosis of schizophrenia', *Soc Sci Med*, 47, 1313–23.
Rollin, H. R. (1990) 'The dark before the dawn', *J Psychopharmacol*, 4, 109–14.
Rosenhan, D.L. (1973) 'On being sane in insane places', *Science*, 179, 250–8.
Rothman, R. B., Baumann, M. H., Dersch, C. M., Romero, D. V., Rice, K. C., Carroll, F. I., et al. (2001) 'Amphetamine-type central nervous system stimulants release norepinephrine more potently than they release dopamine and serotonin', *Synapse*, 39, 32–41.
Royal College of Psychiatrists (2004) 'Mental health and growing up' (pamphlet).
Royal Commission (1926) 'Report of the royal commission on lunacy and mental disorders', Rep. No. Cmd. 2700 (London: Stationery Office).
Ruhrmann, S., Bechdolf, A., Kuhn, K. U., Wagner, M., Schultze-Lutter, F., Janssen, B., et al. (2007) 'Acute effects of treatment for prodromal symptoms for people putatively in a late initial prodromal state of psychosis', *Br J Psychiatry Suppl*, 51, s88–s95.
Rummel-Kluge, C., Komossa, K., Schwarz, S., Hunger, H., Schmid, F., Lobos, C. A., et al. (2010) 'Head-to-head comparisons of metabolic side effects of second generation antipsychotics in the treatment of schizophrenia: a systematic review and meta-analysis', *Schizophr Res*, 123, 225–33.
Rush, A. J., Wisniewski, S. R., Zisook, S., Fava, M., Sung, S. C., Haley, C. L., et al. (2012) 'Is prior course of illness relevant to acute or longer-term outcomes in depressed out-patients? A STAR*D report', *Psychol Med*, 42, 1131–49.
Rushton, P. (1988) 'Lunatics and idiots: mental disability, the community, and the poor law in North-East England, 1600–1800', *Med Hist*, 32, 34–50.
Ryan, M. C., Collins, P. and Thakore, J. H. (2003) 'Impaired fasting glucose tolerance in first-episode, drug-naive patients with schizophrenia', *Am J Psychiatry*, 160, 284–9.
Sacher, J., Mossaheb, N., Spindelegger, C., Klein, N., Geiss-Granadia, T., Sauermann, R., et al. (2008) 'Effects of olanzapine and ziprasidone on glucose tolerance in healthy volunteers', *Neuropsychopharmacology*, 33, 1633–41.
Sacks, O. (1990) *Awakenings*, revised edn (New York: Vintage Books).
Sadler, W. S. (1953) *Practice of Psychiatry* (London: Henry Kimpton).
Sagara, Y. (1998) 'Induction of reactive oxygen species in neurons by haloperidol', *J Neurochem*, 71, 1002–12.
Sainz, A. A. (1956) 'Considerations on the cerebral action of Reserpine', in Kline, N. S. (ed.) *Psychopharmacology. A Symposium Held by the Section on Medical Sciences of the American Association for the Advancement of Science and*

the *American Psychiatric Association*, pp. 59–63 (Washington DC: American Association for the Advancement of Science).

Sakel, M. (1958) *Schizophrenia* (New York: Philosophical Library).

Salgado-Pineda, P., Baeza, I., Perez-Gomez, M., Vendrell, P., Junque, C., Bargallo, N., et al. (2003) 'Sustained attention impairment correlates to gray matter decreases in first episode neuroleptic-naive schizophrenic patients', *Neuroimage*, 19, 365–75.

Salokangas, R. K., Vilkman, H., Ilonen, T., Taiminen, T., Bergman, J., Haaparanta, M., et al. (2000) 'High levels of dopamine activity in the basal ganglia of cigarette smokers', *Am J Psychiatry*, 157, 632–4.

Samaha, A. N., Seeman, P., Stewart, J., Rajabi, H. and Kapur, S. (2007) '"Breakthrough" dopamine supersensitivity during ongoing antipsychotic treatment leads to treatment failure over time', *J Neurosci*, 27, 2979–86.

Sankaranarayanan, J. and Puumala, S. E. (2007) 'Antipsychotic use at adult ambulatory care visits by patients with mental health disorders in the United States, 1996–2003: national estimates and associated factors', *Clin Ther*, 29, 723–41.

Sartorius, N., Jablensky, A. and Shapiro, R. (1977) 'Two-year follow-up of the patients included in the WHO International Pilot Study of Schizophrenia', *Psychol Med*, 7, 529–41.

Sarwer-Foner, G. J. (1960) 'The role of neuroleptic medication in psychotherapeutic interaction', *Compr Psychiatry*, 1, 291–300.

Sawamoto, N., Hotton, G., Pavese, N., Piccini, P. and Brooks, D. J. (2005) 'Frontal endogenous dopamine release detected with [11C]-raclopride PET during a visual search task in healthy subjects and Parkinson's disease patients', *Neurology*, 64, A274.

Scherk, H. and Falkai, P. (2006) 'Effects of antipsychotics on brain structure', *Curr Opin Psychiatry*, 19, 145–50.

Schizophrenia Commission (2012) 'The abandoned illness: a report from the schizophrenia commission' (London: Rethink Mental Illness).

schizophrenia.com (2012) 'Worldwide early diagnosis and tretament centres for schizophrenia', available at: http://www.schizophrenia.com/earlypsychosis. htm (accessed 16 April 2013).

Schleifer, J. J. (2011) 'Management of acute agitation in psychosis: an evidence based approach in the USA', *Adv Psychiatr Treat*, 17, 91–100.

Schmeid, K. and Ernst, K. (1983) ['Isolation and forced injection in the opinion of affected patients and patient care personnel. An accompanied quarter year sample'], *Arch Psychiatr Nervenkr*, 233, 211–22 [in German].

Schmidt, W. R. and Jarcho, L. W. (1966) 'Persistent dyskinesias following phenothiazine therapy. Report of five cases and a review of the literature', *Arch Neurol*, 14, 369–77.

Schneider, L. S., Dagerman, K. S. and Insel, P. (2005) 'Risk of death with atypical antipsychotic drug treatment for dementia: meta-analysis of randomized placebo-controlled trials', *JAMA*, 294, 1934–43.

Schneider, L. S., Dagerman, K. and Insel, P. S. (2006) 'Efficacy and adverse effects of atypical antipsychotics for dementia: meta-analysis of randomized, placebo-controlled trials', *Am J Geriatr Psychiatry*, 14, 191–210.

Schoenecker, M. (1957) ['Paroxysmal dyskinesia as the effect of megaphen']. *Nervenarzt*, 28, 550–3 [in German].

Schooler, N. R., Goldberg, S. C., Boothe, H. and Cole, J. O. (1967) 'One year after discharge: community adjustment of schizophrenic patients', *Am J Psychiatry*, 123, 986–95.

Schooler, N., Rabinowitz, J., Davidson, M., Emsley, R., Harvey, P. D., Kopala, L., et al. (2005) 'Risperidone and haloperidol in first-episode psychosis: a long-term randomized trial', *Am J Psychiatry*, 162, 947–53.

Scull, A. (1993) *The Most Solitary of Afflictions* (New Haven, CT: Yale University Press).

Scull, A. (1994) 'Somatic treatments and the historiography of psychiatry', *Hist Psychiatry*, 5, 1–12.

Sedgwick, P. (1982) *Psychopolitics* (London: Harper & Row).

Sengupta, S., Parrilla-Escobar, M. A., Klink, R., Fathalli, F., Ying, K. N., Stip, E., et al. (2008) 'Are metabolic indices different between drug-naive first-episode psychosis patients and healthy controls?', *Schizophr Res*, 102, 329–36.

Serenace advertisement (1965a) Advertisement, *Br J Psychiatry*, 111, January xiii.

Serenace advertisement (1965b) Advertisement, *Br J Psychiatry*, 111, July viii.

Sernyak, M. J., Leslie, D. L., Alarcon, R. D., Losonczy, M. F. and Rosenheck, R. (2002) 'Association of diabetes mellitus with use of atypical neuroleptics in the treatment of schizophrenia', *Am J Psychiatry*, 159, 561–6.

Sheitman, B. B., Lee, H., Strous, R. and Lieberman, J. A. (1997) 'The evaluation and treatment of first-episode psychosis', *Schizophr Bull*, 23, 653–61.

Shepherd, M. (1994) 'Neurolepsis and the psychopharmacological revolution: myth and reality', *Hist Psychiatry*, 5, 89–96.

Shepherd, M., Goodman, N. and Watt, D. C. (1961) 'The application of hospital statistics in the evaluation of pharmacotherapy in a psychiatric population', *Comp Psychiatry*, 2, 11–19.

Shopsin, B., Klein, H., Aaronsom, M. and Collora, M. (1979) 'Clozapine, chlorpromazine, and placebo in newly hospitalized, acutely schizophrenic patients: a controlled, double-blind comparison', *Arch Gen Psychiatry*, 36, 657–64.

Shorter, E. (1997) *A History of Psychiatry. From the Era of the Asylum to the Age of Prozac* (New York: John Wiley).

Sigwald, J. and Bouttier, D. (1953) ['3-Chloro-10-(3'-dimethylaminopropyl)-phenothiazine hydrochloride in current neuro-psychiatry'], *Ann Med Interne (Paris)*, 54, 150–82.

Sigwald, J., Bouttier, D., Raymondeaud, C. and Piot, C. (1959) ['4 cases of facio-bucco-linguo-masticatory dyskinesis of prolonged development following treatment with neuroleptics'], *Rev Neurol (Paris)*, 100, 751–5.

Singh, S. P., Wright, C., Burns, T., Joyce, E. and Barnes, T. R. E. (2003) 'Developing early intervention services in the NHS: a survey to guide workforce and training needs', *The Psychiatrist*, 27, 254–8.

Smieskova, R., Fusar-Poli, P., Allen, P., Bendfeldt, K., Stieglitz, R. D., Drewe, J., et al. (2009) 'The effects of antipsychotics on the brain: what have we learnt from structural imaging of schizophrenia?—a systematic review', *Curr Pharm Des*, 15, 2535–49.

Smith Kline & French Laboratories (1955) *Chlorpormazine and Mental Health: Proceedings Held Under the Auspices of Smith Kline & French Laboratories* (Philadelphia, PA: Lea & Febiger).

Smith, R. C., Lindenmayer, J. P., Hu, Q., Kelly, E., Viviano, T. F., Cornwell, J., et al. (2010) 'Effects of olanzapine and risperidone on lipid metabolism in chronic schizophrenic patients with long-term antipsychotic treatment: a randomized five month study', *Schizophr Res*, 120, 204–9.

Smythies, J. R. (1973) 'Drug treatment of schizophrenia', in Forrest, A. (ed.) *Companion to Psychiatric Studies, Volume 2*, pp. 250–88 (Edinburgh: Churchill Livingstone).

Snyder, S. H. (1972) 'Catecholamines in the brain as mediators of amphetamine psychosis', *Arch Gen Psychiatry*, 27, 169–79.

Snyder, S. H. (1974) 'Stereoselective features of catecholamine dispostion and their behavioral implications', *J Psychiatr Res*, 11, 31–9.

Snyder, S. H. (1980) 'Basic science of psychopharmacology', in Kaplan, H. I., Freedman, A. M. and Sadock, B. J. (eds) *Comprehensive Textbook of Psychiatry*, 3rd edn, pp. 154–65 (Baltimore, MD: Williams & Wilkins).

Snyder, S. H., Banerjee, S. P., Yamamura, H. I. and Greenberg, D. (1974) 'Drugs, neurotransmitters, and schizophrenia', *Science*, 184, 1243–53.

Soreff, S. M. and Bazemore, P. H. (2006) 'Confronting chaos', *Behav Healthc*, 26, 16–20.

Spielmans, G. I. (2009) 'The promotion of olanzapine in primary care: an examination of internal industry documents', *Soc Sci Med*, 69, 14–20.

Spielmans, G.I. and Parry P.I. (2010) 'From evidence-based medicine to marketing-based medicine: evidence from internal industry documents', *J Bioethic Inq*, 7, 13–29.

Spitzer, R. L. (1975) 'On pseudoscience in science, logic in remission, and psychiatric diagnosis: a critique of Rosenhan's "On being sane in insane places"', *J Abnorm Psychol*, 84, 442–52.

Spivak, B., Mester, R., Abesgaus, J., Wittenberg, N., Adlersberg, S., Gonen, N., et al. (1997a) 'Clozapine treatment for neuroleptic-induced tardive dyskinesia, parkinsonism, and chronic akathisia in schizophrenic patients', *J Clin Psychiatry*, 58, 318–22.

Spivak, B., Mester, R., Wittenberg, N., Maman, Z. and Weizman, A. (1997b) 'Reduction of aggressiveness and impulsiveness during clozapine treatment in chronic neuroleptic-resistant schizophrenic patients', *Clin Neuropharmacol*, 20, 442–6.

Stahl, S. M. (2008) *Antipsychotics and Mood Stablizers* (Cambridge: Cambridge University Press).

Stark, J. (2011) 'McGorry aborts teen drug trial', *Sydney Morning Herald*, 21 Aug.

Stawarz, R. J., Hill, H., Robinson, S. E., Setler, P., Dingell, J. V. and Sulser, F. (1975) 'On the significance of the increase in homovanillic acid (HVA) caused by antipsychotic drugs in corpus striatum and limbic forebrain', *Psychopharmacologia*, 43, 125–30.

Steck, H. (1954) ['The extra-pyradmial and di-encephalic syndrome during treatment with largactil and serpasil'], *Annales Médico-psychologiques*, 112, 737–43.

Stelazine advertisement (1959a) Advertisement, *J Mental Sci*, 105, January, i.

Stelazine advertisement (1959b) Advertisement, *J Mental Sci*, 105, April, i

Stelazine advertisement (1965a) Advertisement, *Br J Psychiatry*, 111, September, xiv.

Stelazine advertisement (1965b) Advertisement. *Br J Psychiatry*, 111, June, xiv.

Stengers, I. (1995) ['The physician and the quack'], in Nathan, T. and Stengers, I. (eds), *[Doctors and Sorcerers]*, pp. 115–61 (Paris: Les Empecheurs de Penser en Rond) [in French].

Stepnisky, J. (2007) 'The biomedical self: hermeneutic considerations', *Soc Theory Health*, 5, 187–207.

Storey, P. B. (1966) 'Lumbar air encephalography in chronic schizophrenia: a controlled experiment', *Br J Psychiatry*, 112, 135–44.

Straus, S. M., Bleumink, G. S., Dieleman, J. P., van der, L. J., 't Jong, G. W., Kingma, J. H., et al. (2004) 'Antipsychotics and the risk of sudden cardiac death', *Arch Intern Med*, 164, 1293–7.

Strudwick, P. (2012) 'How a stressful job lead to my bipolar diagnosis', *The Times*, 26 May.

Sullivan, E. V., Shear, P. K., Lim, K. O., Zipursky, R. B. and Pfefferbaum, A. (1996) 'Cognitive and motor impairments are related to gray matter volume deficits in schizophrenia', *Biol Psychiatry*, 39, 234–40.

Suppes, T., Baldessarini, R. J., Faedda, G. L. and Tohen, M. (1991) 'Risk of recurrence following discontinuation of lithium treatment in bipolar disorder', *Arch Gen Psychiatry*, 48, 1082–8.

Sussman, N. (2009) 'General principles of psychopharmacology', in Saddock, B. J., Saddock, V. A. and Ruiz, P. (eds), 9th edn, pp. 2965–88 (Philadelphia, PA: Wolters Kluwer/Lippincott Williams & Wilkins).

Swazey, J. (1974) *Chlorpromazine in Psychiatry* (Cambridge, MA: Massachusetts Institute of Technology).

Szasz, T. (1970) *Ideology and Insanity; Essays on the Psychiatric Dehumanization of Man* (New York: Anchor Books).

Szasz, T. S. (1957) 'Some observations on the use of tranquilizing drugs', *AMA Arch Neurol Psychiatry*, 77, 86–92.

Tamminga, C. A., Thaker, G. K., Moran, M., Kakigi, T. and Gao, X. M. (1994) 'Clozapine in tardive dyskinesia: observations from human and animal model studies', *J Clin Psychiatry*, 55(Suppl B), 102–6.

Tandon, R., Mazzara, C., DeQuardo, J., Craig, K. A., Meador-Woodruff, J. H., Goldman, R., et al. (1991) 'Dexamethasone suppression test in schizophrenia: relationship to symptomatology, ventricular enlargement, and outcome', *Biol Psychiatry*, 29, 953–64.

Tarsy, D. (1983) 'History and definition of tardive dyskinesia', *Clin Neuropharmacol*, 6, 91–9.

Taylor, D., Paton, C. and Kapur, S. (2009) *The Maudsley Prescribing Guidelines* (London: Informa Healthcare).

Thomas, K. (2012) 'J&J fined $1.2 billion in drug case. New York Times', available at: http://www.nytimes.com/2012/04/12/business/drug-giant-is-fined-1-2-billion-in-arkansas.html (accessed 17 April 2013).

Thorup, A., Petersen, L., Jeppesen, P., Ohlenschlaeger, J., Christensen, T., Krarup, G., et al. (2005) 'Integrated treatment ameliorates negative symptoms in first episode psychosis—results from the Danish OPUS trial', *Schizophr Res*, 79, 95–105.

Thuillier, J. (2000) 'Ten years that changed psychiatry', in Healy, D. (ed.) *The Psychopharmacologists Volume III*, pp. 543–59 (London: Arnold).

Tien, A. Y. and Eaton, W. W. (1992) 'Psychopathologic precursors and sociodemographic risk factors for the schizophrenia syndrome', *Arch Gen Psychiatry*, 49, 37–46.

Tiihonen, J., Walhbeck, K., Lonnqvist, J., Klaukka, T., Ioannidis, J. P., Volavka, J., et al. (2006) 'Effectiveness of antipsychotic treatments in a nationwide cohort of patients in community care after first hospitalisation due to schizophrenia and schizoaffective disorder: observational follow-up study', *BMJ*, 333, 224.

Tiihonen, J., Lonnqvist, J., Wahlbeck, K., Klaukka, T., Niskanen, L., Tanskanen, A., et al. (2009) '11-year follow-up of mortality in patients with schizophrenia: a population-based cohort study (FIN11 study)', *Lancet*, 374, 620–7.

Time Magazine (1954) 'Wonder drug of 1954', *Time Magazine*, 14 Jun.

Time Magazine (1955) 'Pills for the mind', *Time Magazine*, 7 Mar.

Timimi, S., Gardner, N. and McCabe, B. (2011) *Myth of Autism* (Basingstoke: Palgrave Macmillan).

Tohen, M., Baker, R. W., Altshuler, L. L., Zarate, C. A., Suppes, T., Ketter, T. A., et al. (2002) 'Olanzapine versus divalproex in the treatment of acute mania', *Am J Psychiatry*, 159, 1011–17.

Tohen, M., Calabrese, J. R., Sachs, G. S., Banov, M. D., Detke, H. C., Risser, R., et al. (2006) 'Randomized, placebo-controlled trial of olanzapine as maintenance therapy in patients with bipolar I disorder responding to acute treatment with olanzapine', *Am J Psychiatry*, 163, 247–56.

Tohen, M., Sanger, T. M., McElroy, S. L., Tollefson, G. D., Chengappa, K. N., Daniel, D. G., et al. (1999) 'Olanzapine versus placebo in the treatment of acute mania. Olanzapine HGEH Study Group', *Am J Psychiatry*, 156, 702–9.

Tohen, M., Goldberg, J. F., Gonzalez-Pinto Arrillaga, A. M., Azorin, J. M., Vieta, E., Hardy-Bayle, M. C., et al. (2003) 'A 12-week, double-blind comparison of olanzapine vs haloperidol in the treatment of acute mania', *Arch Gen Psychiatry*, 60, 1218–26.

Torniainen, M., Suvisaari, J., Partonen, T., Castaneda, A. E., Kuha, A., Suokas, J., et al. (2012) 'Cognitive impairments in schizophrenia and schizoaffective disorder: relationship with clinical characteristics', *J Nerv Ment Dis*, 200, 316–22.

Torrey, E. F. (2002) 'Studies of individuals with schizophrenia never treated with antipsychotic medications: a review', *Schizophr Res*, 58, 101–15.

TREC Collaborative Group (2003) 'Rapid tranquillisation for agitated patients in emergency psychiatric rooms: a randomised trial of midazolam versus haloperidol plus promethazine', *BMJ*, 327, 708–13.

Tyhurst, J. S. and Richman, A. (1955) 'Clinical experience with psychiatric patients on reserpine—preliminary impressions', *Can Med Assoc J*, 72, 458–9.

Tyrer, P. (2012) 'From the Editor's desk', *Br J Psychiatry*, 201, 168.

Tyrer, P. and Kendall, T. (2009) 'The spurious advance of antipsychotic drug therapy', *Lancet*, 373, 4–5.

Tyrer, P., Oliver-Africano, P. C., Ahmed, Z., Bouras, N., Cooray, S., Deb, S., et al. (2008) 'Risperidone, haloperidol, and placebo in the treatment of aggressive challenging behaviour in patients with intellectual disability: a randomised controlled trial', *Lancet*, 371, 57–63.

Uhrbrand, L. and Faurbye, A. (1960) 'Reversible and irreversible dyskinesia after treatment with perphenazine, chlorpromazine, reserpine and electroconvulsive therapy', *Psychopharmacologia*, 1, 408–18.

Ukai, W., Ozawa, H., Tateno, M., Hashimoto, E. and Saito, T. (2004) 'Neurotoxic potential of haloperidol in comparison with risperidone: implication of Akt-mediated signal changes by haloperidol', *J Neural Transm*, 111, 667–81.

United States Department of Justice (2009) 'Pharmaceutical company Eli Lilly to pay record $1.415 billion for off label drug marketing', available at: http://www.justice.gov/usao/pae/News/2009/jan/lillyrelease.pdf (accessed 25 April 2013).

United States Department of Justice (2010) 'Pharmaceutical giant AstraZeneca to pay $520 million for off label drug marketing', available at: http://www.justice.gov/opa/pr/2010/April/10-civ-487.html (accessed 25 April 2013).

Unsworth, C. (1987) *The Politics of Mental Health Legislation* (Oxford: Oxford University Press).

USA Today (2009) 'Experts raise concerns over Seroquel to treat depression', available at: http://usatoday30.usatoday.com/news/health/2009-04-08-fda-seroquel_N.htm?csp=34 (accessed 17 April 2013).

Van Praag, H. M. and Korf, J. (1975) 'Neuroleptics, catecholamines, and psychoses: a study of their interrelations', *Am J Psychiatry*, 132, 593–7.

van Rossum, J., van der, S. C. H. O. and Hurkmans, J. A. (1962) 'Mechanism of action of cocaine and amphetamine in the brain', *Experientia*, 18, 229–31.

van Rossum, J. M. (1966a) 'The significance of dopamine-receptor blockade for the mechanism of action of neuroleptic drugs', *Arch Int Pharmacodyn Ther*, 160, 492–4.

van Rossum J.M. (1966b) 'The significance of dopamine receptor blockade for the action of neuroleptic drugs', in Brill, H. (ed.) *Neuro-psycho-pharmacology*, pp. 321–9 (Amsterdam: Excerpta Medica Foundation).

Van Voris, R. and Lawrence, J. (2010) 'Pfizer told to pay $142.1 million for Neurontin marketing fraud', available at: http://www.bloomberg.com/apps/news?pid=email_en&sid=a_9aVylZQGjU (available at 17 April 2013).

Venkatasubramanian, G., Jayakumar, P. N., Gangadhar, B. N. and Keshavan, M. S. (2008) 'Automated MRI parcellation study of regional volume and thickness of prefrontal cortex (PFC) in antipsychotic-naive schizophrenia', *Acta Psychiatr Scand*, 117, 420–31.

Verdoux, H. and Cougnard, A. (2006) 'Schizophrenia: who is at risk? Who is a case?', *Int Clin Psychopharmacol*, 21(Suppl. 2), S17–19.

Verdoux, H., Tournier, M. and Begaud, B. (2010) 'Antipsychotic prescribing trends: a review of pharmaco-epidemiological studies', *Acta Psychiatr Scand*, 121, 4–10.

Verhoeff, N. P., Kapur, S., Hussey, D., Lee, M., Christensen, B., Psych, C., et al. (2001) 'A simple method to measure baseline occupancy of neostriatal dopamine D2 receptors by dopamine in vivo in healthy subjects', *Neuropsychopharmacology*, 25, 213–23.

Vernaleken, I., Kumakura, Y., Cumming, P., Buchholz, H. G., Siessmeier, T., Stoeter, P., et al. (2006) 'Modulation of [18F]fluorodopa (FDOPA) kinetics in the brain of healthy volunteers after acute haloperidol challenge', *Neuroimage*, 30, 1332–9.

Vernon, A. C., Natesan, S., Modo, M. and Kapur, S. (2011) 'Effect of chronic antipsychotic treatment on brain structure: a serial magnetic resonance imaging study with ex vivo and postmortem confirmation', *Biol Psychiatry*, 69, 936–44.

Vigen, C. L., Mack, W. J., Keefe, R. S., Sano, M., Sultzer, D. L., Stroup, T. S., et al. (2011) 'Cognitive effects of atypical antipsychotic medications in patients with Alzheimer's disease: outcomes from CATIE-AD', *Am J Psychiatry*, 168, 831–9.

Volavka, J., Czobor, P., Nolan, K., Sheitman, B., Lindenmayer, J. P., Citrome, L., et al. (2004) 'Overt aggression and psychotic symptoms in patients with schizophrenia treated with clozapine, olanzapine, risperidone, or haloperidol', *J Clin Psychopharmacol*, 24, 225–8.

Volkow, N. D., Brodie, J. D., Wolf, A. P., Angrist, B., Russell, J. and Cancro, R. (1986) 'Brain metabolism in patients with schizophrenia before and after acute neuroleptic administration', *J Neurol Neurosurg Psychiatry*, 49, 1199–202.

Volz, A., Khorsand, V., Gillies, D. and Leucht, S. (2007) 'Benzodiazepines for schizophrenia', *Cochrane Database Syst Rev*, CD006391.

Voruganti, L. N. and Awad, A. G. (2006) 'Subjective and behavioural consequences of striatal dopamine depletion in schizophrenia—findings from an in vivo SPECT study', *Schizophr Res*, 88, 179–86.

Waddington, J. L., Youssef, H. A. and Kinsella, A. (1990) 'Cognitive dysfunction in schizophrenia followed up over 5 years, and its longitudinal relationship to the emergence of tardive dyskinesia', *Psychol Med*, 20, 835–42.

Waddington, J. L., O'Callaghan, E., Larkin, C. and Kinsella, A. (1993) 'Cognitive dysfunction in schizophrenia: organic vulnerability factor or state marker for tardive dyskinesia?', *Brain Cogn*, 23, 56–70.

Waddington, J. L., Youssef, H. A. and Kinsella, A. (1998) 'Mortality in schizophrenia. Antipsychotic polypharmacy and absence of adjunctive anticholinergics over the course of a 10-year prospective study', *Br J Psychiatry*, 173, 325–9.

Wade, J. B., Taylor, M. A., Kasprisin, A., Rosenberg, S. and Fiducia, D. (1987) 'Tardive dyskinesia and cognitive impairment', *Biol Psychiatry*, 22, 393–5.

Waldmeier, P. C. and Delini-Stula, A. A. (1979) 'Serotonin–dopamine interactions in the nigrostriatal system', *Eur J Pharmacol*, 55, 363–73.

Walker, E. F., Cornblatt, B. A., Addington, J., Cadenhead, K. S., Cannon, T. D., McGlashan, T. H., et al. (2009) 'The relation of antipsychotic and antidepressant medication with baseline symptoms and symptom progression: a naturalistic study of the North American Prodrome Longitudinal Sample', *Schizophr Res*, 115, 50–7.

Wallace, M. (1994) 'Schizophrenia—a national emergency: preliminary observations on SANELINE', *Acta Psychiatr Scand Suppl*, 380, 33–5.

Warner, R. (2004) *Recovery from Schizophrenia: Psychiatry and Political Economy*, 3rd edn (Hove: Brunner-Routledge).

Warner, R. (2005) 'Problems with early and very early intervention in psychosis', *Br J Psychiatry Suppl*, 48, s104–7.

Waters, F., Woodward, T., Allen, P., Aleman, A. and Sommer, I. (2010) 'Self-recognition Deficits in Schizophrenia Patients With Auditory Hallucinations: A Meta-analysis of the Literature', *Schizophr Bull*, 38, 741–750.

Watts, G. (2012) 'Critics attack DSM-5 for overmedicalising normal human behaviour', *Br Med J*, 344, e1020.

Weinmann, S., Read, J. and Aderhold, V. (2009) 'Influence of antipsychotics on mortality in schizophrenia: systematic review', *Schizophr Res*, 113, 1–11.

Weisler, R., Joyce, M., McGill, L., Lazarus, A., Szamosi, J. and Eriksson, H. (2009) 'Extended release quetiapine fumarate monotherapy for major depressive disorder: results of a double-blind, randomized, placebo-controlled study', *CNS Spectr*, 14, 299–313.

Wen, P. (2009) 'Psychiatric drug sought on streets', *Boston Globe* 13 Jul.

Wen, P. (2010) 'Father convicted of 1st degree murder in death of Rebecca Riley', *Boston Globe* 26 Mar.

Wescott, P. (1979) 'One man's schizophrenic illness', *Br Med J*, 1, 989–90.

Whitaker, R. (2002) *Mad in America* (Cambridge, MA: Perseus Publishing).

Whitaker, R. (2010) *Anatomy of an Epidemic* (New York: Crown Publishers).

Whitty, P. F., Owoeye, O. and Waddington, J. L. (2009) 'Neurological signs and involuntary movements in schizophrenia: intrinsic to and informative on systems pathobiology', *Schizophr Bull*, 35, 415–24.

Wilson, M. (1993) 'DSM-III and the transformation of American psychiatry: a history', *Am J Psychiatry*, 150, 399–410.

Wilson, I. C., Garbutt, J. C., Lanier, C. F., Moylan, J., Nelson, W. and Prange, A. J., Jr (1983) 'Is there a tardive dysmentia?', *Schizophr Bull*, 9, 187–92.

Wilson, M. P., Pepper, D., Currier, G. W., Holloman, G. H., Jr and Feifel, D. (2012) 'The psychopharmacology of agitation: consensus statement of the american association for emergency psychiatry project Beta psychopharmacology workgroup', *West J Emerg Med*, 13, 26–34.

Winkelman, N. W., Jr (1954) 'Chlorpromazine in the treatment of neuropsychiatric disorders', *JAMA*, 155, 18–21.

Winokur, G. (1975) 'The Iowa 500: heterogeneity and course in manic-depressive illness (bipolar)', *Compr Psychiatry*, 16, 125–31.

Winterer, G. (2006) 'Cortical microcircuits in schizophrenia—the dopamine hypothesis revisited', *Pharmacopsychiatry*, 39(Suppl. 1), S68–71.

Wise, C. D., Baden, M. M. and Stein, L. (1974) 'Post-mortem measurement of enzymes in human brain: evidence of a central noradrenergic deficit in schizophrenia', *J Psychiatr Res*, 11, 185–98.

Wolf, M. E., Ryan, J. J. and Mosnaim, A. D. (1983) 'Cognitive functions in tardive dyskinesia', *Psychol Med*, 13, 671–4.

Wolkowitz, O. M. and Pickar, D. (1991) 'Benzodiazepines in the treatment of schizophrenia: a review and reappraisal', *Am J Psychiatry*, 148, 714–26.

Wong, D. F., Wagner, H. N., Jr., Tune, L. E., Dannals, R. F., Pearlson, G. D., Links, J. M., et al. (1986) 'Positron emission tomography reveals elevated D2 dopamine receptors in drug-naive schizophrenics', *Science*, 234, 1558–63.

Woodberry, K. A., Giuliano, A. J. and Seidman, L. J. (2008) 'Premorbid IQ in schizophrenia: a meta-analytic review', *Am J Psychiatry*, 165, 579–87.

Woods, S. W., Morgenstern, H., Saksa, J. R., Walsh, B. C., Sullivan, M. C., Money, R., et al. (2010) 'Incidence of tardive dyskinesia with atypical versus conventional antipsychotic medications: a prospective cohort study', *J Clin Psychiatry*, 71, 463–74.

Woolley, D. W. and Campbell, N. K. (1962a) 'Exploration of the central nervous system serotonin in humans', *Ann N Y Acad Sci*, 96, 108–17.

Woolley, D. W. and Campbell, N. K. (1962b) 'Serotonin-like and antiserotonin properties of psilocybin and psilocin', *Science*, 136, 777–8.

Woolley, D. W. and Shaw, E. (1954) 'A biochemical and pharmacological suggestion about certain mental disorders', *Proc Natl Acad Sci U S A*, 40, 228–31.

Wozniak, J., Mick, E., Waxmonsky, J., Kotarski, M., Hantsoo, L. and Biederman, J. (2009) 'Comparison of open-label, 8-week trials of olanzapine monotherapy and topiramate augmentation of olanzapine for the treatment of pediatric bipolar disorder', *J Child Adolesc Psychopharmacol*, 19, 539–45.

Wright, D. (1997) 'Getting out of the asylum: understanding the confinement of the insane in the nineteenth century', *Soc Hist Med*, 10, 137–55.

Wright, P., Stern, J. and Phelan, M. (2012) *Core Psychiatry*, 3rd edn (Edinburgh: Saunders Elsevier).

Wunderink, L., Nienhuis, F. J., Sytema, S., Slooff, C. J., Knegtering, R. and Wiersma, D. (2007) 'Guided discontinuation versus maintenance treatment in remitted first-episode psychosis: relapse rates and functional outcome', *J Clin Psychiatry*, 68, 654–61.

Wyatt, R. J. (1991) 'Neuroleptics and the natural course of schizophrenia', *Schizophr Bull*, 17, 325–51.

Wyatt, R. J. (1995) 'Early intervention for schizophrenia: can the course of the illness be altered?', *Biol Psychiatry*, 38, 1–3.

Yilmaz, Z., Zai, C. C., Hwang, R., Mann, S., Arenovich, T., Remington, G., et al. (2012) 'Antipsychotics, dopamine D(2) receptor occupancy and clinical improvement in schizophrenia: a meta-analysis', *Schizophr Res*, 140, 214–20.

Yood, M. U., DeLorenze, G., Quesenberry, C. P., Jr, Oliveria, S. A., Tsai, A. L., Willey, V. J., et al. (2009) 'The incidence of diabetes in atypical antipsychotic users differs according to agent—results from a multisite epidemiologic study', *Pharmacoepidemiol Drug Saf*, 18, 791–9.

Young, D. and Scoville, W. B. (1938) 'Paranoid psychosis in narcolepsy and the possible dangers of benzedrine treatment', *Med Clin N Am*, 22, 637–46.

Youssef, H. A. and Waddington, J. L. (1988) 'Involuntary orofacial movements in hospitalised patients with mental handicap or epilepsy: relationship to developmental/intellectual deficit and presence or absence of long-term exposure to neuroleptics', *J Neurol Neurosurg Psychiatry*, 51, 863–5.

Yu, X. (2011) 'Three professors face sanctions after Harvard medical school inquiry', *The Harvard Crimson*, 2 Jul.

Yung, A. R., McGorry, P. D., McFarlane, C. A., Jackson, H. J., Patton, G. C. and Rakkar, A. (1996) 'Monitoring and care of young people at incipient risk of psychosis', *Schizophr Bull*, 22, 283–303.

Zakzanis, K. K. and Hansen, K. T. (1998) 'Dopamine D2 densities and the schizophrenic brain', *Schizophr Res*, 32, 201–6.

Zeeberg, B. R., Gibson, R. E. and Reba, R. C. (1988) 'Elevated D2 dopamine receptors in drug-naive schizophrenics', *Science*, 239, 789–91.

Index

CPSIA information can be obtained at www.ICGtesting.com
Printed in the USA
LVOW10*1715230514

387111LV00009B/268/P